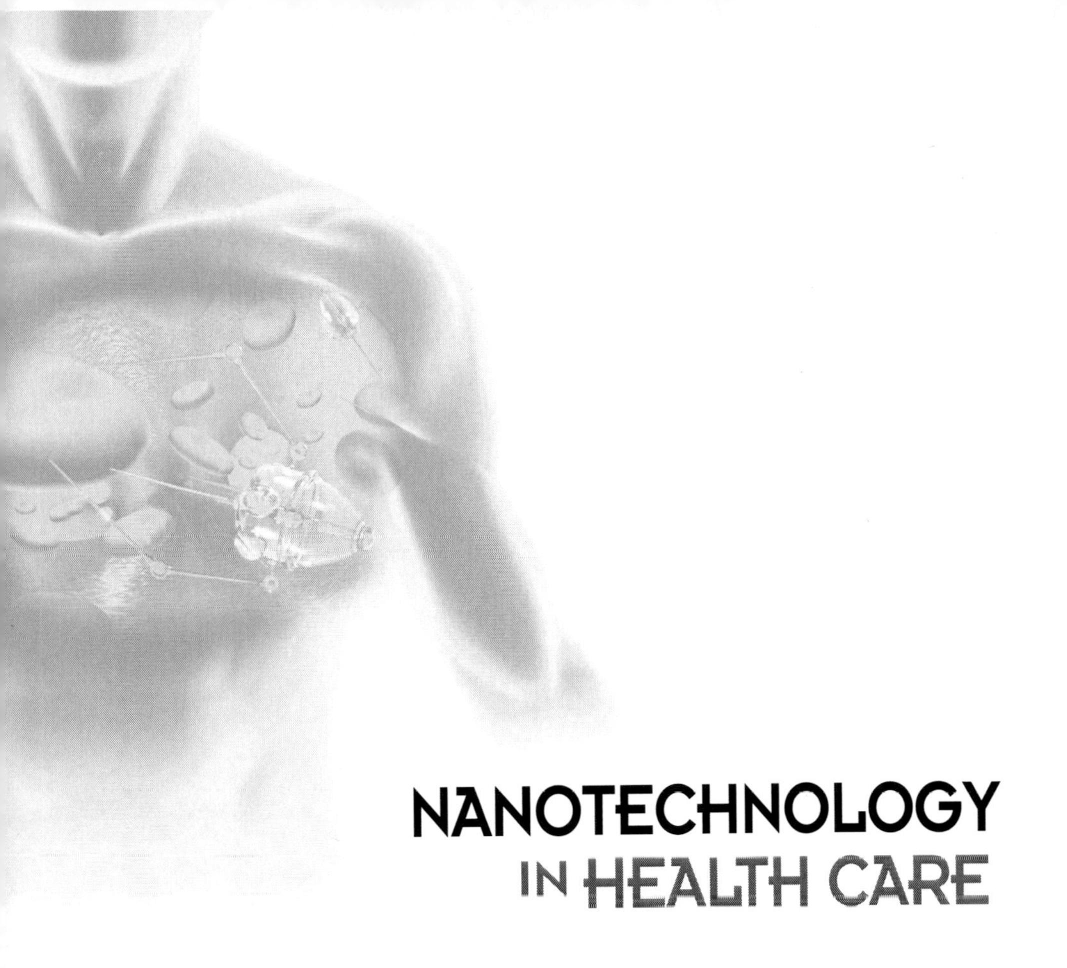

NANOTECHNOLOGY IN HEALTH CARE

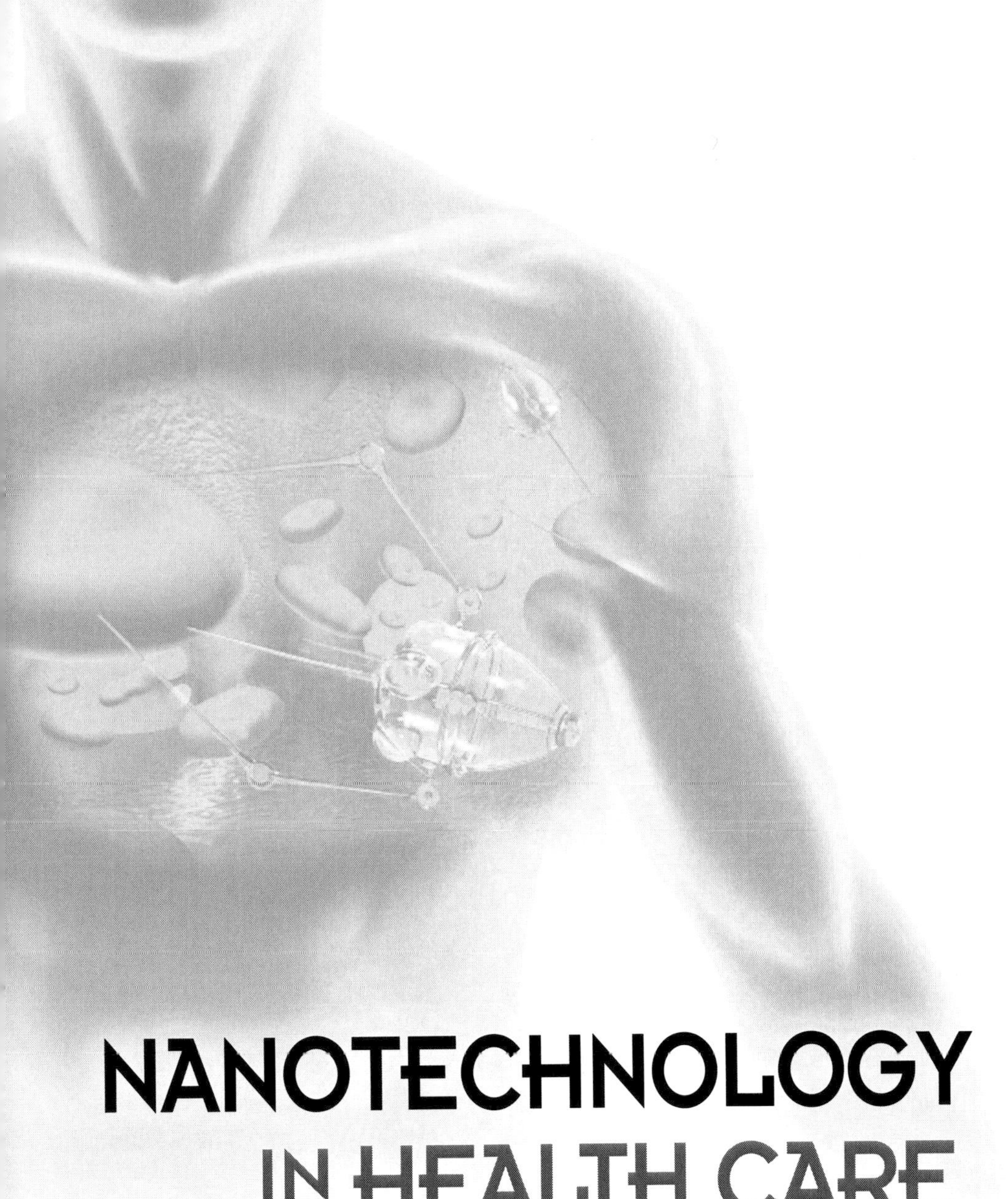

NANOTECHNOLOGY IN HEALTH CARE

Sanjeeb K. Sahoo

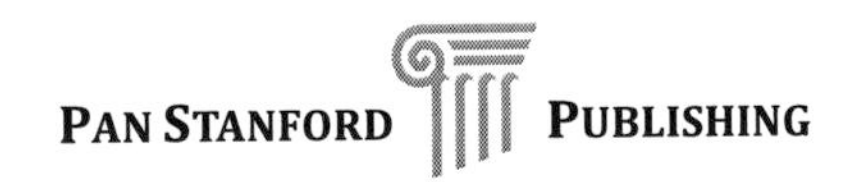

Published by

Pan Stanford Publishing Pte. Ltd.
Penthouse Level, Suntec Tower 3
8 Temasek Boulevard
Singapore 038988

Email: editorial@panstanford.com
Web: www.panstanford.com

British Library Cataloguing-in-Publication Data
A catalogue record for this book is available from the British Library.

Nanotechnology in Health Care

ISBN 978-981-4267-21-2 (Hardcover)
ISBN 978-981-4267-35-9 (eBook)

Printed in the USA

Contents

Preface

The newly recognized research thrust on "nanomedicine," that is, the application of nanotechnology in human health care, is expected to have a revolutionary impact on the future of health care. To advance nanotechnology research for cancer prevention, diagnosis, and treatment, many countries have established alliances for nanotechnology in cancer—for example, United States National Cancer Institute (NCI). Several approaches have been exploited for the development of nanotechnology for cancer molecular medicine. Nanoparticles offer some unique advantages as drug delivery and image enhancement agents. Different varieties of nanoparticulate systems are available, including nanoparticles, micelles, dendrimers, liposomes nanoassemblies, and polymer conjugates, which not only serve as a better platform for drug delivery to tumor sites but have also emerged as an advantageous regime over conventional chemotherapy.

This book focuses on various nanotechnological strategies which show great promise for imaging and treatment of cancer by targeted delivery of drugs to tumor sites and alleviation of the side effects of chemotherapeutic agents. Multifunctional nanosystems also offer the opportunity for combining more than one drug or drug with imaging agents for wide-spectrum application. Contributions from world-renowned authorities proficient in their subjects are brought together here to provide a comprehensive treatise on the subject. The intended audience includes researchers active in nanoscience and technology in industry and academia, medical professionals, government officials responsible for research, and industrialists in pharmaceutical and biomedical technology. I hereby express my gratitude to all of the contributing authors for helping me successfully transmute the concept of the book into reality.

Sanjeeb K. Sahoo
June 2012

Chapter 1

Nanomedicine: Emerging Field of Nanotechnology to Human Health

Chandana Mohanty, Mallaredy Vandana, Abhalaxmi Singh, and Sanjeeb K. Sahoo

Institute of Life Sciences, Nalco Square, Bhubaneswar, India, 751023
sanjeebsahoo2005@gmail.com

1.1 Introduction

Advancing edges of research continue to fuel the development of new fields. Among them, the most prominent and rapidly emerging field is nanotechnology. It is receiving a lot of attention with a never-seen before enthusiasm because of its potential to literally revolutionize each field in which it is being exploited. Nanotechnology is an area of science devoted to the manipulation of atoms and molecules, leading to the construction of structures in the nanometer-scale-size range (often 100 nm or smaller), which maintain distinct properties. Interestingly, bulk properties of materials break down at these length scales, showing unique phenomena. For example, nano materials such as carbon nanotubes (CNTs) and gold nanoparticles (AuNPs) have physical properties that are different from their bulk counterparts. Therefore, such

Nanotechnology in Health Care
Edited by Sanjeeb K. Sahoo

ISBN 978-981-4267-21-2 (Hardcover), 978-981-4267-35-9 (eBook)
www.panstanford.com

technologies generate new opportunities and applications. However, nano-scale particles are nothing new. They occur naturally and are also formed in combustion processes Nanomaterials and devices provide unique opportunities in the field of medicine. The application of nanotechnology to medicine is referred to as "nanomedicine" or "nanobiomedicine." This technological advancement has the most apparent role in the field of human health care and is expected to pervade further and revolutionize the practice of medicine. It encompasses all fields of science, engineering, and technology that involve imaging, measuring, modeling, and manipulating matter at the nano-scale and may well have important applications spanning all aspects of disease, diagnosis, prevention, treatment, and tissue engineering (Fig. 1.1). Besides, the availability of more durable and better prosthetics, new drug delivery systems are of great invention and scientific interest, which give hope for human health care. Herein, we will be describing these applications of nanotechnology in the field of nanomedicine, followed by future expectations and hurdles that must be overcome before these systems can be translated to clinical use.

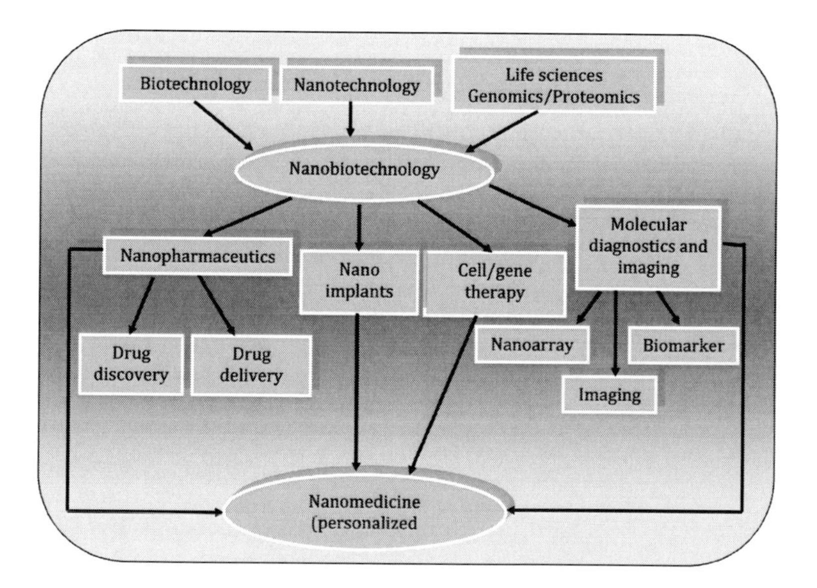

Figure 1.1 A scheme showing the interrelationship of various technologies that contribute to nanomedicine under the concept of personalized medicine.

1.2 Nanotechnology Approach to Nanomedicine

Nanotechnology stands to fabricate momentous scientific and technological advances in fields of medicine and physiology, giving shape to nanomedicine. Nanomedicine is based on molecular knowledge of the human body, and it involves molecular tools for the diagnosis and treatment of different diseases. Since nanotechnology began as a futuristic endeavor, it started by applying mainly nanomechanical concepts to the body. The size domains of components involved with nanotechnology are similar to that of biological structures. Because of this similarity in scale and certain functional properties, nanotechnology is a natural progression of many areas of health-related research, such as synthetic and hybrid nanostructures, that can sense and repair biological lesions and damages just like biological nanostructures (e.g., white blood cells and wound-healing molecules). A series of nanotechnological tools are used individually or in combination to make products and applications for better understanding in medical sciences. These materials and devices can be designed to interact with cells and tissues at a molecular (i.e., subcellular) level with a high degree of functional specificity, thus allowing a degree of integration between technology and biological systems not previously attainable.

There are various nanotechnological tools like the atomic force microscope (AFM), the scanning tunneling microscope (STM), molecular modeling software, and various production technologies that help in the visualization and manipulation of items at the nano-scale level for a better understanding of the nature of science. In a broad spectrum, nanomaterials are classified as raw nanomaterials, nanostructured materials and nanotubes, and fullerenes. Raw nanomaterials such as NPs and nanocrystalline materials are readily manufactured and can be substituted for less performed bulk materials. They are generally used as biocompatible materials or coatings in drug encapsulation, bone replacements, prostheses, and implants. On the other hand, nanostructured materials are typically processed forms of raw nanomaterials providing special shapes or functionality. These include quantum dots (nanostructures that force atoms to occupy discrete energy states as in biological markers) and dendrimers (branched polymers used for drug delivery, filtration, and chemical markers). While still in the developmental stage, the first "wonder materials" of nanotechnology, nanotubes and fullerenes, are the new forms of carbon molecules that can be safely used in some medical applications. They are capable of producing materials that are 100 times stronger than steel and one-sixth of its weigh and more conductive than copper. The range of applications includes artificial muscles, injection needles for individual cells, and drug delivery systems.

Over the past several years, research into nanomedicine has gained momentum. With the surplus funding, research into new technology areas is underway. Recent advances in engineering nanotechnological devices that include micro devices (like microelectromechanical systems [MEMS], microfluidics, microarrays, and biocompatible electronic devices) along with nanodevices have a significant potential for improving the treatment of many disorders. Another progression of nanomedicine is the development of technologies and informatics tools to enable minimally invasive detection, diagnosis, and management of disease and injury using technology platforms for biomolecular sensors that can function in the living body to measure, analyze, and manipulate molecular processes. In oncology, nanomedicine provides oncologists with new tools for tracking and targeting cell surface receptors and other molecules. Also, the development of nano-scale reporters (devices) provides near real-time data and enables clinicians to determine within hours or days of treating a patient if an experimental drug is killing tumor cells as intended.

Thus, nanomedicine is one promising path by which medicine can advance in favor of the new treatment options for certain diseases, better imaging techniques, and other diagnostic tools. These add significantly to the currently available arsenal of therapies and medicines, raising similar ethical and societal concerns as did the medical advances of the past. Like all disease-oriented research, nanomedicine requires public forethought on which diseases should be prioritized in the context of global health care.

1.3 Application of Nanotechnology and Its Impact on Human Health/Nanomedicine

Nanotechnology is an extremely powerful emerging technology expected to have a substantial impact on medical technology now and in the near future. The current research and its application in the field of nanomedicine are broadly summarized in following sections.

1.3.1 Pharmaceutical and Therapeutics

The potential impact of novel nanomedical applications on disease therapy and prevention is foreseen to change health care in a fundamental way. Therapeutic selection can increasingly be tailored to each patient's profile. The following sections present the promising approaches of nanotechnology for therapeutics.

1.3.1.1 Drug delivery

In recent years, there has been a rapid increase in nanotechnology applications to medicine in order to prevent and treat diseases in the human body. Conventional drug delivery techniques have some common limitations in systemic biodistribution, including toxicity to nontarget tissues, difficulty in maintaining drug concentrations within therapeutic doses, and metabolism and excretion of drugs, all of which can reduce drug efficacy. Moreover, literature states that about 60% of all drugs are poorly soluble. Poor solubility in water correlates with poor bioavailability. If there is no way to improve drug solubility, it will not be absorbed from the gastrointestinal tract into the bloodstream and reach the site of action. Nanotechnology-based delivery systems could mitigate these problems and additionally provide tissue- or organ-specific targeting with therapeutic action. Nanomaterial, the gift of nanotechnology, acts as drug-delivery and drug-targeting systems. Due to the smallness of nanomaterials, these are not recognized by the human body; they migrate through cell membranes beneath a critical size and are able to pass and, hence, developed as nano-scaled ferries, which transport high-potential pharmaceutics precisely to their destination. There are different kinds of NPs that are suitable for drug deliveries and are categorized as liposomes, polymer NPs (nanospheres and nanocapsules), solid-lipid NPs, nanocrystals, polymer therapeutics such as dendrimers, and inorganic NPs (e.g., Au and magnetic NPs), as depicted in Fig. 1.2 [1]. This nanocarrier improves the solubility, stability, and absorption of several drugs, avoiding the reticuloendothelial system (RES), thus protecting the drug from premature inactivation during its transport [2].

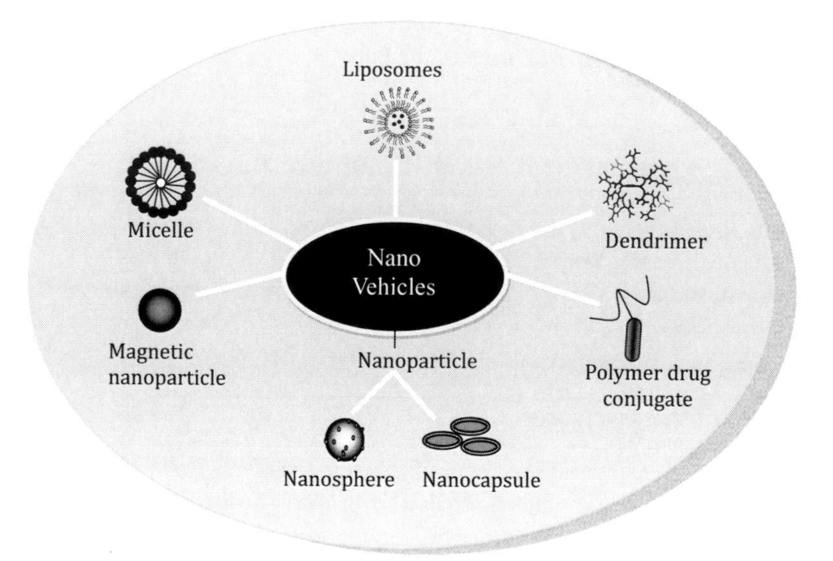

Figure 1.2 Different nanovehicles for drug targeting.

NPs are solid colloidal particles consisting of macromolecular substances that vary in size from 10 nm to 1,000 nm. The drug of interest is dissolved, entrapped, adsorbed, attached, or encapsulated into the NP matrix. Depending on the method of preparation NP, nanospheres, or nanocapsules can be obtained with different properties and release characteristics for the encapsulated therapeutic agent. This provides advantages like small size, which enable them to penetrate through smaller capillaries, easily taken up by the cell, making it efficiently accessible at the target site [3]. Beside this, the biodegradable material of NPs preparation allows sustained drug release to the target site over a period of days or even weeks. Similarly, ceramic NPs are very stable and their surface can be easily conjugated to a variety of ligands for effective targeting. Besides NPs, the other researched nanocarriers are liposomes. These are the first type of nanovehicles to be used to create therapeutic agents with novel characteristics. These are small spherical artificial vesicles that can be produced from natural nontoxic phospholipids and cholesterol. Liposomes have become very versatile tools in biology, biochemistry, and medicine and are widely used to treat infectious diseases and to deliver anticancer drugs either by endocytic pathway or by the fusion of liposomal surfaces with the cell membrane. Among the other drug carriers used for controlled delivery, micelle has also drawn the attention for the systemic delivery of water-insoluble drugs and better thermodynamic stability in physiological solution by its low critical micellar concentration. This makes the polymer more stable and prevents rapid dissociation *in vivo*. Effective targeting of the disease site can be achieved by the association of different ligands to the micelle. The resulting multifunctional micelle shows a tremendous role in delivering a high concentration of drugs to the target site [4].

Research has already shown that drugs can be encapsulated in NPs or conjugated to well-defined multivalent macromolecules, such as dendrimers (highly branched polymers) [5]. These mechanisms can improve the bioavailability of drugs and enable continued release, thereby controlling the initial dose, improving effectiveness, and widening the therapeutic window. Potential targets include proliferating smooth muscle cells, neoplastic cells, inflammatory mediators, proteins expressed in viral infections, and even distinct subcellular localizations such as mitochondria and other cytoplasmic organelles [6, 7]. Specific targeting of drugs can mitigate systemic toxicity, and encapsulating or conjugating drugs to nano-scale carriers can protect them from systemic metabolism or excretion. In addition, nanoparticulate or macromolecular targeting systems can be used to give triggered release in response to internal triggers such as pH or to externally administered signals such as ultrasound, near-infrared (NIR) light, magnetic fields, or radiofrequency pulses [8]. For example, magnetic microparticles or NPs that bind to specific cells could be heated with an alternating magnetic field to kill neighboring cells thermally. It has been recognized that fullerenes and CNTs are key building blocks for nano-scale materials and their further applications to medicine could be inevitable. Fullerenes have unique properties as drug candidates; for example modified C_{60} fullerenes were found to have antiprotease activity and were recommended for the treatment of human immunodeficiency virus (HIV) and acquired immunodeficiency symdrome (AIDS) [9, 10]. C_{60} fullerenes also have powerful antioxidant properties and are being incorporated into drugs designed for the treatment of neurodegenerative disorders, including amyotrophic lateral sclerosis, also known as Lou Gehrig disease, and Parkinson disease [11, 12]. Experts believe that the nanodelivery system will become the order of the day and may be available for clinical use in near future to eradicate different diseases, starting from polio to cancer, and thus revolutionize the medical field.

Nanofabrication and microfabrication approaches based on integrated circuit processing may be used to fabricate controlled-release drug delivery devices. Using photolithographic and integrated circuit processing methods, silicon-based microchips have been fabricated that can release single or multiple chemicals on demand using electrical stimuli. These engineered microdevices can be used to maintain biological activity of the drugs and facilitate the local, accurate, and controlled release of potentially complex drug-release profiles. In addition to silicon-based devices, polymeric-based microfabricated devices have been made that can release drugs based on the degradation of polymeric reservoir covers. Microfabrication techniques have also been used to develop transdermal drug delivery approaches based on microneedles. The recent emerging technology that has gained the attention of the pharmaceutical research is cell encapsulation. Microencapsulated living genetically engineered cells can be used as drug delivery vehicles for immunotherapy and engineered tissues [13]. People envisage the use of encapsulated cells in clinical treatments, like type I diabetes, central nervous system regeneration, and tumor therapy. The implantation of microencapsulated recombinant cells has great potential for gene therapy where therapeutic proteins can be sustained and, in the long-term, delivered by microencapsulated cells [14]. The technology of cell microencapsulation represents a strategy in which cells that secrete therapeutic products are immobilized and immunoprotected within polymeric and biocompatible devices [13]. Based on this concept, a wide spectrum of cells and tissues may be immobilized, enhancing the potential applicability of this strategy to the treatment of numerous diseases [15]. One potential impact of this drug delivery approach is that the administration of immunosuppressants and implementation of strict immunosuppressive protocols can be eliminated; therefore, the serious risks associated with these drugs can also be avoided.

1.3.1.2 Gene delivery

Nanotechnology progress in the fields of medicine, predominantly in gene therapy, holds great promise for therapeutics and health care. It is a therapeutic modality designed to introduce an extraneous gene into the patient's cells to produce a specific protein, which can potentially treat a variety of inherited and acquired diseases. Gene medicines are composed of a gene expression vector that encodes a therapeutic protein and a gene delivery system that delivers the gene to the desired tissue and subcellular compartments. The specific and efficient delivery of DNA to the diseased sites and to the nuclei of particular cell populations is the key for successful gene therapy. The gene delivery system is usually mediated by viral vectors such as retro virus, adenovirus, adeno-associated viruses, and popular viral vectors [16]. The problem associated with the viral vector is the toxicity, immune and inflammatory responses, gene control, and targeting issue; additionally, there is always the fear that the virus will recover to cause disease. To overcome this, much interest has been shown for a non-viral-mediated gene transfer technique. The most widely used nonviral nanodelivery systems are liposome-mediated cationic polymers and NPs. The physical properties of NPs, including their morphology, size, charge, density, and colloidal stability, are important parameters to determine the overall efficacy of NPs to act as potential nonviral gene delivery vehicles.

As mentioned earlier, magnetic NPs (MNPs), which include iron oxide particles, can be attracted and guided by an external magnetic field for drug and gene delivery and further they act as a potential tool for diagnosis. In this regard, the magnetic iron oxide NPs coated with polyethyleneimine (PEI), a polymer, serve as a potential gene carrier with high transfection efficacy for cancer gene therapy. The NPs were tested as gene vectors with *in vitro* transfection models. Tumor necrosis factor-related apoptosis-inducing ligand (TRAIL) induces apoptosis (or cell death) in cancer cells. The magnetic NPs were used as gene carriers to transfect TRAIL gene into MCF-7 cells, a breast cancer cell line [17]. In addition, many inorganic materials, such as calcium phosphate, Au, carbon materials, silicon oxide, iron oxide, and layered double hydroxide (LDH), have been studied as a candidate for gene delivery [18]. Inorganic NPs show low toxicity and promise for controlled delivery properties, thus presenting a new alternative to viral carriers and cationic carriers. Similarly, protein particles can be designed in such a way that one can afford to control the size and shape and preserve the protein's biofunctionality, stability, solubility, and concentration while minimizing interparticle forces that cause aggregation. Various proteins are used for drug and gene delivery processes; a few examples are albumin NPs and gelatin NPs where proteins serve as an ideal gene delivery vehicle

[19]. In this regard, Mo *et al.* revealed that the corneal intrastromal injection of albumin-based NPs shows sustained antiangiogenic gene expression and provides potential effects in corneal angiogenesis in a mouse model [20]. Similarly, $\alpha v\beta 3$ integrin is a potential pharmacological target for antiangiogenic therapy. A recent report describes the use of $\alpha v\beta 3$-targeted NPs successfully delivering a gene to tumor vasculature, resulting in substantial tumor regression in several experimental mouse tumor models [21].

Another well-researched modality is novel cationic solid-lipid NPs as lipids. These are important components of cellular membranes. Lipid-based NPs serving as gene delivery are seen in human nonsmall cell lung cancer tumors in mice where these lipid NPs drastically reduce the number and size of the tumors. FUSI is a novel tumor suppressor gene identified in the human chromosome. The loss of expression and deficiency of posttranslational modification of FUSI protein have been found in a majority of human lung cancers. For dual gene therapy, both p53 (well-known tumor suppressor gene) and FUSI protein were wrapped in the NPs. The FUSI works with p53 to force the lung cancer cells to kill themselves — a process known as apoptosis. The positively charged NPs are delivered to the negatively charged cancer cell membrane, accumulating mainly in the tumoregenic lungs cell, where the genes repeatedly express either p53 or FUSI tumor-suppressing proteins [22]. Similarly polymeric NPs (both synthetic and natural) have the advantage of sustaining the release of the encapsulated therapeutic agents over a period of time. Different polymeric NPs can also be used as gene delivery agents. However, recently, a polymer termed C32, derived from poly (β-amino ester), was developed, which was capable of delivering genes to cancer cells more efficiently and with less toxicity than other screened polymers that have been tested [23]. Polymers like poly(lactide-co-glycolic acid) (PLGA), poly lactic acid (PLA), and chitosan are under investigation to deliver genes in cancer therapy. In a study conducted by Prabha *et al.* (2004), the antiproliferative activity of NPs loaded with wild-type p53 gene in the breast cancer cell line was depicted [24]. Cells transfected with wild type p53 DNA–loaded NPs demonstrated sustained and significantly greater antiproliferative effect than those treated with naked p53 DNA [25]. Hence, studies suggest that gene delivery having the nanotechnology approach is suitable for the therapeutic application in human diseases.

1.3.1.3 Vaccine delivery

Over the past several years, the immunization and treatment of infectious diseases have undergone a paradigm shift. Diseases such as measles, mumps, rubella, diphtheria, tetanus, pertussis, haemophilus influenzae type b (Hib) disease, polio, and yellow fever are now under control because of vaccination [26]. Smallpox has been completely eradicated [26, 27], and polio is on the verge of elimination. Other diseases, including influenza, hepatitis B virus (HBV), and pneumococcal infection are being at least partially controlled by vaccines, but there is still much that needs to be done to eliminate many such diseases, even in the developed world. A vaccine is any preparation intended to produce immunity to a disease by stimulating the production of antibody vaccines, which include suspensions of killed or attenuated microorganisms or products or derivatives of microorganisms. The most common method of administering vaccines is by inoculation, but some are given by mouth or nasal spray. Indeed, many of the vaccines available, including protein antigens and DNA vaccines, are very unstable and need to be protected from degradation in the biologic environment. In addition, vaccines for many infectious diseases are poorly developed or simply unavailable and their efficacy is limited by their poor capacity to cross biologic barriers to reach the target sites. Nanotechnology is an attractive methodology for optimizing vaccine development to constitute an effective vaccine by integrating into particle design and affording optimal immune responses to specific pathogens. As a consequence, the design of appropriate antigen carriers that could help to mitigate these problems coupled with vaccine delivery becomes easy.

To circumvent discussed problems, much research is currently focused on developing new adjuvants and delivery systems. Microparticles and NPs offer the possibility of enhancement of vaccine uptake by appropriate cells through the manipulation of their surface properties. Such crucial vaccine components could facilitate the development of novel vaccines for viral and parasitic infections, such as hepatitis, HIV, malaria, and cancer. Vaccine-delivery systems are generally particulate (e.g., emulsions, microparticles, and liposomes) and have dimensions comparable to that of the pathogens that the immune system evolved to fight. Particulate systems of micron size offer several advantages for vaccine delivery [28, 29]. For example, microparticles are approximately the same size as many pathogens that the immune system is equipped to attack [30]. Additionally, larger particles generally provide sustained release of antigens than equivalent smaller ones [31]. Moreover, microparticles have been shown to elicit both vigorous cellular [41] and humoral immunity [10]. Smaller particles (10–1,000 nm in size) can also serve as vaccine delivery systems and adjuvants. These nanosystems for vaccine delivery can be potentially used against many diseases as compared to traditional vaccination. For example, the novel aerosol version of the common tuberculosis (TB) vaccine, administered directly to the lungs as an oral mist, offers significantly better protection against the disease in experimental animals than a comparable dose of the traditional injected vaccine. In the aerosol vaccine, particles formed at micrometer and nanometer (nm) scales and in spherical and elongated shapes appeared to improve dispersal in the mouth. Spray-drying of the vaccine is much lower in cost than Bacille Calmette-Guérin (BCG) (the vaccine for TB), easily scalable for manufacturing, and ideal for needle free use, such as via inhalation [32].

New-generation vaccines, particularly those based on recombinant proteins and DNA, are likely to be less reactogenic than traditional vaccines and are also less immunogenic. Therefore, there is an urgent need for the development of new and improved vaccine adjuvants and delivery vehicles approximately nano-scale (1,000 nm) in size. These novel immunopotentiators, like immunostimulating complex (ISCOMs), Montanide™ ISA51, MF59, Monophosphoryl lipid AMPL® and delivery vehicles, are able to elicit humoral, cellular, and mucosal immunity [32]. This component facilitates the targeting and/or controlled release of the antigen to antigen presenting cells. Enhancement of adjuvant activity through the use of micro- and nanoparticulate delivery systems is particularly exciting as synergistic effects are often seen resulting in immune responses stronger than those elicited by the adjuvant or delivery system alone. Thus, through the judicious selection of the nanocarrier systems and the vaccine antigen, optimal immunization and protection can be induced.

1.3.2 Molecular Imaging and Diagnostic Tools

1.3.2.1 Molecular imaging

Molecular imaging is a new discipline that unites molecular biology and *in vivo* imaging. It enables the visualization of the cellular function and the follow-up of the molecular process in living organisms without perturbing them. The multiple and numerous potentialities of this field are applicable to the earlier and precise diagnosis of diseases, improving the treatment of these disorders by optimizing preclinical and clinical tests.

Various exogeneous agents like lanthanide chelates and organic fluorophores are being used to visualize key subcellular compartments [33]. However, these materials have several disadvantages as organic fluorophores are prone to photobleaching and lanthanide chelates are prone to nonselective localization in extravascular space. The shortcomings of the conventional imaging agents have limited their applications as biomedical diagnostic tools. Nanotechnology offers a new imaging technology that provides high-quality images, which is not possible with current devices. Different nanomaterials, such as magnetic NPs, quantum dots, and AuNPs, are being used as contrasting agents. These nanomaterials are optimal diagnostic tools since they eliminate most of the vulnerabilities of the conventional imaging agents.

1.3.2.1.1 *Magnetic resonance imaging*

The human body is mainly composed of water molecules, which contain protons. Magnetic resonance imaging (MRI) is a noninvasive diagnostic tool that applies magnetic fields to the heterogeneous composition of water in organisms [34–36]. The water protons of different cells show different relaxivity rates, which get translated into different contrasting images. Different MRI images can be enhanced by reducing the longitudinal and transverse relaxation time of the water protons [37]. Enhancement is often observed on the use of contrasting agents such as gadolinium chelates [37] and superparamagnetic iron oxide, among which gadoliniumdiethyltriaminepentaacetic acid (Gd-DTPA) is the most widely used contrasting agent [33]. In this reagent, the contrasting agent GdIII is complexed with DTPA, which is the chelating ligand that minimizes the leaching of the cytotoxic, ionic GdIII into the cellular milieu. AuNPs have been utilized as a delivery vehicle to convey multiple Gd-DTPA complexes into selective cellular targets and to avoid rapid renal clearance.

Researchers at the University of Michigan are developing nanoprobes that can be used with MRI. NPs with a magnetic core are attached to a cancer antibody that attracts cancer cells. The NPs are also linked with a dye that is highly visible in MRI. When these nanoprobes latch onto cancer cells, they can be detected in MRI, which then can be treated by different ways. Applications of nanotechnology have revolutionized the pathologies related to cardiovascular, nephrological, and even neurological diseases. Molecular MRI of macrophages in atherosclerosis has been accomplished using ultrasmall particles of iron oxide or paramagnetic immunomicelles. Hyafil *et al.* have shown the possibility to image macrophages in atherosclerotic plaques with computed tomography imaging using N1177, a nanoparticulate formulation of iodine [38]. Several multimodality molecular imaging studies of cardiovascular disease–related processes, including apoptosis after myocardial infarction and the overexpression of cell adhesion molecules in atherosclerosis, have been realized using superparamagnetic cross-linked iron oxide NPs that were additionally labeled for fluorescence or nuclear imaging. These studies revealed the significance of integrating multiple properties within one NP to allow the exploitation of the strengths of the different imaging modalities used. Diseases of the nervous system are a challenge to the medical field as direct access to the central nervous system is difficult. Ultrasmall superparamagnetic iron oxide (USPIO) is a potential contrasting agent for MRI in brain imaging as it can avoid the blood–brain barrier [39]. Harisinghani *et al.* showed that highly lymphotropic superparamagnetic NPs, which gain access to lymph nodes by means of interstitial lymphatic fluid transport, allow the high-resolution MRI of clinically occult lymph-node metastases in patients with prostate cancer, which previously were not detectable by any other noninvasive approaches.

1.3.2.1.2 *X-ray-computed tomography*

X-ray-computed tomography is another noninvasive diagnostic method that generates three-dimensional (3-D) images of different cells based on a series of two-dimensional (2-D) X-ray images compiled around a single rotating axis. Contrasting agents are often utilized to enhance the contrast between cells because of their affinity to absorb X-rays. Miniature wireless devices are being developed with nanotechnology for providing high-quality images not possible with traditional devices. MediRad has developed a miniature X-ray device that can be inserted into the body. They are attempting to make CNTs into a needle-shaped cathode that can generate electron emissions to create extremely small X-ray doses directly targeting an area without damaging the surrounding normal tissue.

One of the widely used contrasting agents in X-ray computed tomography is called Ultravist (iopromide), an iodinated small molecule dye [40]. But it has several shortcomings, like renal toxicity [41, 42], vascular permeation, and limited imaging interval due to rapid renal excretion [43]. These limitations can now be overcome by the use of AuNPs. AuNPs present several advantages over the current contrasting agents, such as higher X-ray absorption coefficients [44], versatility in surface modification, and regulated control of the size and shape. Kim and colleagues (2007) used AuNPs coated with poly-ethylene glycol (PEG) [45–51] as antibiofouling agents to test *in vivo* applications as computed tomography contrast agents for angiography and hepatoma detection. X-ray absorption coefficient measurements *in vitro* revealed PEG-coated AuNPs have 5.7 times more attenuation, four hours of longer blood circulation time, and about twofold contrast enhancement than the conventional Ultravist. These results showed the feasibility of AuNPs as a computed tomography contrast agent *in vivo*.

1.3.2.1.3 *Optical imaging*

Optical imaging is an imaging technique that takes the advantage of the luminescent properties of different materials to visualize the biomolecules. AuNPs are the most utilized contrasting agents that permit light scattering or absorption at the NIR spectrum (700–1,000 nm) [52]. Light penetration at this range is at the maximum, with minimum loss to hemoglobin and water absorption, thereby permitting deep imaging of the cells [53]. Also, AuNPs are the most tolerable and compatible materials with the cellular environment [54–57]. AuNPs show a strong absorption band in the visible region due to surface plasmon resonance (SPR). The colorimetric contrast observed within the AuNP-treated cells could be controlled by size, shape, or even surface modification of the AuNPs [58]. When excited, the SPR of AuNPs could scatter and/or absorb light in the visible or the NIR spectrum [59], an extremely useful property for *in vivo* optical imaging techniques such as photoacoustic [52] and two-photon luminescence imaging [60]. Besides AuNPs, other materials are also being tried for photo imaging. Due to unique photoluminescent properties, quantum dots are being extensively studied for imaging purposes. Synthesized quantum dots have significant advantages over traditional fluorescent dyes due to better stability, stronger fluorescent intensity, and different colors, which are adjusted by controlling the size of the dots. In addition, quantum dots do not fade when exposed to ultraviolet (UV) light and the stability of their fluorescence allows longer periods of observation. Experiments have shown that the highly emissive, low-energy anthryl defect sites in an aggregated poly(p-phenylene ethynylene) (PPE) emit green fluorescence [61]. The incorporation of anthryl sites into polymers led to the development of crude solution-state and solid-state sensors, which, upon exposure to water, exhibited a visually noticeable blue-to-green fluorescence color change.

1.3.2.2 Diagnostic tools

Diagnostic tools provide detection and characterization of the changes seen in healthy persons that may be at the individual cell level or at the molecular level or even minor changes in blood that differentiate a healthy person from a diseased person.

1.3.2.2.1 *Genetic testing*

The present-day normal genetic testing involves many steps with a lot of challenges. In addition, current assay technologies use fluorescent dyes to label molecules and require expensive equipment such as a laser to light up biological interactions and an optical microscope to detect the binding sites. But fluorescent dyes are not always precise or sufficiently sensitive to detect every gene. Nanotechnology has helped to face these challenges in the process of genetic testing.

For example, at Genicon, AuNP probes or nanostrings are being used that will cling to target genetic materials and illuminate when the sample is exposed to light. Chand Mirkin used AuNP probes coated with a string of nucleotides that complement one end of a target sequence in the sample and another set of nucleotides complementing the other end, attached to a surface between two electrodes. If the target sequence is present, it anchors the nanoprobes to the surface like little balloons, and when treated with a silver solution, they create a bridge between the electrodes and produce a current. Quantum Dot Corp. uses quantum dots to detect biological material. The potential to get multiple colors from the quantum dots by changing the size of the dots has increased the efficiency of quantum dots to detect even very low amounts and low levels expressing genes in comparison to fluorescent dyes.

Another application of nanotechnology in molecular diagnostics falls under the category of biochips/microarrays, currently also known as nanochips and nanoarrays. DNA microarrays typically perform one type of analysis thousands of times. This is like a lab-on-a-chip in which there are nanofluidic devices that can integrate mixing, moving, incubation, separation, detection, and data processing in a small portable device. At the micro- and nano-scale, fluids move through pipes in laminar flow, as opposed to turbulent flow at the macrolevel. This provides the opportunity to exploit certain physical behaviors. For example, two liquids can separately circulate through micro pipelines and valves without mixing with each other. The combination of arrays and fluidic capabilities can greatly increase the speed and accuracy of various genetic testing. Microarrays contain thousands of spots. With continued miniaturization beyond microlevel, the possibility exists to greatly increase the number of spots on a single chip, with the ultimate objective of including the entire genome. Measuring the presence or activity of selected biomolecules using nanomaterials as tags or labels can result in faster, more sensitive, and more flexible testing. In the drug discovery and diagnostic fields, microfluidic devices in the form of nanoarrays or lab-on-a-chip technologies could allow the production of more efficient and disposable DNA and protein sequencers for drug discovery and diagnostic kits.

1.3.2.2.2 *Biosensors*

Biosensors employ biological molecules such as antibodies, enzymes, carbohydrates, and nucleic acids to identify or follow the course of any biological phenomena of interest [62, 63]. Interactions, such as hydrogen bonding and charge–charge transfers between the ligand and receptor molecules, coupled with read-out techniques such as colorimetry, fluorescence, and biomagnetic signals, are used for sensing specific biochemical events [62] and have applications in food processing, environmental monitoring, and clinical diagnostics, for example, for measuring blood glucose levels [62, 64]. Different nanomaterials like AuNPs, magnetic NPs, and quantum dots are widely used in biosensors. AuNPs due to their flexibility in changing the imaging contrast are the most favorable materials. But in comparison with an AuNP-conjugating probe, the Au nanowire-functionalized probe could prevent the leakage of biomolecules from the composite film and enhances the stability of the sensor [65]. It is well known that well-dispersed solutions of AuNPs display red color while aggregated NPs appear blue in color. Based on this phenomenon, Jena *et al.* established an AuNP-based biosensor to quantitatively detect polyionic drugs such as protamine and heparin [66]. Wei *et al.* described a simple and sensitive aptamer-based colorimetric sensor using AuNP probes to sense alpha-thrombin protein [67]. AuNPs in biosensors can also provide a biocompatible microenvironment for biomolecules, greatly increasing the amount of immobilized biomolecules on the electrode surface and thus improving the sensitivity of the biosensor.

MNPs, due to their special magnetic properties, have been widely explored as biosensors. Zhang *et al.* prepared a magnetic dextran microsphere (MDMS) by cross-linking iron NPs and dextran. Then, HRP was immobilized on the MDMS-modified glassy carbon electrode. On the basis of the immobilized HRP-modified electrode with hydroquinone as mediator, an H_2O_2 biosensor was fabricated [68] (Fig. 1.3). Zhang *et al.* prepared a magnetic chitosan microsphere (MCMS) using carbon-coated MNPs and chitosan on which hemoglobin can be immobilized with the cross-linking of glutaraldehyde [68].

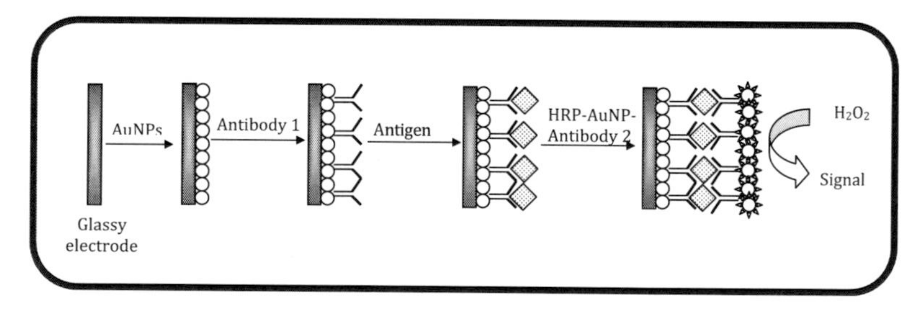

Figure 1.3 The immunoassay procedure of an AuNP-modified immunosensor using HRP–AuNPs–Ab2 conjugates as a label.

Quantum dots have been subjected to intensive investigations because of their unique photoluminescent properties and potential applications. Quantum dots provide a new functional platform for bioanalytical sciences and biomedical engineering. For example, CdTe quantum dots led to an increased effective surface area for the immobilization of enzymes and their electrocatalytic activity promoted electron transfer reactions and catalyzed the electro-oxidation of thiocholine, thus amplifying the detection sensitivity [69]. Besides, still many other nanomaterials, such as metals, metal-oxides, and polymers, could be used in biosensors. For example, hollow nanospheres CdS were first used to study the direct electrochemical behavior of hemoglobin and the construction of nitrite biosensors. Metal NPs, like nano-Cu, due to a large surface area and high surface energy, are used as electron conductors and show a good catalytic ability to reduce H_2O_2. Platinum NPs have also been widely used in biosensors. Nano-scale metal-oxides have also been widely used in the immobilization of proteins and enzymes for bioanalytical applications. Cheng *et al.* reported a nano-TiO_2-based biosensor for the detection of LDH [70].

Although few sensors based on nanomaterials work at commercial applications, nanomaterial-based biosensors exhibit fascinating prospects. Compared with traditional biosensors, nanomaterial-based biosensors have marked advantages such as enhanced detection sensitivity and specificity and possess great potential in applications such as the detection of DNA, RNA, proteins, glucose, pesticides, and other small molecules from clinical samples, food industrial samples, as well as environmental monitoring [71].

1.3.3 Tissue Engineering

Tissue engineering combines biology, medicine, engineering, and materials science to develop tissues that restore, maintain, or enhance tissue function [72]. To date, most tissue engineering studies are focused on the investigations of macrolevel structures (i.e., super cellular structures greater than 100 μm and cellular structures greater than 10 μm) to build the tissue or organ system. Engineering the functional units of the tissue, not only at the supercellular- and cellular-scale structures but also at the subcellular-scale structures (1–10 μm) and nanostructures (1–100 nm) need to be constructed to control cellular environment, cell-molecular interactions, and cell-cell interaction [73]. Herein, the application of nanotechnology in tissue engineering is discussed in terms of three aspects: biomaterial scaffolding, biomolecular manipulation, and cellular engineering.

The tissue-engineering strategy involves the isolation of healthy cells from a patient, followed by their expansion *in vitro*. These expanded cells are then seeded onto a 3-D biodegradable scaffold that provides structural support. The scaffold gradually degrades with time, to be replaced by newly grown tissue from the seeded cells [74]. The convergence of nanotechnology for constructing nanofabricated and microfabricated tissue-engineering scaffolds has the potential to direct cell fate as well as regulate processes such as angiogenesis and cell migrations. In addition, it brings unpredictable new properties to the materials, such as mechanical (stronger), physical (lighter and more porous), optical (tunable optical emission), electronic (more electrical conductivity), and magnetic properties (superparamagnetics) [75]. Other advantages include enhanced biocompatibility, improved contact guidance, reduced friction and therefore wear for joint applications, reduced need for revision surgery, and altered physical or chemical characteristics of the scaffold, promoting tissue growth around the implants.

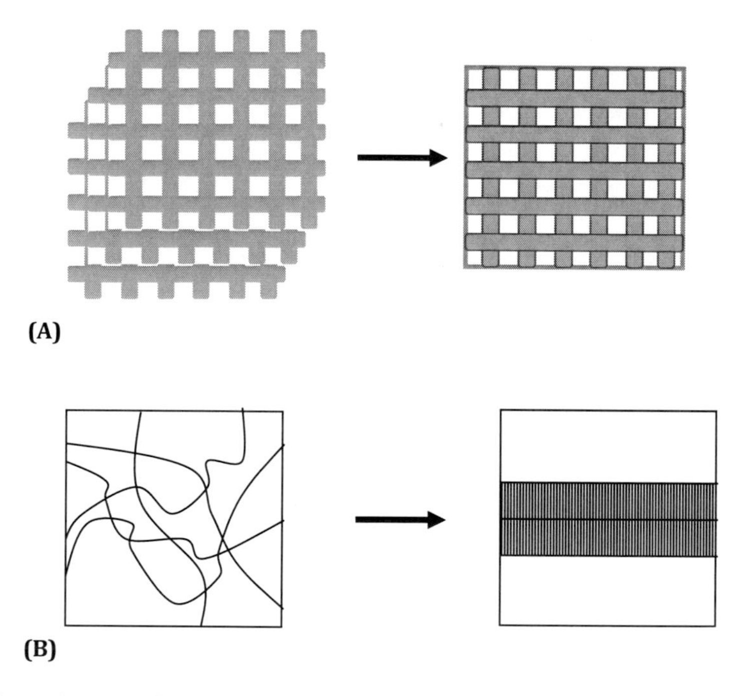

Figure 1.4 A schematic representation of the (A) top-down and (B) bottom-up approaches of nanotechnology to tissue engineering. (A) Nanofabrication approaches can be used to generate 3-D tissue-engineering scaffolds. (B) Nanotechnology can also be used to generate tissue-engineering scaffolds from the self-assembly of nanomaterials, such as nanofibers.

Both top-down and bottom-up technologies have been used to incorporate nano-scale control for tissue-engineering scaffolds (Fig. 1.4). These approaches have been used for fabricating control pore geometry, size, distribution, and spatial geometry. For example, microfabricated approaches have been used to directly engineer the microvasculature within tissue-engineering scaffolds by micromolding biocompatible polymers such as PLGA and poly(glyceride sebacate) (PGS) [76]. In this approach, networks of microfluidic channels that mimic the tissue microvasculature are fabricated from PLGA or PGS. By stacking multiple layers of these microfabricated plates, tissue-engineered scaffolds can be fabricated with nano-scale control. Other approaches, such as the layer-by-layer deposition of cells and proteins using microfluidic channels [77], microsyringe deposition of PLGA polymer [78], and photopolymerization within microfluidic channels [79] have been used to generate 3-D structures with controlled geometries and properties. The miniaturization of these technologies can be performed to generate scaffolds with sub-100 nm features, such as grooves, pores, and surface patterns.

More recently, nanofiber-based scaffolding systems are being explored as scaffolds for nanomedicine, controlled drug release, and tissue engineering [80]. There are several scaffold fabrication techniques, namely electrospinning (random, aligned, vertical, and core shell nanofibers), self-assembly, phase separation, melt-blown, and template synthesis utilized for the preparation of nanofibrous materials. These techniques are used for the preparation of nanofibers and macroporous scaffolds intended for drug delivery and tissue engineering. The main objective is to fabricate artificial extracellular matrix (ECM) and to accommodate cells and guide their growth for tissue regeneration. Another successful achievement is constructing composite nanofibers. A number of merits are conceivable with the new composite nanofibers, as they provide better hydrophilicity (wettability), improved mechanical properties, and so on. Biologically, the incorporation of bioactive macromolecules (e.g., collagenous protein and growth factors) into the synthetic components could promote cell surface recognition and also promote or control many aspects of cell physiology, such as adhesion, spreading, activation, migration, proliferation, and differentiation [81]. Due to the size of nanofibers, such effects are being augmented or made more effective because of the high surface area for cells to access. So, the biomimetic composite nanofiber provides controlled and sustained delivery of growth factor for successful tissue engineering. Its core-sheath structure could perform controlled and effective delivery of bioactive molecules purely from nanofibrous scaffolds without using extra delivery devices. Using nanotechnologies, NPs, nanofibers, nanopores, nanotubes, and dendrimers loaded with these molecules can also be embedded into the scaffolds. This technology also allows the incorporation of very tiny biocomputer chip into the scaffold design; for example, nano-scale transistors and sensors can be used to mimic a brain circuit for the treatment of Alzheimer's disease [82].

Cell shape and its ECM have been shown to influence the cell behavior [81]. Changes in the cell shape alter the cell cytoskeleton and influence cell fate decisions such as apoptosis, proliferation, and differentiation [81]. The cellular microenvironment using nanopatterning and micropatterning may be controlled for directing cell fate for tissue-engineering applications. It is envisioned that the incorporation of such patterning approaches can be used to direct cell behavior to induce stem cell (SC) differentiation and generate desired cell types or regulate cell behavior within 3-D scaffolds. In addition, microtopology and nanotopology can influence cell gene expression and migration and thus can be incorporated into microfabricated tissue-engineering scaffolds. For example, topographically patterned PLGA surfaces have been shown to induce alignment and elongation of smooth muscle cells and enhance the adhesion of several cell types such as endothelial cells and smooth muscle cells. The application of nanotechnology in tissue engineering to study cellular behavior includes cell movement, migration, tracing, and identification; for example, nanofabricated structures can be used to measure the force generated by individual cells. Neumann *et al.* have measured the mechanical properties of isolated thick filaments from muscle using nanofabricated cantilever force transducers. Not only the force generated by the cells can be measured, cell deformability and flow behavior of cell can also be examined [83]. Similarly, NPs (quantum-dot, i.e., CdSe, ~8 nm) can be used to label varieties of cellular targets. For example, if the cell is allowed to ingest quantum dot dyes, the cell movement can be monitored for days without photo-bleaching the quantum dot dyes [84]. Moreover, this can also be used to trace cancer cell and SC. It is becoming increasingly obvious that in the near future, the already ongoing amalgamation of nanotechnology and tissue engineering will bring even more exciting and valuable results.

1.3.4 Stem Cell Research

Stem Cells (SCs) have the remarkable potential to develop into many different cell types in the body during early life and growth. In many tissues, they serve as a sort of internal repair system, dividing essentially without limit to replenish other cells as long as the person or animal is alive. The approach of nanotechnology and SCs will dramatically advance our ability to understand and control SC-fate decisions and develop novel SC technologies, which will eventually lead to SC-based therapeutics for the prevention, diagnosis, and treatment of human diseases [85]. Advancement in nanotechnology in SC research augers well for SC microenvironment research, SC transfection, isolation and sorting, tracking and imaging, tissue engineering, and molecular detection [86].

A key challenge in the SC microenvironment research is to develop an *in vitro* system that accurately recapitulates functions of the *in vivo* microenvironment. Nanotechnology can be utilized to create *in vivo*-like SC microenvironment and help to determine mechanisms underlying the conversion of an undifferentiated cells into different cell types. For example, micro/nanopatterned surface for the study of SC response to topography, micro-/nano-scale mechanical study, NPs to control release growth factors and biochemicals, nanofibers to mimic ECM, a self-assembly peptide system to mimic signal clusters of SCs, lab-on-a-chip with nanoreservoir to study environmental cues, nanowires to study intra- and intercellular biological processes, laser-fabricated nanogrooves to study cell-cell interactions, and nanophase thin film to study cell adhesion and proliferation. Similarly, gene delivery is essential for genetic manipulation in SCs. Efficient gene delivery to SCs is required for studies of gene function, control of SC differentiation, cellular labeling and purification, and cellular secretion of therapeutic drugs. Because of safety issues, nonviral gene delivery to SCs (so-called SC transfection) is highly sought. A key challenge in SC transfection is to deliver genes to SCs with high efficiency and low cytotoxicity. Nanotechnology provides invaluable tools for SC transfection. For example, NPs for *in vivo* gene delivery, nanoneedles for gene delivery to SCs, a self-assembly peptide system for SC transfection, nanowires for gene delivery to SCs, and micro/nanofluidic devices for SC electroporation [87]. There is great promise in the use of SCs to replace lost function of organs. Essential prerequisites for successful approaches in SC-based regenerative medicine are the reliable identification of SCs and their sorting from heterogeneous populations as well as the safe expansion of SCs *in vitro* without altering their differentiation potential. To this end, nanotechnology-based approaches are well explored for example, magnetic or fluorescent NPs are used to label SCs, followed by magnetic force or flow cytometry sorting and separation [88].

SCs act as attractive tools in regenerative medicine and tissue engineering due to their ability to be committed along several lineages either through chemical or physical stimulation. The combination of SCs with tissue-engineering principles enables the development of the SC-based therapeutic strategy to human diseases. Various micro-/nanofabrication technologies have been introduced to guide SCs to develop into 3-D tissue constructs. For example, nanofibers are able to provide an *in vivo*-like extracellular scaffolding to promote the regeneration of specific tissues. Nanopatterned or nanostructured scaffolds are designed to trigger SCs to become specific cell types, compromising the tissues and organs in the body [89].

In addition, nanofiber has also been used for nerve regeneration, vascular grafts, bone tissue engineering, etc. Similarly, to better understand SC biology and realize the full potential of SC therapy, it is essential to monitor the trafficking of labeled SCs by molecular and cellular imaging. Nanotechnology enables the labeling of SCs using magnetic and fluorescent probes, which can be monitored by MRI or fluorescence imaging. For example, superparamagnetic iron oxide NPs are used for SC labeling, MRI tracking, and the detection of transplanted SCs and diagnostics. Moreover, a variety of imaging modalities are widely used, like quantum dots for SC tracking, fluorophore nanocrystal for SC imaging, nanoprobes for SC detection, photothermal nanospectroscopy to identify SC in the body, and nanotube for SC near-IR fluorescence. In addition, to detect labeled SCs, it is of paramount importance to detect particular molecules in the SC pathway at the cellular level. Nanotechnology provides advanced probes and devices for molecular detection. For example, carbon nanotube optical probes for single molecule detection in living cells, carbon nanotube nanoelectrode array for deep-brain stimulation, nanosphere for neurochemical detection and biosensors, nanowires for molecular detection in SCs, self-assembly polymeric micelle-based bioassay, nanofluidic device for single-cell genomic analysis on a chip, and nanoarrays in mass spectrometry for proteomic applications [90]. Although SC nanotechnology is still in its infancy, this exciting frontier will definitely accelerate the discovery in SCs and the development of better SC technology.

1.3.5 Implant and Prosthesis in Nanomedicine

1.3.5.1 Assembly fabrication of implantable and prosthetic devices

The recent surge in biomedical engineering is largely driven by the potential to improve health care quality while reducing health care costs. Nanotechnology bestows remarkable possibilities of developing new innovative products in the field of medical applications. This fabrication allows for a wide variety of probe shapes and configurations. Many revolutionary applications, such as novel sensing technologies, surface modifications, and implant technologies are currently being developed. For applications to medicine and physiology, prosthetic devices and implantable systems can be designed to interact with cells and tissues at a molecular (i.e., subcellular) level with a high degree of functional specificity, allowing a degree of integration between technology and biological systems not previously attainable. These nanoengineered materials and devices are synthesized using different synthetic methods that can accommodate precursors from solid, liquid, or gas phases. In general, synthetic methods can be classified into two main approaches — "top down" and "bottom up" — and combinations thereof. Top-down techniques begin with a macroscopic material or group of materials and incorporate smaller-scale details into them. Bottom-up approaches, on the other hand, begin by designing and synthesizing custom-made molecules that have the ability to self-assemble or self-organize into higher-order meso-scale and macro-scale structures (Fig. 1.5). The driving force behind the construction of such complex devices out of nanometer-scale components are the biomaterials used and their physiochemical properties. These biomaterials can be synthetic or natural in origin like ceramics, metals, collagen, and polymers, with unusual properties of strength, hardness, reduced friction, and improved biocompatibility.

The chip-scale integration of electronics, photonics, and microelectromechanical systems/nanoelectromechanical systems (MEMS/NEMS) have been enabled by top-down fabrication techniques based on photolithography, whereas the bottom-up nanofabrication technique is based on molecular self-assembly processes that mimic biology that produces complex systems out of simple molecules. For example, CNTs and inorganic nanotubes are developed by electric arc discharge, laser ablation, and chemical vapor deposition techniques. Nanowires can be synthesized using a large variety of materials, such as metals (e.g., Ag), semimetals (e.g., Bi), semiconductors (e.g., CdS), and superconductors using various synthesis methods like template-assisted synthesis, vapor and electrochemical deposition, and vapor-liquid-solid growth. The creation of dendrimers using specifically designed chemical

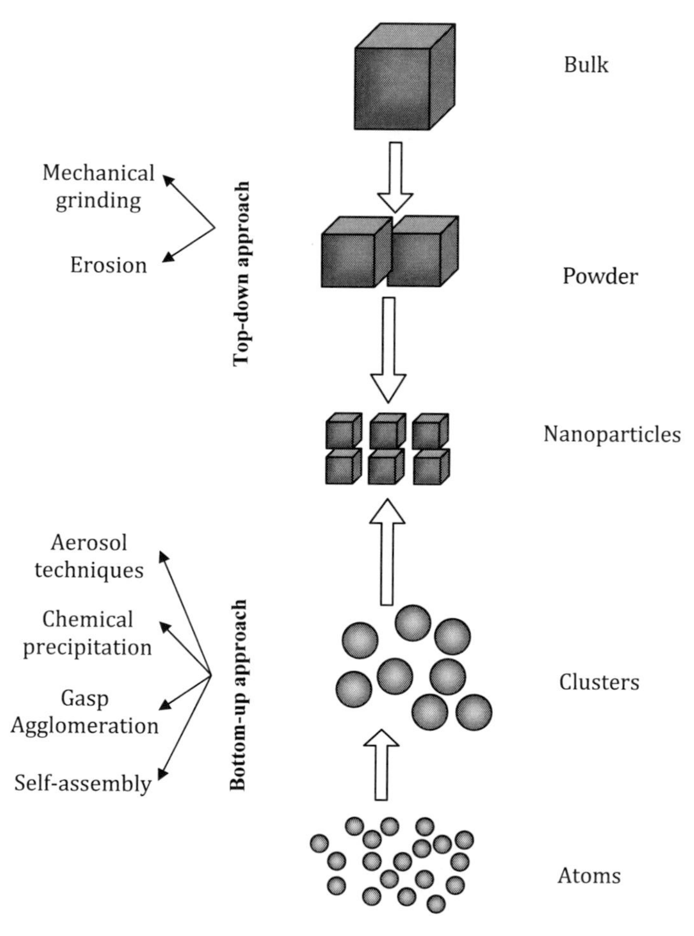

Figure 1.5 A schematic representation of the bottom-up and top-down synthesis processes of nanomaterials with the popular techniques that are used.

reactions is one the best examples of controlled hierarchical synthesis, an approach that allows the bottom-up creation of complex systems. The functional end groups can be modified for various purposes, including sensing, catalysis, or biochemical activity.

Other advanced methods of nanotechnology in medicine are the UV-photolithography, reactive ion etching, chemical vapor deposition, electron beam evaporation, etc., that can be used for the fabrication of silicon-based chips.

1.3.5.2 Biological applications

In the present scenario, medical implantable devices such as stents and catheters represent a large and critical market in the health care industry. Focus is growing on a variety of unmet needs in the medical device industry that can potentially be addressed by engineered nanomaterials. Medical devices such as catheters, stents, and orthopedic implants are often infected with opportunistic bacteria and other infectious microorganisms. Such infections can result in serious illness and require the removal of the devices. More than half of all nosocomial infections are caused by implanted medical devices.

Consequently, nanotechnology offers opportunities to enhance prosthetic devices and implantable systems used for human functioning using nanoengineered materials. At the nano-scale stage, NPs can attach to certain cells or tissues and providing healing of their location and structure.

1.3.5.3 Implant coatings

Nanotechnology brings a variety of biocompatible nanomaterials that are developed with improved coating techniques to increase the surface area, adhesion, durability, and lifespan of implants. Nanoceramic materials such calcium phosphate (hydroxyapatite, or HAP) are made into orthopedic implant coatings, which enhances the implant's potential when in contact with bone surface to improve bone growth. The nanocomposite hydroxyapatite/PMMA/carbon nanotube coatings on the dental implants and prostheses improve its mechanical properties. Similarly, in case of the implanted stents that become fat clogged after implantation and slowly release chemicals through a biodegradable polymer coating, nanostructured materials offer the opportunity to enhance the surface areas of medical devices to address these problems. New types of nanomaterials are also being evaluated as implant coatings to develop interface properties. Nanopolymers such as polyvinyl alcohol (PVA) can be used to coat implantable devices that are in contact with blood (e.g., artificial hearts, vascular grafts, and catheters) for dispersing clots or preventing their formation.

1.3.5.4 Implantable medical devices

Implantable medical devices that are greater than 1 mm in diameter might unfavorably alter the functions of surrounding tissue. Smaller implantable devices with nonintrusive or minimally intrusive systems will likely contain nano-scale materials and smaller systems approaching the nano-scale level. Progress at the juncture of matter science and nanotechnology has led to the development of implantable devices that sense and respond to their surroundings like temperature, pressure, illumination, electricity, or various stimuli. These artificially generated impulses could reach the brain and produce sensitivity. With the advent of nanotechnology, a new generation of smaller and more powerful implants made from nanomaterials has developed, which are intended to offer better quality sound and vision for people who are deaf and blind. Remarkable approaches are made by various research groups in this regard for the treatment of deafness due to cochlear defects and degenerative diseases of the retina, such as retinitis pigmentosa.

There has been significant development in dental implants and devices using nanomaterials for dental treatment. Various applications like nanoindentation of orthodontic archwires by varying the elastic modulus and hardness within a stainless steel wire and replacing upper enamel layers of the tooth with a fracture-resistant nanostructured composite material such as sapphire or diamond with embedded CNTs for more durability and improved appearance using nanomedicine has brought smiles to many [91, 92].

Additionally, reconstructive bone surgeries, such as hip replacements, use titanium implants. In many cases, the muscle tissue does not adhere well to titanium's smooth surface, causing the implants to fail after a period of time. A team of Brown University engineers, led by Thomas Webster, placed human osteoblasts, or bone-forming cells, on anodized titanium covered by CNTs. Studies showed that osteoblast cells grew faster and also made significantly more calcium — the essential ingredient for healthy bones. This approach has drawn closer to making a successful nanostructured orthopedic implant with minimal side effects.

The lack of a comprehensible scientific perceptive of the functional mechanism for a host of different neurological disorders, such as Parkinson's disease, has paved the way for nanomedicine to provide greater insight into the complexity of the brain, enabling a positive approach for its treatment. A novel method has been developed via carbon nanofibers (CNFs) precisely grown on underlying electronic circuits using techniques compatible with Si microfabrication by the researchers at Aalborg University in Denmark. It provides real-time feedback of neurological processes upon electrical stimulation, which can improve implantable devices currently employed for the deep-brain-stimulation treatment of neurological disorders.

With a view toward more long-term applications, University of Texas researchers have demonstrated that networks of nanotubes can transmit electrical signals to neurons, opening up the possibility of using nanotubes as an electrical interface between neural prosthetics and the body. And a group at Brown University has shown that nanotubes combined with adult SCs can effectively deliver the cells to damaged regions of animal brains and facilitate differentiation of the cells into neurons.

With the expansion of new production methods, nanostructures are now being fabricated using active biological components. Current efforts to couple biology and microfabrication are extending the individual strengths and raising expectations. The precise structure of natural materials endows them with impressive functionality, such as selective recognition and catalysis, whereas the ability to manipulate structure controllably (i.e., to alter sequence) allows properties to be engineered for specific functions. Biology creates molecules and macromolecules with an unparalleled level of structural control (Table 1.1). For example, proteins, and nucleic acids are biosynthesized with a precise control of sequence, linkage, and molecular weight — a level of control that is unachievable through chemical synthesis.

Unfortunately, the two are not fully compatible because they do not share a common energy currency and often use different signals. If these incompatibilities can be bridged, it might be possible to fabricate implantable devices that are powered by metabolic energy or to engineer biomolecular interfaces that communicate in two directions. Potentially, biofabrication — the marriage between biology and microfabrication — will emerge as the standard for construction at the nano-scale.

Table 1.1 Characteristics of biological materials that endow them with useful capabilities for fabrication

Characteristics of biological materials	Examples of materials	Fabrication capabilities
Precisely controlled structures	Nucleic acids	Templates for nanowires; molecular lithography
	Proteins	Fusion tails to direct assembly
Physiological properties	Lipids	Self-assembly (vesicles and membranes)
	Nucleic acids	Electrophoresis; layer-by-layer assembly
	Elastin-like peptides	Stimuli-responsive assembly
Molecular-recognition-based self-assembly	Integrins	Cell binding
	Nucleic acids	Novel macromolecular architectures; molecular machines
	Microtubules	Nanowires
	Virus particles	Nanocavities

1.4 Risks of Nanotechnology in Human Health Care

Although at this time, the benefits of nanotechnology dominate our thinking, the potential for undesirable human health outcomes should not be overlooked. Because of their small size, large proportions of the atoms that make up a NP are exposed to the exterior of the particle and would be free to participate in many chemical processes. Hence, concerns over safety issues for the use of nanotechnology in medical and human health are heightened.

In relation to human health, NPs can enter the human body in several ways: (i) via the lungs, where rapid translocation through the blood stream to vital organs is possible, including by crossing the blood-brain barrier; (ii) the intestinal tract; and (iii) the skin. Thus, biocompatibility of the material is important for its use in nanotechnology. Noble metals such as Au, platinum, and palladium are biocompatible and silver is moderately biocompatible. Titanium being biocompatible is widely used in implants, while single-crystal silicon is not biocompatible. Luminescent semiconducting quantum dots are biocompatible, but they often contain toxic metals like arsenic and cadmium. Exceptions are the indium gallium phosphide (InGaP) quantum dots produced by Evident Technologies. There is also the need for minimizing the generation of waste during the production of nanomaterials. Bottom-up nanotechnology can be intrinsically more atom efficient since products can be built atom by atom, or molecule by molecule, in self-repairing assembly processes and without generating waste. Carbon forms being the basis of many nanoparticulates (including carbon black, fullerenes, and nanotubes) can be obtained from renewable biomass, an important issue at least for large-volume nanomaterials such as composite fibers [93].

NPs provide only a glimpse of some toxic paradigms that compel us to ponder the adverse effects against the beneficial effects. There are different types of CNTs, including single-walled CNT (SWCNTs) and multiwalled carbon nanotubes (MWCNTs), that lead to substantial production volumes and consequently to increased emissions into the environmental compartments air, groundwater, and soil. The large surface area of CNTs may cause other molecules to adhere to and potentially pick up pollutants and transport these throughout the environment [94]. In an aqueous environment, SWCNTs can clump together to form aggregates in the micrometer range. The functionalization, coating, length, and agglomeration state of CNTs are influenced by the external environmental conditions during their production, use, and disposal stages. This suggests a possible accumulation along the food chain and high persistence. CNTs produce a toxic response upon reaching the lungs in sufficient quantity, which is produced in a time- and dose-dependent manner [95].

Hence, the identification of possible risks to human health and environment is a prerequisite for a successful introduction of nanotechnology in future applications. The development of safety guidelines by the government for the nanotechnology industries, including manufacturing, monitoring of worker exposure, the ambient release of NPs, and risk evaluations, is mandatory to promote nanotechnology for its economic incentives and medicinal applications. However, the escalating number of patent applications filed and the regulatory issues at the US Food and Drug Administration (USFDA) with respect to safety guidelines regarding nanotechnology can hold back the commercialization of nanomedicine products.

1.5 Future Prospective of Nanotechnology in Human Health Care

It is widely anticipated that nanotechnology will continue to evolve and expand in areas of nanomedicine. The scientific innovations achieved with nanotechnology are a welcome strategy for enhancing and encouraging results already achieved in biomedical and tissue-engineering fields. But extensive research is needed before the launch of these innovations for health care purposes. For example, a more detailed understanding of the interaction of cells with nanofibrous scaffolds, especially based on the structural and functional similarity between nanofibers and native, is significant for the growth of tissue engineering. It is envisioned that new nanomaterials may provide proper signals and environmental cues to cells as well as generate 3-D microenvironments that may be advantageous over today's polymers. Nano-scale structures such as surface topography and patterning could be used to direct cell behavior. The incorporation of these strategies within tissue-engineering scaffolds could further enhance their functions. For drug delivery, the design and testing of novel methods for controlling the interaction of nanomaterials with the body are some of the current barriers in translating these technologies to therapies. Methods of targeting these nanomaterials to specific sites of the body while ensuring that they are not captured by organs such as the liver and spleen are major challenges that need to be addressed.

There are several other exciting proposals for practical applications of nanomechanical tools into the clinical practice in the short term. It has also been hypothesized that nanomachines could distribute drugs within the patient's body. Such nanoconstructions could deliver medicines to particular sites, making more adequate and precise treatment possible. Similar machines equipped with specific "weapons" could be used to remove obstructions in the circulatory system or even identify and kill cancer cells. Nanorobots may be modified bacteria and viruses that already have most of the motorization and target delivery of genetic information. Moreover, they can operate in the human body, monitor levels of different compounds, and store that information in internal memory. They could be used to rapidly examine a given tissue location, surveying its biochemistry, biomechanics, and histometric characteristics in greater detail. This would help in better disease diagnosing. The use of nanodevices would give the additional benefits of reduced intrusiveness, increased patient comfort, and greater fidelity of results, since the target tissue can be examined in its active state in the actual host environment.

With respect to current advancements in the drug delivery field, certain anionic surface-modified dendrimers are proving to function as safe and effective topical nanodrugs against HIV and genital herpes. These dendrimer-based nanopharmaceutics are in the final stages of human clinical testing in the USFDA approval process [96]. Nanomedicine also aims to learn from nature to understand the structure and function of biological devices and to use the same for biomimetic nanostructures by exploiting the concept of self-assembly. Some products of nanomedicine, like miniaturized nanofluidic devices and systems that transport fluids more efficiently to the site of delivery, preventing turbulence and mixing (because fluids move with laminar flow through micro/nanochannels), will appear in the distant future. We expect that in the coming years, significant research will be undertaken with greater funding and coordination efforts from multiple agencies and international cooperation will be required to deliver the benefits that nanotechnology promises.

1.6 Conclusion

Applications of nanotechnology to medical sciences are a milestone on the road to pioneering technologies adopted for the diagnostics and treatment of various diseases that were once considered grave. But numerous bottlenecks like complexity of clinical trials along with the hesitancy that the radical technologies adopted in biomedical sciences may hinder the progress of nanomedicine. Another immediate apprehension in nanomedicine is to evaluate the potential toxicological effects of different nanomaterials. Hence, significant resources must be invested for managing these technologies. Advancement in delivering nanotherapies (combined with related advances in surgery, therapeutics, diagnostics, and computerization) in conjunction with the miniaturization of analytic tools substantiates high optimism for the promising task of nanomedicine in the treatment of diseases. Only the upcoming years will reveal whether nanomedicine in relation to human health is augmented or revolutionized.

References

1. Sahoo, SK, and V Labhasetwar: Nanotech approaches to drug delivery and imaging. *Drug Discov. Today*, **8**, 1112–1120 (2003).
2. Parveen, S, and SK Sahoo: Nanomedicine: clinical applications of polyethylene glycol conjugated proteins and drugs. *Clin. Pharmacokinet*, **45**, 965–988 (2006).
3. Sahoo, SK, F Dilnawaz, and S Krishnakumar: Nanotechnology in ocular drug delivery. *Drug Discov. Today*, **13**, 144–151 (2008).
4. Wang, YC, XQ Liu, TM Sun, MH Xiong, and J Wang: Functionalized micelles from block copolymer of polyphosphoester and poly(epsilon-caprolactone) for receptor-mediated drug delivery. *J. Control. Release*, **128**, 32–40 (2008).
5. Kolodgie, FD, M John, C Khurana *et al.*: Sustained reduction of in-stent neointimal growth with the use of a novel systemic nanoparticle paclitaxel. *Circulation*, **106**, 1195–1198 (2002).
6. Savic, R, L Luo, A Eisenberg, and D Maysinger: Micellar nanocontainers distribute to defined cytoplasmic organelles. *Science*, **300**, 615–618 (2003).
7. Smith, RA, CM Porteous, AM Gane, and MP Murphy: Delivery of bioactive molecules to mitochondria *in vivo*. *Proc. Natl. Acad. Sci. USA*, **100**, 5407–5412 (2003).
8. Lee, ES, K Na, and YH Bae: Polymeric micelle for tumor pH and folate-mediated targeting. *J. Control. Release*, **91**, 103–113 (2003).
9. Eldridge, JH, JK Staas, JA Meulbroek, TR Tice, and RM Gilley: Biodegradable and biocompatible poly(DL-lactide-co-glycolide) microspheres as an adjuvant for staphylococcal enterotoxin B toxoid which enhances the level of toxin-neutralizing antibodies. *Infect. Immun.*, **59**, 2978–2986 (1991).

10. Men, Y, H Tamber, R Audran, B Gander, and G Corradin: Induction of a cytotoxic T lymphocyte response by immunization with a malaria specific CTL peptide entrapped in biodegradable polymer microspheres. *Vaccine*, **15**, 1405–1412 (1997).

11. Borges, O, G Borchard, JC Verhoef, A de Sousa, and H.E., Junginger: Preparation of coated nanoparticles for a new mucosal vaccine delivery system. *Int. J. Pharm.*, **299**, 155–166 (2005).

12. Johansen, P, C Raynaud, M Yang, MJ Colston, RE Tascon, and DB Lowrie: Antimycobacterial immunity induced by a single injection of M. leprae sp65-encoding plasmid DNA in biodegradable microparticles. *Immunol. Lett.*, **90**, 81–85 (2003).

13. Orive, G, RM Hernandez, AR Gascon *et al.*: Cell encapsulation: promise and progress. *Nat. Med.*, **9**, 104–107 (2003).

14. Wang, W, XD Liu, YB Xie *et al.*: Microencapsulation using natural polysaccharides for drug delivery and cell implantation. *J. Mater. Chem.*, **16**, 3252–3267 (2006).

15. Chang, TM: Therapeutic applications of polymeric artificial cells. *Nat. Rev. Drug Discov.*, **4**, 221–235 (2005).

16. Ferber, D: Gene therapy: safer and virus-free? *Science*, **294**, 1638–1642 (2001).

17. Weizhong, W, X Chunfang, W Hua: Use of PEI-coated magnetic iron oxide nanoparticles as gene vectors. *J. Huazhong Univ. Sci. Technol. - Med. Sci.*, **24**, 618–620 (2004).

18. Slowing, II, BG Trewyn, SV Giri, and SY Lin: Mesoporous silica nanoparticles for drug delivery and biosensing applications. *Adv. Funct. Mater.*, **17**, 1225–1236 (2007).

19. Kommareddy, S, and M Amiji: Poly(ethylene glycol)-modified thiolated gelatin nanoparticles for glutathione-responsive intracellular DNA delivery. *Nanomedicine*, **3**, 32–42 (2007).

20. Mo, Y, ME Barnett, D Takemoto, H Davidson, and UB Kompella: Human serum albumin nanoparticles for efficient delivery of Cu, Zn superoxide dismutase gene. *Mol. Vis.*, **13**, 746–757 (2007).

21. Reynolds, AR, S Moein Moghimi, and K Hodivala-Dilke: Nanoparticle-mediated gene delivery to tumour neovasculature. *Trends Mol. Med.*, **9**, 2–4 (2003).

22. Roth, DM, NC Lai, MH Gao *et al.*: Nitroprusside increases gene transfer associated with intracoronary delivery of adenovirus. *Hum. Gene Ther.*, **15**, 989–994 (2004).

23. Zucates, GT, SR Little, DG Anderson, and R Langer: Poly(β-amino ester)s for DNA delivery. *Israel J. Chem.*, **45**, 477–485 (2005).
24. Prabha, S, and V Labhasetwar: Nanoparticle mediated wildtype p53 gene delivery results in sustained antiproliferative activity in breast cancer cells. *Mol. Pharm.*, **1**, 211 (2004).
25. He, Q, J Liu, X Sun, and ZR Zhang: Preparartyion and characteristics of DNA nanoparticles targeting to hepatocarcinoma cells. *World J. Gastroenterol.*, **10**, 660 (2004).
26. Plotkin, SA: Vaccines: past, present and future. *Nat. Med.*, **11**, S5–S11 (2005).
27. Ravanfar, P, A Satyaprakash, R Creed, and N Mendoza: Existing antiviral vaccines. *Dermatol. Ther.*, **22**, 110–128 (2009).
28. Jiang, W, RK Gupta, MC Deshpande, and SP Schwendeman: Biodegradable poly(lactic-co-glycolic acid) microparticles for injectable delivery of vaccine antigens. *Adv. Drug Deliv. Rev.*, **57**, 391–410 (2005).
29. Singh, M, A Chakrapani, and D OH: Nanoparticles and microparticles as vaccine-delivery systems. *Expert Rev. Vaccines*, **6**, 797–808 (2007).
30. Sharma, S, TK Mukkur, HA Benson, and Y Chen: Pharmaceutical aspects of intranasal delivery of vaccines using particulate systems. *J. Pharm. Sci.*, **98**, 812–843 (2009).
31. O'Hagan, DT, M Singh, and JB Ulmer: Microparticle-based technologies for vaccines. *Methods*, **40**, 10–9 (2006).
32. Garcia-Contreras, L, YL Wong, P Muttil *et al.*: Immunization by a bacterial aerosol. *Proc. Natl. Acad. Sci. USA*, **105**, 4656–4660 (2008).
33. Sharma, P, S Brown, G Walter, S Santra, and B Moudgil: Nanoparticles for bioimaging. *Adv. Colloid Interface Sci.*, **123–126**, 471–485 (2006).
34. Caravan, P, AV Astashkin, and AM Raitsimring: The gadolinium(III)-water hydrogen distance in MRI contrast agents. *Inorg. Chem.*, **42**, 3972–3974 (2003).
35. Langereis, S, HA Kooistra, MH van Genderen, and EW Meijer: Probing the interaction of the biotin-avidin complex with the relaxivity of biotinylated Gd-DTPA. *Org. Biomol. Chem.*, **2**, 1271–1273 (2004).
36. Weissleder, R, and U Mahmood: Molecular imaging. *Radiology*, **219**, 316–333 (2001).
37. Caravan, P, JJ Ellison, TJ McMurry, and RB Lauffer: Gadolinium(III) chelates as MRI contrast agents: structure, dynamics, and applications. *Chem. Rev.*, **99**, 2293–2352 (1999).

38. Hyafil, F, JC Cornily, JE Feig *et al.*: Noninvasive detection of macrophages using a nanoparticulate contrast agent for computed tomography. *Nat. Med.*, **13**, 636–641 (2007).

39. Jain, KK: Role of nanotechnology in developing new therapies for diseases of the nervous system. *Nanomedicine*, **1**, 9–12 (2006).

40. Kim, DK, M Mikhaylova, and W FH: Starch-coated superparamagnetic nanoparticles as MR contrast agents. *Chem. Mater.*, **15**, 4343–4351 (2003).

41. Haller, C, and I Hizoh: The cytotoxicity of iodinated radiocontrast agents on renal cells *in vitro*. *Invest. Radiol.*, **39**, 149–154 (2004).

42. Hizoh, I, and C Haller: Radiocontrast-induced renal tubular cell apoptosis: hypertonic versus oxidative stress. *Invest. Radiol.*, **37**, 428–434 (2002).

43. Kim, D, Park S, and L JH: Antibiofouling polymer-coated gold nanoparticles as a contrast agent for in vivo X-ray computed tomography imaging. *J. Am. Chem. Soc.*, **129**, 7661–7665 (2007).

44. Hainfeld, JF, DN Slatkin, TM Focella, and HM Smilowitz: Gold nanoparticles: a new X-ray contrast agent. *Br. J. Radiol.*, **79**, 248–253 (2006).

45. Allen, TM, C Hansen, F Martin, C Redemann, and A Yau-Young: Liposomes containing synthetic lipid derivatives of poly(ethylene glycol) show prolonged circulation half-lives *in vivo*. *Biochim. Biophys. Acta*, **1066**, 29–36 (1991).

46. Ballou, B, BC Lagerholm, LA Ernst, MP Bruchez, and AS Waggoner: Noninvasive imaging of quantum dots in mice. *Bioconjug. Chem.*,**15**, 79–86 (2004).

47. Herrwerth, S, W Eck, S Reinhardt, and M Grunze: Factors that determine the protein resistance of oligoether self-assembled monolayers–internal hydrophilicity, terminal hydrophilicity, and lateral packing density. *J. Am. Chem. Soc.*, **125**, 9359–9366 (2003).

48. Kohler, N, GE Fryxell, and M Zhang: A bifunctional poly(ethylene glycol) silane immobilized on metallic oxide-based nanoparticles for conjugation with cell targeting agents. *J. Am. Chem. Soc.*, **126**, 7206–7211 (2004).

49. Lee, H, E Lee, K Kim do, NK Jang, YY Jeong, and S Jon: Antibiofouling polymer-coated superparamagnetic iron oxide nanoparticles as potential magnetic resonance contrast agents for *in vivo* cancer imaging. *J. Am. Chem. Soc.*, **128**, 7383–7389 (2006).

50. Papahadjopoulos, D, TM Allen, A Gabizon *et al.*: Sterically stabilized liposomes: improvements in pharmacokinetics and antitumor therapeutic efficacy. *Proc. Natl. Acad. Sci. USA*, **88**, 11460–11464 (1991).
51. Zheng, M, F Davidson, and X Huang: Ethylene glycol monolayer protected nanoparticles for eliminating nonspecific binding with biological molecules. *J. Am. Chem. Soc.*, **125**, 7790–7791 (2003).
52. Agarwal, A, Huang SW, and OD M: Targeted gold nanorod contrast agent for prostate cancer detection by photoacoustic imaging. *J. Appl. Phys.*, **102**, 700–701 (2007).
53. Mahmood, U, and R Weissleder: Near-infrared optical imaging of proteases in cancer. *Mol. Cancer Ther.*, **2**, 489–496 (2003).
54. Connor, EE, J Mwamuka, A Gole, CJ Murphy, and MD Wyatt: Gold nanoparticles are taken up by human cells but do not cause acute cytotoxicity. *Small*, **1**, 325–327 (2005).
55. Pan, Y, S Neuss, A Leifert *et al.*: Size-dependent cytotoxicity of gold nanoparticles. *Small*, **3**, 1941–1949 (2007).
56. Shukla, R, V Bansal, M Chaudhary, A Basu, RR Bhonde, and M Sastry: Biocompatibility of gold nanoparticles and their endocytotic fate inside the cellular compartment: a microscopic overview. *Langmuir*, **21**, 10644–10654 (2005).
57. Tkachenko, AG, H Xie, D Coleman *et al.*: Multifunctional gold nanoparticle-peptide complexes for nuclear targeting. *J. Am. Chem. Soc.*, **125**, 4700–4701 (2003).
58. Khlebtsov, NG, LA Trachuk, and AG Mel'nikov: The effect of the size, shape, and structure of metal nanoparticles on the dependence of their optical properties on the refractive index of a disperse medium. *Opt. Spectrosc.*, **98**, 83–90 (2005).
59. Jain, PK, KS Lee, IH El-Sayed, and MA El-Sayed: Calculated absorption and scattering properties of gold nanoparticles of different size, shape, and composition: applications in biological imaging and biomedicine. *J. Phys. Chem. B*, **110**, 7238–7248 (2006).
60. Durr, NJ, T Larson, DK Smith, BA Korgel, K Sokolov, and A Ben-Yakar: Two-photon luminescence imaging of cancer cells using molecularly targeted gold nanorods. *Nano Lett.*, **7**, 941–945 (2007).
61. Satrijo, A, and TM Swager: Anthryl-doped conjugated polyelectrolytes as aggregation-based sensors for nonquenching multicationic analytes. *J. Am. Chem. Soc.*, **129**, 16020–16028 (2007).
62. McFadden, P: Tech. Sight. Biosensors. Broadband biodetection: holmes on a chip. *Science*, **297**, 2075–2076 (2002).

63. Otsuka, H, Y Akiyama, Y Nagasaki, and K Kataoka: Quantitative and reversible lectin-induced association of gold nanoparticles modified with alpha-lactosyl-omega-mercapto-poly(ethylene glycol). *J. Am. Chem. Soc.*, **123**, 8226–8230 (2001).

64. Li, H, and L Rothberg: Colorimetric detection of DNA sequences based on electrostatic interactions with unmodified gold nanoparticles. *Proc. Natl. Acad. Sci. USA*, **101**, 14036–14039 (2004).

65. Patolsky, F, BP Timko, G Zheng, and CM Lieber: Nanowire-based nanoelectronic devices in the life sciences. *MRS Bull*, **32**, 142–149 (2007).

66. Jena, BK, and CR Raj: Optical sensing of biomedically important polyionic drugs using nano-sized gold particles. *Biosens. Bioelectron.*, **23**, 1285–1290 (2008).

67. Wei, H, B Ling, J Li, E Wang, and S Dong: Simple and sensitive aptamer-based colorimetric sensing of protein using unmodified gold nanoparticle probes. *Chem. Commun.*, 3735–3737 (2007).

68. Zhang, HL, GS Lai, DY Han, and AM Yu: An amperometric hydrogen peroxide biosensor based on immobilization of horseradish peroxidase on an electrode modified with magnetic dextran microspheres. *Anal. Bioanal. Chem.*, **390**, 971–977 (2008).

69. Du, D, S Chen, D Song, H Li, and X Chen: Development of acetylcholinesterase biosensor based on CdTe quantum dots/gold nanoparticles modified chitosan microspheres interface. *Biosens. Bioelectron.*, **24**, 475–479 (2008).

70. Cheng, J, J Di, J Hong *et al.*: The promotion effect of titania nanoparticles on the direct electrochemistry of lactate dehydrogenase sol-gel modified gold electrode. *Talanta*, **76**, 1065–1069 (2008).

71. Kusakari, A, M Izumi, and H Ohnuki: Preparation of an enzymatic glucose sensor based on hybrid organic-inorganic Langmuir-Blodgett films: adsorption of glucose oxidase into positively charged molecular layers. *Colloids Surf.*, **321**, 47–51 (2008).

72. Roth, CC, and BP Kropp: Recent advances in urologic tissue engineering. *Curr. Urol. Rep.*, **10**, 119–125 (2009).

73. Ashammakhi, N, A Ndreu, L Nikkola, I Wimpenny, and Y Yang: Advancing tissue engineering by using electrospun nanofibers. *Regen. Med.*, **3**, 547–574 (2008).

74. Langer, R, and JP Vacanti: Tissue engineering. *Science*, **260**, 920–926 (1993).

75. Mele, E, and D Pisignano: Nanobiotechnology: soft lithography. *Prog. Mol. Subcell. Biol.*, **47**, 341–358 (2009).

76. Lee, WB, CH Weng, FY Cheng, CS Yeh, HY Lei, and GB Lee: Biomedical microdevices synthesis of iron oxide nanoparticles using a microfluidic system. *Biomed. Microdevices*, **11**, 161–171 (2009).

77. Tan, W, and TA Desai: Layer-by-layer microfluidics for biomimetic three-dimensional structures. *Biomaterials*, **25**, 1355–1364 (2004).

78. Vozzi, G, A Previti, D De Rossi, and A Ahluwalia: Microsyringe-based deposition of two-dimensional and three-dimensional polymer scaffolds with a well-defined geometry for application to tissue engineering. *Tissue Eng.*, **8**, 1089–1098 (2002).

79. Burdick, JA, A Khademhosseini, and R Langer: Fabrication of gradient hydrogels using a microfluidics/photopolymerization process. *Langmuir*, **20**(13), 5153–5156 (2004).

80. Ma, PX, and R Zhang: Synthetic nano-scale fibrous extracellular matrix. *J. Biomed. Mater. Res.*, **46**, 60–72 (1999).

81. Reed, CR, L Han, A Andrady *et al.*: Composite tissue engineering on polycaprolactone nanofiber scaffolds. *Ann. Plast. Surg.*, **62**, 505–512 (2009).

82. Lu, K, J Jacob, P Thiyagarajan, VP Conticello, and DG Lynn: Exploiting amyloid fibril lamination for nanotube self-assembly. *J. Am. Chem. Soc.*, **125**, 6391–6393 (2003).

83. Neumann, T, M Fauver, and GH Pollack: Elastic properties of isolated thick filaments measured by nanofabricated cantilevers. *Biophys. J.*, **75**, 938–947 (1998).

84. Levi, V, and E Gratton: Exploring dynamics in living cells by tracking single particles. *Cell Biochem. Biophys.*, **48**, 1–15 (2007).

85. Jain, KK: Applications of nanobiotechnology in clinical diagnostics. *Clin. Chem.*, **53**, 2002–2009 (2007).

86. Seifulla, RD, AB Timofeev, ZG Ordzhonikidze *et al.*: Nanotechnology applications in pharmacology. *Eksp. Klin. Farmakol.*, **71**, 61–69 (2008).

87. Hromadka, M, C Reed, L Han, T Andrady, KK Kolappa, and JA van Aalst: Nanofiber technology for burn care. *J. Burn Care Res.*, (2008).

88. Radisic, M, RK Iyer, and SK Murthy: Micro- and nanotechnology in cell separation. *Int. J. Nanomedicine*, **1**, 3–14 (2006).

89. Qi, L, S Pal, P Dutta, M Seehra, and M Pei: Morphology controllable nanostructured chitosan matrix and its cytocompatibility. *J. Biomed. Mater. Res. A*, **87**, 236–244 (2008).

90. Hoover, DK, EJ Lee, EW Chan, and MN Yousaf: Electroactive nanoarrays for biospecific ligand mediated studies of cell adhesion. *Chembiochem*, **8**, 1920–1923 (2007).

91. Alcock, J, AJ Ireland, RJ Sandy, and ME Barbour: Nanoindentation of orthodontic archwires: variation of elastic modulus and hardness within a stainless steel wire. *Int. J. Nano Biomater.*, **1**, 128–137 (2007).

92. Jackson, MJ, W Ahmed, H Sein, and H Taylor: Diamond coated molybdenum dental tools for machining orthodontic bridgework materials. *Int. J. Nano Biomater.*, **1**, 184–199 (2007).

93. Albrecht, MA, CW Evans, and CL Raston: Green chemistry and the health implications of nanoparticles. *Green Chem.*, **8**, 417–432 (2006).

94. Kleiner, K, and J Jenny Hogan: How safe is nanotech? *New Scientist*, **177** (2003).

95. Helland, A, P Wick, A Koehler, K Schmid, and C Som: Reviewing the environmental and human health knowledge base of carbon nanotubes. *Environ. Health Perspect.*, **115**, 1125–1131 (2007).

96. McCarthy, TD, P Karellas, SA Henderson *et al.*: Dendrimers as drugs: discovery and preclinical and clinical development of dendrimer-based microbicides for HIV and STI prevention. *Mol. Pharm.*, **2**, 312–318 (2005).

Chapter 2

Nanomedicines Impacts in Ocular Delivery and Targeting

Yadollah Omidi, Jaleh Barar, and Hossein Hamzeiy

Research Centre for Pharmaceutical Nanotechnology, Faculty of Pharmacy, Tabriz University of Medical Sciences, Tabriz, Iran
yomidi@tbzmed.ac.ir

2.1 Introduction

For a perfect functionality of the visual cells, the integrity of the cells/tissues in anterior and posterior segments is of essence. In fact, the tight cellular membranes and barriers that control the transport of fluids and solutes within the segments play a key role in ocular homeostasis, maintenance, and diseases. Figure 2.1 shows the fluorescein angiograms in a healthy eye — panel (A), a fluorescein angiogram with some leakage — panel (B), and a detachment in the retina — panel (C). Nevertheless, intense drug delivery challenges are demanded to circumvent such biological protective barriers and access the target cells/tissue (Macha and Mitra, 2003).

Within the eye, the retina and the vitreous are separated from the systemic circulation and the vitreous body by the inner and outer blood–retinal barriers (BRB), thus resulting in lessened convection of molecules between them. Basically, ophthalmic drug delivery and

Nanotechnology in Health Care
Edited by Sanjeeb K. Sahoo

ISBN 978-981-4267-21-2 (Hardcover), 978-981-4267-35-9 (eBook)
www.panstanford.com

targeting tackles various objectives, (a) to improve drug permeation (e.g., using techniques such as iontophoresis), (b) to control the release rate of a designated drug (e.g., using appropriate delivery system such as micro/nanosuspension, liposomes, and intraocular implants), and (c) to target designated cellular biomarkers (e.g., using immunpharmaceuticals), the reader is directed to see Sahoo *et al.*, (2008). Of these, prolonged action dosage forms may modestly increase the bioavailability and length of drug function; however, these systems are yet to be improved from different viewpoints such as patients' compliance, the ocular absorption, which is architecturally limited due to the presence of the ocular barriers, and the tissue irritation and damage caused by penetration enhancers and collagen shields (Sahoo *et al.*, 2008; Urtti, 2006).

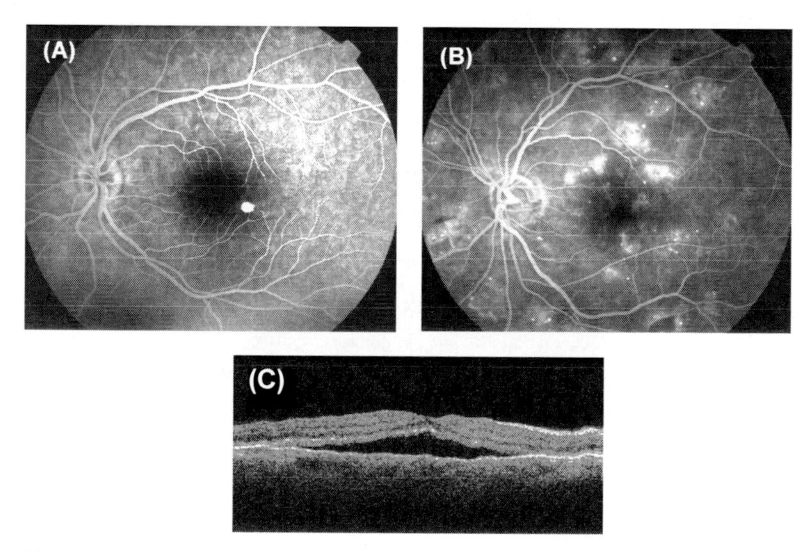

Figure 2.1 Fluorescein angiograms. (A) A healthy eye. (B) An eye with a resolution of leakage. (C) Retinal detachment. The image is from our unpublished work.

In fact, due to the anatomical architectural hallmarks of the eye, topical dosage forms are the most used medications, which are routinely administered from the anterior segment (i.e., the cornea, the conjunctiva, the sclera, and the anterior uvea). However, most of these medications can be easily drained away from the ocular surface. Such function usually results in low bioavailability; thus, the fluid-based dosage forms often fail to reach the posterior segments (the retina and the vitreous). This, together with the selective functionality of the ocular barriers, makes drug delivery to the posterior segment a challenging issue, while the current strategies to treat ocular diseases reveal limited successes (Mitra *et al.*, 2006; Macha and Mitra, 2003). Drug therapy via intravitreal injection seems to be the remaining option as reported for the treatment of age-related macular degeneration (AMD) with the antivascular endothelial growth factor (VEGF) therapies, for example, pegaptanib (Macugen®), ranibizumab (Lucentis®), and bevacizumab (Avastin®) (El-Beik and Elligott, 2007; Bakri and Kaiser, 2006). Nevertheless, it is an invasive strategy that can be exacerbated with repeated injections and may inevitably cause adverse consequences. Systemic administrations are also considered a suitable approach for some pharmaceuticals that possess appropriate physicochemical and biopharmaceutical characteristics. The ocular diseases therapy via subconjunctival and periocular (sub-Tenon's and peribulbar) routes is deemed to provide prolonged pharmacologic impacts with lower toxicity (Chastain, 2003).

In general, despite possessing many advantages, conventional dosage forms are not devoid of many pitfalls, such as repetitive use resulting in poor patient compliance, difficulty of insertion in the case of ocular inserts, and being invasive when injected/implanted that is also associated with some tissue damage. In contrast, novel nanosystems are deemed to shed some light on the ocular drug therapy by efficiently crossing the related barriers with minimal inadvertent side effects (Cai *et al.*, 2008).

Nanomedicines, depending on their architecture, provide controlled drug release and accordingly prolonged therapeutic impacts. To obtain such goals, for example, an ocular particulate nanosystem needs to be localized and retained within the cul-de-sac, where the entrapped drug should be released from the nanosystem. The utility of nanoparticles as an ocular drug delivery system (DDS) is deemed to largely depend on various factors (Visor, 1994), including (a) lipophilic-hydrophilic properties of the polymer-drug system, (b) the rates of biodegradation in the precorneal pocket, and (c) the retention efficiency in the precorneal pocket (Kothuri *et al.*, 2003). To achieve an optimized effect, it is highly desirable to engineer bioadhesive nanoparticles, which can enhance the retention time of the particles in the ocular cul-de-sac to prevent their fast elimination (Visor, 1994). This can be attained using either polymeric solutions or particulate systems, in which it has been shown that natural bioadhesive polymers are able to improve the ocular bioavailability.

Some biodegradable and/or bioadhesive polymers appear to optimize the particulate ocular DDSs. The biodegradable polymers were shown to be the most safe and biocompatible/genocompatible polymers for molecular therapy. Of these, smart nanoformulations can be exploited to target the specific biomarkers within the retinal pigment epithelium (RPE) or choroidal vasculature. The modified (e.g., PEGylated) nanomedicines may also be administered intravenously and reach the target sites via blood stream (Sanders *et al.*, 2007). For more efficient therapy, futuristic molecular Trojan delivery systems are deemed to be developed exploiting more specific cellular characteristics of carrier-/receptor-mediated transport machineries of the eye. Such battle has already begun as a frontier paradigm using genetically engineered antibodies and modified oligonucleotides (Pardridge, 2007; Shen *et al.*, 2006; Boado *et al.*, 2008).

To achieve such goals, better understanding of the biological membranes and barriers of the ocular system is clearly demanded. Here, we will provide an overview of the ocular drug delivery and targeting towards the implementation of nanomedicines in the ocular diseases regarding the main biological aspects of the eye.

2.2 Topical Absorption of Ocular Drug

Corneal and/or noncorneal routes are the main routes for the local drug therapy of the eye. However, it should be noticed that in the eye cul-de-sac, the medications are subjected to some physiological/biological barriers. First, the administered pharmaceuticals may be carried away by the lacrimal fluids. Second, inevitable systemic absorption occurs through the conjunctival sac as well as the nasal cavity (Leeming, 1999; Urtti *et al.*, 1994; Chiou *et al.*, 1991).

The corneal route represents the main absorption path for most of the ophthalmic therapeutics. However, corneal absorption is also considered to be a rate-limited process due to the presence of the corneal epithelium (Macha and Mitra, 2003; Ghate and Edelhauser, 2006).

The second path involves penetration across the conjunctiva and sclera into the intraocular tissues; however, this path appears to be less productive due to the presence of the local capillary beds that remove the drug from target sites to the general circulation. Despite this drawback, poor corneal permeability compounds such as timolol maleate, gentamicin, and prostaglandin $PGF_2\alpha$ were shown to reach the intraocular section through diffusion across the conjunctiva and sclera (Lee *et al.*, 1986; Lee, 1990; Lehr *et al.*, 1994). Thus, the absorption mechanism depends mostly on the physiochemical characteristics of the compounds and the biological membranes and barriers of the target tissue (Huang *et al.*, 1983a; Schoenwald and Huang, 1983).

2.3 Ocular Membranes, Barriers, and Transporters

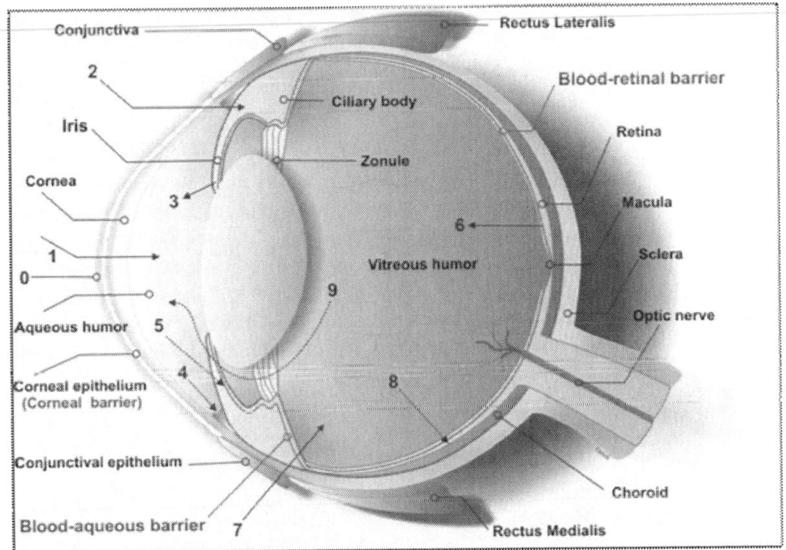

Figure 2.2 A schematic illustration of the eye and its biological barriers. The tear film functions against installed drugs as the physiologic impediment (0). Topical therapies are delivered through the cornea to the anterior chamber (1). Macromolecules and hydrophilic drugs can be delivered via the conjunctival/scleral route (2). Small compounds penetrate from the iris blood vessels into the anterior chamber after systemic administration (3). The administered drugs can be carried from the anterior chamber away either by aqueous humor outflow (4) or by venous blood flow after diffusing across the iris surface (5). The retinal pigment epithelium (RPE) and the retinal capillary endothelium are the main barriers for systemically administered drugs (6). Intravitreal injection to reach the vitreous (7). Drugs can be removed from the vitreous away through the blood–retinal barrier (8) and/or diffusion into the anterior chamber (9). The image was adapted from our work with permission (Barar *et al.*, 2008). See also Color Insert.

Figure 2.2 shows a schematic representation of the eye and the routinely used routes for administration of drugs and barratries. To reach the desired target sites of the eye, the administered drugs need to cross the tear film and lacrimal fluid and pass through the controlling membranes and barriers located in the cornea, the conjunctiva, the iris-ciliary body, and the retina. These biological structures are able to selectively control the traverse of substances within the eye, where mainly the epithelial and/or endothelial cells are sealed by the tight junctional constituents (Sunkara and Kompella, 2003).

2.3.1 Tear Film

A healthy ocular surface (cornea and conjunctiva) is largely dependent on the amount and composition of the tear film, which is tightly controlled by the regulation of the orbital glands and ocular surface epithelial secretions (Dartt *et al.*, 2006). The lightly buffered aqueous fluid as tear film (pH ~ 7.2–7.5) possesses a turnover rate of 15–30% per minute under normal/therapeutic conditions, and the restoration of the normal tear volume takes 2–3 minutes. This results in the loss of most of the administered eyedrops within the first 15–30 seconds, causing poor drug penetration through membranes and accordingly poor bioavailability (less than 5% for topically applied drugs) (Ahmed, 2003) through the flow of lacrimal fluid (Urtti and Salminen, 1993b) and inevitable systemic absorption by the conjunctival sac and the nasal cavity (Leeming, 1999; Urtti *et al.*, 1994; Chiou *et al.*, 1991). These physiologic impediments have led researchers to exploit more robust medications (e.g., nanosuspension) that remain within the local target tissues for a longer period of time. The tear film, having provided the optimal levels of various factors (e.g., nutrients, electrolytes, proteins, lipids, mucin, and pH), maintains the health of the cornea and conjunctiva. Of these, tear proteins (e.g., lysozyme, secretory immunoglobulin IgA, lactoferrin, lipocalin, and peroxidase) prevent bacterial and viral infections of the eye (Fullard and Tucker, 1994). Thus, to circumvent these physiologic impediments, more robust medications such as gel-forming timolol (Timoptol®-LA and Timoptol®-XE, used to treat glaucoma) (Shedden *et al.*, 2001), thermosensitive *in situ* gel-forming systems (Cao *et al.*, 2007), or mucoadhesives (Ludwig, 2005) are required in order to prolong the desired pharmacologic activities.

2.3.2 Cornea and Corneal Route

The clear and avascular cornea consists of five layers: the corneal epithelium, the basement membrane, Bowman's layer, the stroma, Descemet's membrane, and the endothelium. The 35–50 μm thickness corneal epithelium is formed by several cell layers, including superficial, wing, and basal cells, and is maintained by several cell–cell and cell–substrate interactions (Fischbarg, 2006a; Sunkara and Kompella, 2003). Figure 2.3 demonstrates the cornea and its cellular organization of various transport-limiting layers (Barar *et al.*, 2008).

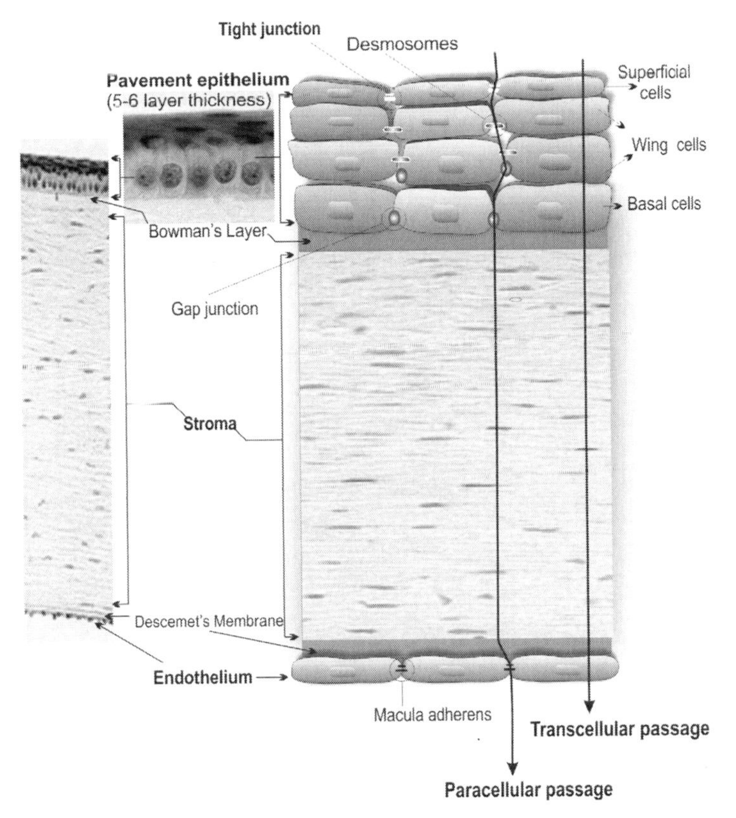

Figure 2.3 The cornea and its cellular organization of various transport limiting layers. The outer superficial epithelial cells possessing tight junctions display the tightest monolayer. The inner endothelial cells displaying macula adherens are more permeable. The image was adapted from our work with permission (Barar *et al.*, 2008).

Drug transport across the cornea is mediated mostly through passive diffusion although carrier/receptor mediated transport systems may also be involved. The partitioning and diffusion potentials of pharmaceuticals within the cellular lipid bilayers are the main driving forces, regardless of the poor bioavailability (less than 5%) of the topically used drugs even for small lipophilic molecules (Kyyronen and Urtti, 1990). The corneal epithelium is a tight barrier for hydrophilic molecules as well as macromolecules, while it may retard traverse of some small lipophilic molecules. The conjunctiva and sclera can provide anterior routes for new potential biotech-drugs and macromolecules such as protein and peptide drugs and gene medicines (Sasaki *et al.*, 1995; Cai *et al.*, 2008).

2.3.3 Corneal Epithelium and Endothelium

The corneal epithelia are formed in the corneoscleral limbus; then they migrate toward the anterior surface of the corneal epithelium and become flattened. Ultimately, the superficial cells adhere to one another through desmosomes and form tight junctions (Klyce and Crosson, 1985). The corneal epithelium barrier selectively controls the traverse of ocular drugs (in particular, hydrophilic compounds), whereas the stroma and the endothelium confer less control on transcorneal permeation (Huang *et al.*, 1983a; Huang *et al.*, 1983b), that is, the stroma is mainly composed of hydrated collagen and functions as a barrier, particularly to highly lipophilic drugs. The corneal endothelial monolayer forms a cellular barrier between the stroma and the aqueous humor, and its selective carrier- and/or receptor-mediated transport functionality favors corneal transparency (Sunkara and Kompella, 2003). These latter membranous transporters confer selective gates for hydrophilic pharmaceuticals as well as macromolecules to be shuttled to the anterior chamber.

Drug penetration across the cornea into the eye largely depends on the physicochemical properties of administered therapeutics (i.e., drug and formulation components), including octanol–water partition coefficient, molecular weight, solubility, and ionization state (Chastain, 2003) — for example, the greater the molecular size, the less the rate of paracellular permeation (Hamalainen *et al.*, 1997). Further, at physiological pH, the corneal epithelium is negatively charged, at which the permeation profile will change with the surface charge of the molecules and pH (Palmgren *et al.*, 2002; Prausnitz and Noonan, 1998). In general, upon permeability as well as Log P and Log D values, lipophilic drugs permeate faster and to a greater extent through the cornea by the transcellular mechanism than by hydrophilic drugs (Prausnitz and Noonan, 1998). For example, the permeability increases with increasing distribution coefficient in the corneal epithelium. However, the permeability of just the endothelial layer of the cornea was shown to be largely dependent on both distribution coefficient and molecular size; that is, both lipophilic pathway across cells (related to the distribution coefficient) and hydrophilic pathway between cells (related to the molecular size) are involved, where the endothelium is not a uniquely rate-limiting barrier, but playing some role in the corneal barrier for lipophilic molecules (Prausnitz and Noonan, 1998). Given that the drug diffuses into the aqueous humor and to the anterior uvea after crossing the corneal impediment, it seems to be unlikely that the locally used pharmaceuticals display the potential to reach the retina and vitreous at sufficient therapeutic concentrations. Nevertheless, some novel approaches appear to provide a promising platform for such implementations (Kurz and Ciulla, 2002; Davis *et al.*, 2004; Myles *et al.*, 2005).

The corneal endothelium is a monolayer of polygonal cells, most of which are hexagonal in shape, with about 20 μm diameter and 4–6 μm thickness. These cells play a key role in maintaining corneal transparency through their transport, synthetic, and secretory functions. In fact, the corneal endothelium has to pump fluid from the stroma to the aqueous. The abundance of endothelial intracellular organelles (e.g., mitochondria) explains that the corneal endothelium is metabolically very active. The endothelial cells, at the apical border, form a characteristic regular array of hexagons; however, they are very different at the basolateral border (Fischbarg, 2006b). The corneal endothelium is polarized so that some crucial transporters are restricted to one of the sides of the cell; for instance, the Na^+ pump is restricted to the lateral membrane. Intriguingly, the transcellular movement of Na^+ takes place in the opposite direction, that is, the amount of Na^+ leaking back into the cell via apical epithelial Na^+ channels is as much as 50–70% of that transported by the Na^+ pumps. The rest of the Na^+ inflow would take place via the cotransporters and exchangers (Kuang *et al.*, 2004). Contrary to corneal epithelial cells, macular occludens, not entirely occlusive junctions, rather than zonula occludens, exist between endothelial cells (Wood *et al.*, 1985; McLaughlin *et al.*, 1985). This results in a leaky barrier between the aqueous humor and the stroma, which allows the passage of large molecules (e.g., up to 70 kDa in size) — the involvement of paracellular or endocytic routes is yet to be uncovered (Fischbarg, 2006b). The leakiness of the corneal endothelia correlates with the transendothelial/epithelial electrical resistance (TEER) (20–60 $\Omega.cm^2$) (Fischbarg, 2006b), while capillary endothelial cell membranes often display significantly higher bioelectrical resistances as reported brain microvasculature endothelial cells (>1500 $\Omega.cm^2$) (Omidi *et al.*, 2003a; Smith *et al.*, 2007). Although the endothelium is leaky, it is the site of the major active ion and fluid transport mechanisms that maintain constant corneal thickness. Gap junctions present on the lateral membranes of the endothelial cells contribute to intercellular communication. In comparison, the immortalized human corneal epithelial cells (Toropainen *et al.*, 2001) and the rabbit primary corneal epithelial cultures (Chang *et al.*, 2000) display TEER of approximately 500 and 5,000 ($\Omega.cm^2$), respectively. On the whole, a topically applied drug diffuses into the aqueous humor and to the anterior uvea after crossing the corneal impediment, but these pharmaceuticals fail to reach the retina and the vitreous at sufficient therapeutic concentrations (Duvvuri *et al.*, 2003).

2.3.4 Noncorneal Route, Conjunctiva, and Sclera

The noncorneal route, the so-called conjunctival/scleral pathway, is a competing and parallel route of absorption, which is a minor absorption pathway compared to the corneal route, but for a few compounds its contribution is significant.

The conjunctiva is a thin and transparent membrane lining the inside of the eyelids continuously with cornea and covers the anterior surface of the sclera (bulbar conjunctiva). The mucous membrane conjunctiva consists of three layers: (a) an outer epithelium, which is a permeability barrier; (b) substantia propria, containing nerves, lymphatics, and blood vessels; and (c) the submucosa, which provides a loose attachment to the underlying sclera. The more firmly adhering segment lining the inside of the eyelids is called the tarsal or palpebral conjunctiva (Ahmed, 2003). Due to its rich vasculature nature, the existence of goblet cells, and the transdifferentiation potential, it is different from the cornea and appears to provide an important noncorneal route for ocular drug delivery, in particular for macromolecules. The conjunctival epithelium plays a key role as a protective barrier by presenting tight junctions at the apical surface of the epithelium, which is of note for the hydrophilic substances permeation and delivery of oligonucleotides (Liaw *et al.*, 2001), peptides, and proteins (Einmahl *et al.*, 2001). Intriguingly, the conjunctival epithelium in rabbits possesses larger pores and a higher pore density than the corneal epithelium, resulting in a significant higher permeability compared to the cornea (Hamalainen *et al.*, 1997). However, a markedly large amount of the administered pharmaceutical is usually carried by the systemic circulation away while crossing the conjunctiva and the remaining drug penetrates across the sclera to reach the posterior parts, that is, the uveal tract, the retina, the choroid, and the vitreous humor (Lee and Robinson, 2004; Robinson *et al.*, 2006; Kothuri *et al.*, 2003).

Further, the conjunctival epithelium plays a key protective role by the tight junctional barrier at the apical surface of the epithelium with a bioelectrical resistance of over 1,500 $\Omega.cm^2$ (Saha *et al.*, 1996), which is of note function for the permeation and delivery of macromolecules in hydrophilic substances (Liaw *et al.*, 2001; Einmahl *et al.*, 2001). A markedly large amount of the administered pharmaceutical is usually carried by the systemic circulation away while crossing the conjunctiva and the remaining drug penetrates across the sclera to reach the posterior parts (i.e., the uveal tract, the retina, the choroid, and the vitreous humor) (Lee and Robinson, 2004; Robinson *et al.*, 2006; Kothuri *et al.*, 2003). Various transporters were shown to be expressed in the conjunctival epithelium. Among them, neutral and cationic amino acids transporter ($ATB^{0,+}$), nucleoside transporter (CNT2), and peptide transporter 1 (PepT1) can be exploited for transporting the associated drugs (e.g., acyclovir) (Hosoya *et al.*, 1998; Hosoya *et al.*, 2005; Ganapathy and Ganapathy, 2005). The functional expression of efflux pumps, including P-glycoprotein (P-gp) and multidrug resistance protein (MRP1), have been reported (Saha *et al.*, 1998; Yang *et al.*, 2007), but the role of the vesicular transport machineries (e.g., clathrin coated pits and caveolae) in the conjunctival epithelium is yet to be fully examined.

The sclera is continuous with the cornea and extends posteriorly from the limbus. Structurally, the sclera is very similar to the corneal stroma containing numerous channels and consists mainly of collagen and mucopolysaccharides (Hamalainen *et al.*, 1997; Kim *et al.*, 2007). The poorly vascularized sclera is significantly more permeable than the cornea but less permeable than the conjunctiva. The sclera was shown to be exploited for antibody delivery (Ambati *et al.*, 2000).

In general, ophthalmic drugs can be absorbed from the conjunctiva and delivered to the eye via the sclera. However, drainage loss through blood vessels of the conjunctiva can greatly impact the conjunctival/scleral pathway. Therefore, this noncorneal route is considered to be nonproductive for most of the ophthalmic drugs, but it should be evoked that the conjunctival epithelium is the most viable route for the ocular delivery of peptides and oligonucleotides (Hamalainen *et al.*, 1997).

2.3.5 Iris, Ciliary Body, and Aqueous Humor Flow

The iris, the ciliary body, and the choroid represent the vascular uveal coat of the eye, where the iris anterior is immersed in the aqueous humor. The ciliary body is formed by several biological regions, including the nonpigmented ciliary epithelium, the pigmented ciliary epithelium, the stroma, and the ciliary muscle. Its fenestrated and leaky capillaries confer intercommunication of the anterior and posterior chambers (Stewart and Tuor, 1994), at which the aqueous humor is secreted into the posterior chamber and flows through the pupil into the anterior chamber. By mechanisms of diffusion, ultrafiltration, and active transport, the aqueous humor is derived from the plasma within the capillary network of the ciliary body. Of these, the active transport processes account for the majority of aqueous humor production, where water-soluble substances of larger size or higher charge are actively transported through the cellular membrane, requiring the expenditure of energy such as Na^+, K^+-ATPase, and glycolytic enzymes (Mitra *et al.*, 2006).

2.3.6 Vitreous Body and Fluid Flow

The space between lens and the retina is filled by the clear and avascular connective tissue of the vitreous (~4 mL and ~4 g in adults) (Lee *et al.*, 1992). The gel-like composition of the vitreous contains water (99.9%), collagen, hyaluronic acid, and ions (Lee *et al.*, 1994b; Lee *et al.*, 1994a). Drug movement in the vitreous is largely dependent on its diffusion rate; and unlike the vitreous composition, the convective flow fails to affect drug diffusion (Mitra *et al.*, 2006). The intravitreal route appears to be the major route of drug administration to the posterior segment, in which the diffusivity potential of the vitreous depends on the pathophysiological state and molecular weight of the administered drugs (Mitra *et al.*, 2006; Raghava *et al.*, 2004).

2.3.7 Blood–Aqueous Barrier

Two discrete cell layers (the endothelium of the iris/ciliary blood vessels and the nonpigmented ciliary epithelium) form the blood–aqueous barrier (BAB) in the anterior part of the eye (see Fig. 2.2), whose functionality controls the traverse of solutes between the posterior and anterior chambers (Bill, 1986; Freddo, 2001). Both these cell layers display tight junctional complexes, by which, inadvertent nonspecific passage of solutes into the intraocular milieu is impeded. This results in maintenance of the transparency and chemical composition of the ocular fluids (Freddo, 2001). However, the barrier functionality of the BAB is not complete even when it is intact. The injected horseradish peroxidase (HRP, 40 kDa) was shown to reach the aqueous humor through the fenestrated capillaries of the ciliary but not via the iris blood vessels, which control the permeation of the plasma proteins into the aqueous humor (Schlingemann *et al.*, 1998).

The traverse of substances from the aqueous humor into systemic circulation through the iris microvasculature endothelia seems to be less restricted. Hence, the drugs dissolved in the aqueous humor can easily penetrate the anterior surface of the iris and be absorbed by the iris pigments; thereafter, they are washed from the anterior chamber away by passage into the iris blood vessels (Mannermaa *et al.*, 2006; Urtti, 2006). The small and lipophilic drugs were shown to enter the uveal blood circulation via the BAB, from where they are eliminated more rapidly than larger and more hydrophilic drugs, which are eliminated by aqueous humor turnover only (Hornof *et al.*, 2005). The passage of drugs from the anterior segment to the posterior segment appears not to be an efficient strategy because of the continuous drainage of the aqueous humor (i.e., a turnover of 2.0–3.0 mL/min). Thus, the locally used ophthalmic therapies fail to provide an efficient pharmacological effect in the posterior segment (e.g., the retina and the vitreous). The novel therapeutic strategies like intravitreal injections and subconjunctival implants seem to grant only limited successes (Mitra *et al.*, 2006).

2.3.8 Retina and Blood–Retinal Barrier

Retina, the light-sensitive part of the eye, is a thin film of tissue that covers the entire inner wall of the eye. The retina is formed from neural cells as well as glial cells (i.e., Müller cells, astrocytes, microglial cells, and oligodendroglial cells) (la Cour and Ehinger, 2006). The outermost part of the retina is a single layer of pigmented cuboidal epithelial cells, the so-called RPE (la Cour and Ehinger, 2006). Although the functions of the RPE and the retina are tightly coupled, the RPE and accordingly the BRB will be our focus due to their important roles in ocular drug therapy. Figure 2.4 shows the retinal cellular organization.

The BRB is located in the posterior part of the eye and consists of two types of cells, including the retinal capillary endothelial (RCE) and RPE cells that form the inner and outer BRB, respectively (Fig. 2.4). Specialized transport processes within the RPE, along with the robust barrier restrictiveness of RPE, control the traverse of nutrients/compounds selectively, at which only selected nutrients are exchanged between the choroid and the retina (Mitra *et al.*, 2006; Duvvuri *et al.*, 2003). The polarized RPE cells display predominant apical localization of Na^+, K^+-ATPase, which regulates intracellular Na^+ and K^+ homeostasis (Lin *et al.*, 1992; Quinn and Miller, 1992). The inner BRB covers the lumen of retinal capillaries and selectively protects the retina from the blood circulating molecules. Unlike the fenestrated choroidal capillary endothelial cells, the RCE cells possess intercellular tight junctions (Fig. 2.4) (Gardner *et al.*, 1999). Regardless of the permeation of lipophilic substances across the RCE cells, this barrier displays poor permeability to proteins and small hydrophilic compounds (Sunkara and Kompella, 2003; Hornof *et al.*, 2005).

Substantial delivery and sufficient pharmacological effects of drugs within the vitreous and the retina necessitate systemic or intravitreal drug administration. A systemic application, via oral or intravenous administration, requires high doses of the drug since blood flow and restrictive functionality of the BRB allow only a very small fraction of the drug to reach the posterior segment. Thus, a large portion of the drug is disseminated in the entire body, leading to inadvertent adverse reactions (Selvin, 1983).

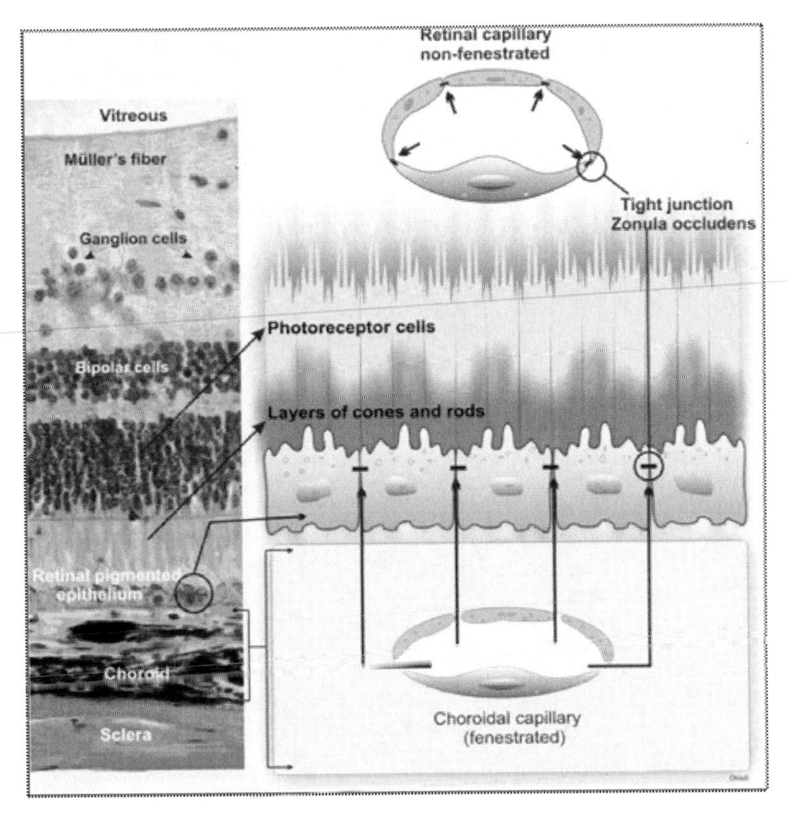

Figure 2.4 The retina and its cellular organization of various transport limiting layers. The outer layer of retinal pigmented epithelium displays a tight barrier due to the presence of a tight junction (zonula occludens). The inner layer retinal capillary endothelial (RCE) cells possessing a tight junction are nonfenestrated compared to choroidal capillary endothelial cells that are fenestrated. The image was adapted from our work with permission (Barar *et al.*, 2008).

2.3.9 Ocular Transport Machineries

Cell membranes impose a barrier to the free movement of molecules through a membranous lipid bilayer and associated transport machineries. A solute, based upon molecular properties, is transported across the cell membranes by passive diffusion and/or carrier/receptor-mediated transport (Omidi and Gumbleton,

2005). Nearly most of the ocular tissue displays Na^+/H^+ exchanger, Na^+/HCO_3^- symporter, and Cl^-/HCO_3^- exchanger that are involved in the regulation of intracellular pH (Jentsch *et al.*, 1985). The Na^+/H^+ exchanger is present at the basolateral membranes of both

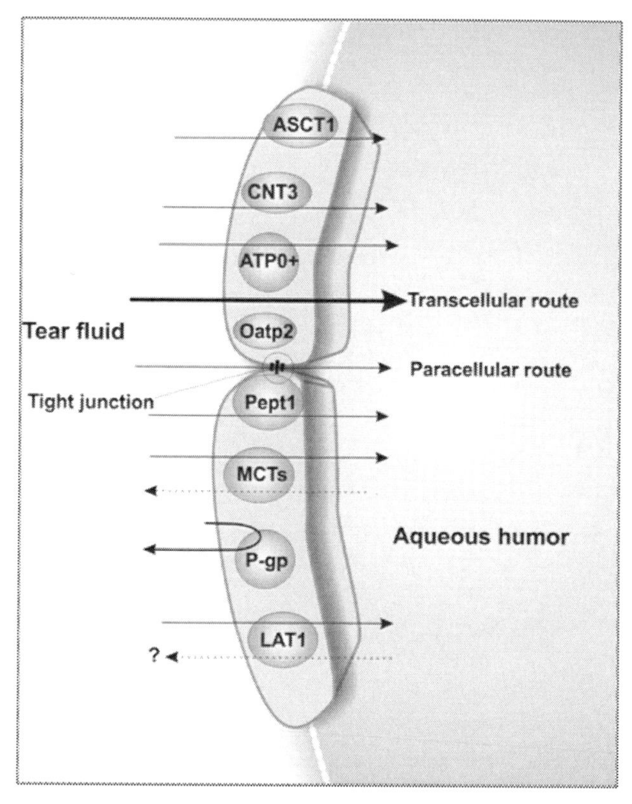

Figure 2.5 A schematic representation of the currently known carrier-mediated transport machineries in the corneal epithelium. ASCT: Na^+-dependent small neutral amino acid transporter (L-alanine); MCTs: onocarboxylate transporters (lactate, pyruvates, and ketones); CNT3: concentrative nucleoside transporter 3 (thymidine); Oatp2: organic anion transporting polypeptides 2 (unknown); LAT1: large neutral amino acids transporter (L-phenylalanine); P-gp: P-glycoprotein (verpamil and fluorescein); ATB^{0+}: concentrative amino acids transporter (carnitine, valacyclovir, and valganciclovir); Pept1: proton-coupled oligopeptide transporter (POT) di/tri peptide transporter 1 (valacyclovir, valganciclovir, glycylsarcosine, and cephalexin). The image was adapted from our work with permission (Barar *et al.*, 2008).

epithelial and endothelial cells, while Na^+/HCO_3^- transporter is predominantly localized at the basolateral side of the corneal endothelium and is faintly expressed in the corneal epithelium. This implies that the distribution pattern of these channel transporters at the apical and basolateral membrane varies depending upon the cellular needs and physiologic functions (Gao *et al.*, 2000; Sun *et al.*, 2000). Figures 2.5 and 2.6 schematically represent the currently known influx/efflux transport machineries of the corneal epithelium and the retinal outer/inner barriers, respectively — the reader is directed to see the following reviews for more details: Mannermaa *et al.*, 2006; Dey and Mitra, 2005; Sunkara and Kompella, 2003. The functional expression, the transport direction, the membrane distribution pattern, and exchange potentials of many of these transporters need to be fully investigated.

The influx and efflux transport machineries are functionally expressed in the main membranous barriers of the eye, that is, the cornea, the conjunctiva, the iris–ciliary body, and the retina (see Figs. 2.5 and 2.6) (Mannermaa *et al.*, 2006). The unidirectional/bidirectional influx transporters such as monocarboxylate transporters (MCTs), glucose transporters (e.g., Glut1), amino acid transporters (LAT1 and LAT2), and PepT1 supply essential nutrient requirements of the cells (Omidi and Gumbleton, 2005). The LAT1 transporter of the brain capillary endothelial cells functions bidirectionally with greater efflux activity (Omidi *et al.*, 2008). However, its functional directionality in the corneal/retinal barriers is yet to be fully investigated and so are most of the carrier-mediated transporters in the eye. For more detailed information, the reader is directed to see the following citations: Shimoyama *et al.*, 2007; Fischbarg *et al.*, 2006; Mannermaa *et al.*, 2006; Dey and Mitra, 2005; Ganapathy and Ganapathy, 2005; Schorderet *et al.*, 2005; Atluri *et al.*, 2004; Hamann, 2002; Gerhart *et al.*, 1999.

In the ATP-binding cassette (ABC) superfamily, the P-gp and multidrug resistance–associated proteins (MRPs) play a key role in the unidirectional efflux of substances. The human and rabbit corneal epithelia were shown to significantly express P-gp (Dey *et al.*, 2003) and MRPs (Karla *et al.*, 2007). Similarly, these efflux pumps have been identified in different tissues of the eye, such as the RCE cells (Holash and Stewart, 1993), the retinal pigmented epithelial cells (Duvvuri *et al.*, 2003), the ciliary nonpigmented epithelium (Wu *et al.*, 1996), the conjunctival epithelial cells (Saha *et al.*, 1998), and the iris and ciliary endothelial cells (Saha *et al.*, 1998). On the ground of the current knowledge about the functional expression of efflux transporters in ocular tissues, useful modification of drug delivery strategies is expected in order to increase ocular bioavailability and to harness ophthalmic diseases in a more efficient way.

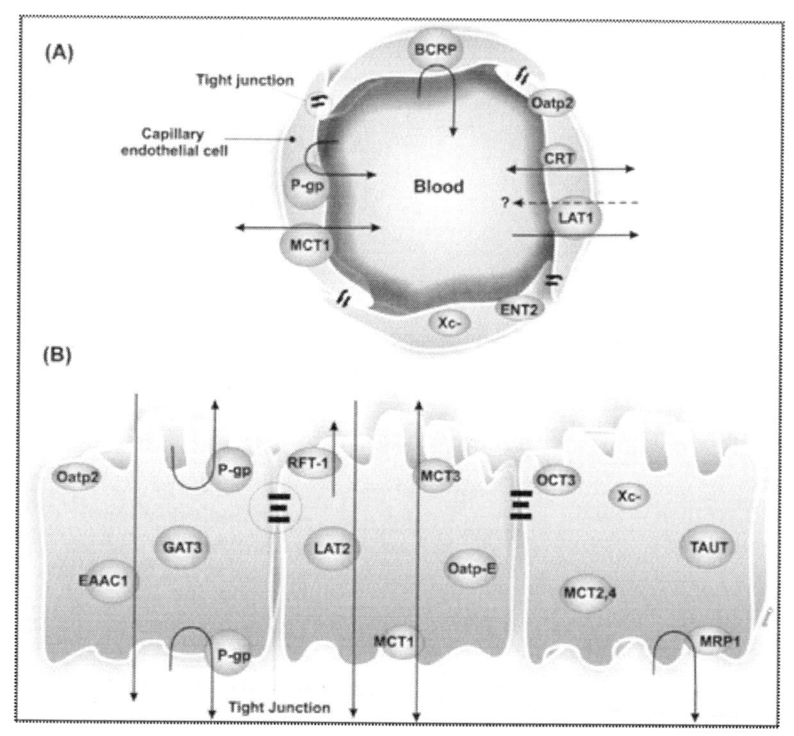

Figure 2.6 A schematic demonstration of the currently known transport machineries in the cellular barriers of the retina. (A) The inner endothelial cells of the retina. (B) The outer pigmented epithelial cells of the retina. MCTs: monocarboxylate transporters (lactate, pyruvates, and ketones); EAAC: glutamate transporter; ENT2: equilibrative nucleoside transporter 2 (thymidine); Oatp2: organic anion transporting polypeptides 2; LAT1: large neutral amino acids transporter (L-phenylalanine); P-gp: P-glycoprotein (verpamil and vincristin); MRP: multidrug resistance proteins; BCRP: breast cancer–related protein; CRT: creatine transporter; GAT3: GABA transporter; OCT: organic cation transporter; RFT: reduced folate/thiamine transporter; X_C^-: glutamate/cysteine exchange transporter; TAUT: taurine transporter. The image was adapted from our work with permission (Barar *et al.*, 2008).

Specialized receptors exist at the ocular barriers to control the passage of xenobiotics. The endocytosis pathway via clathrin-coated and/or caveolae uncoated smooth vesicles are accounted for ocular receptor–mediated transports. The expression of clathrin and the integral protein of the caveolae domain (caveolin-1) have been reported within the ocular tissues (Lo *et al.*, 2004; Bridges *et al.*, 2001; Lo *et al.*, 1991; Hunt *et al.*, 1989; Sabah *et al.*, 2007). Using cultured human retinal pigment epithelial cells (ARPE-19) and a mouse model, Mo *et al.* reported the involvement of caveolae-mediated endocytosis pathways in the uptake of albumin nanoparticles containing Cu/Zn superoxide dismutase gene (Mo *et al.*, 2007). However, Qaddoumi *et al.* showed that the endocytosis of the poly(lactic-co-glycolic) acid (PLGA) nanoparticles in primary cultured rabbit conjunctival epithelial cells occurs mostly independently of clathrin- and caveolin-1-mediated pathways, despite the transcriptome and protein expression of clathrin (Qaddoumi *et al.*, 2003). However, the transport of albumin in the rabbit lens epithelial cells revealed the involvement of a transcellular transport mechanism, employing both clathrin- and caveolae-mediated endocytosis/transcytosis pathways (Sabah *et al.*, 2007). The detection of insulin and insulin-like growth factor (IGF)-1 receptors in the corneal and conjunctival epithelial cells membranes (Rocha *et al.*, 2002), together with the role of transferring in nanoparticle delivery (Kompella *et al.*, 2006), reveal that more investigations are required to resolve the ambiguity of macromolecular (e.g., peptide/protein) trafficking in the eye.

2.4 *In vivo* and *in vitro* Models

For the development of strategies to overcome the ocular barriers for the targeted ocular delivery of drugs, the exploitation of appropriate animal and cell culture models is crucial (Hornof *et al.*, 2005). There are many applications for animal experiments, including pharmacokinetic and pharmacodynamic studies and toxicity evaluations. For example, the Draize test is an acute toxicity test devised in 1944 by Food and Drug Administration (FDA) toxicologist John H. Draize to assess the impact of a 0.5 mL or 0.5 g of a test substance on an animal's eye or skin for four hours (Parascandola, 1991). Of the different animals used for ocular drug delivery examinations, the rabbit is the most commonly used animal model although some other animals (e.g., pigs, dogs, cats, and monkeys) have also been used. Nevertheless, the rabbit eye shows distinct morphologic and biochemical differences from the human eye, including (a) an infrequent blinking rate that significantly decreases precorneal drainage of topically applied solutions and (b) larger corneal and conjunctival surface areas (Urtti and Salminen, 1993a). As a result, the ocular bioavailability of topically applied drugs in the rabbit is less influenced by nonproductive absorption through the conjunctiva (Hornof *et al.*, 2005). Although animal experimentation is deemed to be an essential part of ocular drugs advancement, it has been largely criticized from ethical and economical viewpoints. For example, the model animals must be sacrificed at each time-point in ocular pharmacokinetic studies and a large number of animals must be exploited for a single study. Besides, in the European Union, tight restricted regulations (Council Directive 86/609/EEC) for the protection of animals used in experimental/scientific approaches have been ruled out to minimize such investigations to the least (Hornof *et al.*, 2005).

These issues directed researchers to recruit *in vitro* cell-based models, including primary and immortalized cell culture models, with a particular focus on models serving blood–eye barriers (BEB). For example, the primary isolated corneal epithelial cells cultured onto the fibronectin-/collagen-/laminin-coated membrane with a serum-free medium resulted in a TEER value of 5,000 $\Omega.cm^2$ (Chang *et al.*, 2000). While TEER values of the isolated rabbit cornea (epithelium–stroma–endothelium) were determined to be 3,200–7,500 $\Omega.cm^2$. Of the immortalized corneal epithelial cell lines established from rabbit, rat, hamster and human cells, the immortalized human cell lines (e.g., HCE, HCE-T, and tet HPV16-E6/E7-transduced HCE cell lines) resulting in TEER values of 400–500 $\Omega.cm^2$ are widely used cell culture models (Hornof *et al.*, 2005).

Primary cell culture models of the conjunctival epithelium are from the rabbit and the cow, with TEER values of 1,000–2,000 and 5,000 $\Omega.cm^2$, respectively. The TEER value of excised rabbit conjunctiva was determined to be 1,300 $\Omega.cm^2$ (Hornof *et al.*, 2005). Numerous cell culture models have been established as models of the inner and outer BRB; however, the establishment of an appropriate *in vitro* model for the barrier function of the RPE remains a scientific challenge. Primary cell culture models of the RPE utilizing frog, rat, chick, bovine, and human RPE cells have been described in the literature. Of the immortalized cell lines, Davis *et al.* cloned a spontaneously arising cell line (i.e., D407) from a primary culture of human RPE. These cells were shown to possess most of the metabolic and morphologic characteristics of RPE cells *in vivo* (e.g., epithelial cobblestone morphology, the expression of typical keratins, and the synthesis of retina-specific CRALBP protein), but the model lacked some enzymatic activities (Davis *et al.*, 1995). Another human RPE cell line (i.e., ARPE-19) was established and characterized by Dunn *et al.* in 1996. The cell line was characterized toward its morphology, the expression of retina-specific markers (CRALP and RPE65), and their barrier properties (Dunn *et al.*, 1996). Despite the presence of tight junctional complexes, these cells displayed TEER values of ~100 $\Omega.m^2$. For the retinal capillary endothelium, the second passage of primary isolated bovine retinal capillary endothelial cells (BRCECs) cultured on polycarbonate filters (coated with gelatin, laminin, fibronectin, and collagen) resulted in TEER values of ~150 $\Omega.cm^2$ (Gillies *et al.*, 1995). Recently, a conditionally immortalized rat RCE cell line (TRiBRB) was developed from a transgenic rat harboring the temperature-sensitive SV40 T antigen gene (Hosoya *et al.*, 2001), which showed a very low level of TEER value (30 $\Omega.cm^2$) (Shen *et al.*, 2003). All these cell-based models have provided a valuable platform for investigations on ocular drug targeting through nanomedicines.

2.5 Ocular Pharmacotherapy

The absorption poorness of topically applied ophthalmic drugs is due to the efficient mechanisms, including reflex blinking, lacrimation, tear turnover, and drainage. Such impacts naturally result in the rapid removal of foreign substances from the eye surface; hence, frequent instillations of eyedrops are demanded to maintain a therapeutic drug level in the tear film or at the site of action. This frequent use of medications may expose ocular tissues to highly concentrated drug solutions, inducing toxic side effects and cellular damage at the ocular surface (Gaudana *et al.*, 2009; Baudouin, 1996).

2.5.1 Conventional Pharmaceuticals

Eyedrops, gels, creams, and ointments are the simplest approaches to treat some eye diseases. Of these, sustained drug delivery is achievable though the formulation of a drug in a viscous gel, cream, or ointment, in which the release of drugs is basically governed through both diffusion and partitioning — the lower the solubility of a drug in the vehicle, the higher its chemical potential and the more readily the drug will partition into the release medium. A small drug molecule (e.g., pilocarpine) can move faster than a larger molecule (e.g., peptide/protein) through a highly viscous gel; thus, the delivery of macromolecules can be more sustained in hydrogels, compared to small molecules. Further, it should be also evoked that because of the relatively poor penetration of the topically applied dosage forms into the eye tissue, these ophthalmic drugs usually contain high concentrations of their active ingredients and may induce inadvertent adverse reactions.

In the case of the direct injection of drugs to the intraocular tissues, regularly repeated injections are necessary for the successful treatment, in particular, for drugs such as antibiotics, by which the risk of retinal detachment/hemorrhage seems to be inevitable. Intravitreal injections of antibiotics (along with the adjunctive IV injection of antibiotics) were shown to be the keystone of the management of endophthalmitis even though the usefulness of the adjunctive IV injection of antibiotics appeared to be skeptical. Severe side effects may limit such medication modalities while there is no ideal antibiotic for intravitreal use with a broad spectrum of action and a long half-life in the vitreous yet with no/minimal toxic impacts on the eye (Ashton, 2006).

Of the attempts to improve ocular drug delivery are development of prodrugs, the use of penetration enhancers, and the development of novel drug-delivery such as nanomedicines (Vandervoort and Ludwig, 2007).

In fact, various factors affect the topical ocular drug therapy, including the drainage of the instilled solution, lacrimation and tear turnover, metabolism, tear evaporation, nonproductive absorption/adsorption, limited corneal area and poor corneal permeability, and binding by lacrimal proteins (Mitra *et al.*, 2006). Effective ocular drug absorption requires sufficient corneal penetration and prolonged contact time with the corneal tissue. Hence, various approaches such as iontophoresis, prodrugs, ion pair formation, sustained-release formulations, mucoadhesives, and cyclodextrins have been exploited to enhance ocular drug absorption. Nonetheless, most of the currently used medications for the treatment of the ocular diseases (e.g., glaucoma, conjunctivitis, keratitis, and uveitis) were shown to have bioavailability problems (Mitra *et al.*, 2006).

Further, the treatment of retinal pathologies (e.g., fungal and bacterial endophthalmitis, viral retinitis, and proliferative vitreal retinopathies) requires systemic administration, although it has limited success primarily due to the exclusion of the organ from systemic circulation. For example, foscarnet sodium or ganciclovir is used to treat cytomegalovirus (CMV) retinitis and endophthalmitis as intravenous (Costabile, 1998) or intravitreal injections (Lopez-Cortes *et al.*, 2001). Of these, the intravitreal injection appears to be the mainstay treatment of posterior segment infections/diseases (Mitra *et al.*, 2006), even though it may associate with patient noncompliance and endophthalmitis, cataract, astigmatism, and retinal detachment (Stone and Jaffe, 2000; Cantrill *et al.*, 1989). Thus, to avoid such complications, intravitreal implants (e.g., Vitrasert®) have been developed. Nevertheless, scleral implants and subconjunctival administrations appear to confer limited success, mainly because of the repeated need for surgical intervention associated with the presence of a foreign device within the eye (Mitra *et al.*, 2006).

Taking all these issues together, for intraocular delivery, some major factors have to be considered as follows: (a) how to pass the cornea and reach the site of the action, (b) how to prolong the duration of drug action to minimize the frequency of drug administration, (c) how to selectively target the desired biomarkers and localize the desired pharmacodynamic action, with minimal impacts on nonspecific tissues, and (d) how to cross the BEB (Kothuri *et al.*, 2003). Novel technologies are deemed to favor ocular pharmacotherapy by providing new platforms for more advanced and efficient ocular medications.

2.5.2 Emergence of Novel Technologies

An ophthalmic dosage form should provide suitable biopharmaceutical characteristics as well as an appropriate ocular tolerability. Nowadays, nearly 90% of ocular drug administration includes eyedrops. Despite very easy application of these formulations, the main problem is nonpersistency due to removal via tear drainage. As reported previously, the tight epithelium of the cornea also selectively controls the permeation of drug molecules. Thus, little of the topically applied drug can reach the posterior segment of the eye. Such limited access imposes the administration of some drugs (e.g., antiglaucoma drugs, corticosteroids, and certain antibiotics) by the systemic route, in which because of the restrictive barrier functionality of the BRB, very small fractions of the drug can reach the ocular tissues. The doses required to give a therapeutic effect via this route, however, can lead to considerable side effects; the reader should refer to Barar *et al.* (2008).

Thus, exploiting nanobiotechnology means, novel ophthalmologic formulations are being/have been developed. These nanoscaled formulations can provide longer exposure time at the ocular surface by confronting the clearance mechanisms of the eye, providing more drug concentration and reducing the dose and frequency of drug administration (Vandervoort and Ludwig, 2007).

Similarly, such approach can be exploited for intraocular drug delivery in a controlled manner to reduce the number of injections required and target the site of action with the drug, leading to a decrease in the dose and, therefore, the side effects. Formulation stability, particle size, control of drug release, and large-scale production of sterile formulations are among the major issues in nano-formulations.

Colloidal systems for either hydrophilic or hydrophobic drugs have been shown to provide DDSs for ocular tissues since they are liquid dosage forms and do not interfere with the vision function (Badawi *et al.*, 2008). In a recent study, as an example, indomethacin-loaded chitosan (CS) nanoparticles have been produced using modified ionic gelation of the polymer with tripolyphosphate. The nanoparticles had regular well-identified spherical shapes with a mean size of 280 nm, a zeta potential of +17 mV, and a high loading efficiency of 84.8%. Slight initial burst release during the first hour followed by slow and gradual indomethacin (IM) release of 76% during a 24-hour period have been revealed during *in vitro* studies (Badawi *et al.*, 2008). Moreover, the ability of the nanoparticles to provide slow and gradual release of the drug has been shown in following *in vivo* studies, increasing delivery to both external and internal ocular tissues.

Microemulsion colloidal systems (as transparent liquids) composed of an oil phase, an aqueous phase, and a surfactant and cosurfactant at appropriate ratios may offer a possible solution to the problem of poor delivery to the cornea by sustaining the release of the drug, as well as by providing a higher penetration of the drug into the deeper layers of the eye (Gaudana *et al.*, 2009).

Modified-release liposome formulations for ocular delivery constitute another example of efforts to increase drug consistency, enhance direct delivery, minimize intraocular toxicity, and control ocular delivery by preventing the drug metabolism from the enzymes present at the tear/corneal epithelial surface (Diebold *et al.*, 2007). Sodium diclofenac-loaded lipid nanoparticles have also been prepared by combining the homolipid from a goat (goat fat) and a phospholipid with high encapsulation efficiency using the hot high-pressure-homogenization technique (above 90%). The administration of this formulation in bioengineered human cornea produced a sustained release and improved the permeation through the cornea construct of the drug (Attama *et al.*, 2008).

Diclofenac-loaded biopolymeric nanosuspensions produced using PLGA, poly(alkylcyanoacrylate) (PACA), or poly-e-caprolactone (PCL) have shown no sign of irritation or damaging effects to ocular tissues in rabbit eyes for as long as 24 hours after application (Agnihotri and Vavia, 2009).

In a recent study, the formulation of mucoadhesive microdiscs by emulsification with PLGA as a core material and, in some cases, poly(ethylene glycol) as a mucoadhesion promoter, has been reported to increase preocular residence time. The study demonstrated that the formulation in a dry tablet can achieve a prolonged residence time on the preocular surface and thus is a promising DDS for ophthalmic applications (Choy *et al.*, 2008).

2.5.3 Ocular Implants

A variety of innovative DDSs (implants) have been so far introduced for ophthalmic applications, including Ocusert® (1974) for 1 week constant release of pilocarpine from conjunctiva; Vitrasert® (1996) for 6 months constant release of ganciclovir from the pars plana area of vitreous; and Retisert® (2005) for 2.5 years constant release of fluocinolone acetonide. Further, intravitreally injectable biodegradable (Posurdex®) and nonbiodegradable (Medidur®) implants are currently undergoing phase III clinical trials (Rana and Pearson, 2006; Ashton, 2006). Basically, these devices use a reservoir-type system with a rate-controlling nonbiodegradable polymer membrane. Although these devices demonstrate a relatively constant release rate, they need to be removed after drug release has been completed. Thus, it seems that biodegradable/bioerodible polymers can minimize this drawback; nevertheless, they are subjected to erosion and, thereby, can be used for a short period of time.

2.5.4 Drug-Polymer Nanoformulations

DDSs with biodegradable/bioerodible polymers can provide a significant advantage over the nondegradable system because the entirety is eventually absorbed by the body, eliminating the need for subsequent removal. However, these polymers are predisposed and time dependent due to erosion, which can occur through the following mechanisms: (a) cleavage of the cross-linked or water-soluble backbone in the cross-linked water-soluble macromolecules, (b) hydrolysis, ionization, or protonation of pendant groups in the water-insoluble macromolecules, and (c) hydrolytic cleavage of labile bonds in the polymer backbone high-molecular-weight, water-insoluble macromolecules (Kimura and Ogura, 2001). The pattern of drug release largely depends upon the association of the drug with polymers since two approaches can be undertaken for formulation — a drug core surrounded by a rate-controlling biodegradable membrane and the drug dispersed within polymer(s). Of the polymer-based systems, the nanoparticles are colloidal drug carrier systems with a range in size of 10 to 1,000 nm while nanospheres are solid matricial structures with drug molecules within the matrices and/or adsorbed on the surfaces of the colloidal carriers and nanocapsules are small capsules with a central core surrounded by a polymeric shell with dissolved/ adsorbed drug molecules in the core/surface interface. Almost most of nanoparticles used for ocular investigations appeared to be mucoadhesive and biocompatible; nevertheless, polystyrene (PS), Eudragit® RL100 (ERL), and RS100 (ERS) are not biodegradable. Figure 2.7 represents the scanning electron micrographs of the piroxicam nanoparticles formulated with ERS.

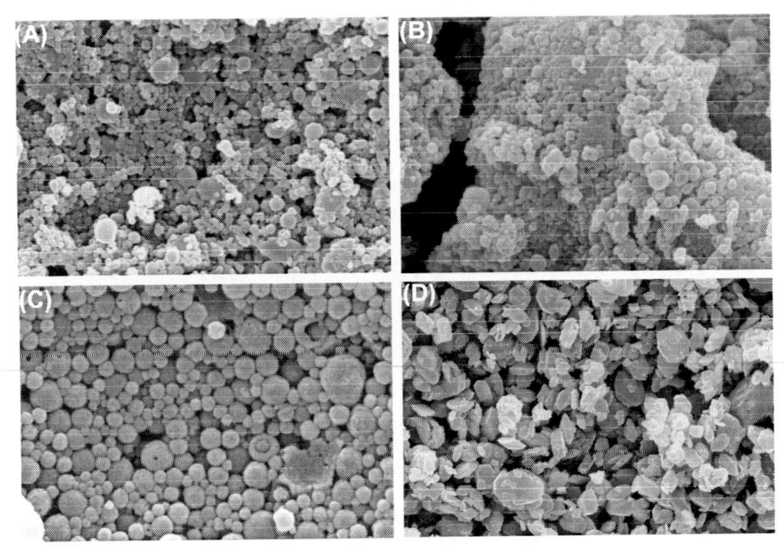

Figure 2.7 Scanning electron micrographs of piroxicam formulations. (A) Piroxicam: ERS nanoparticles at the ratios of 1:2.5. (B) Piroxicam: ERS nanoparticles at the ratios of 1:10. (C) Treated ERS. (D) Treated piroxicam. Bar equals 2 μm. ERS: Eudragit® RS100. The image was adapted from our work with permission (Adibkia *et al.*, 2007b).

According to our literature survey, the most commonly used polymers in the ophthalmic drug formulations are poly(alkyl cyanoacrylates), PCL, and poly(lactic acid)/poly(lactic-co-glycolic acid) (PLA, PGA, PLGA). Moreover, some others, such as CS, ERL/ERS, PS, and poly(acrylic acid) (PAA) as well as bovine serum albumin (BSA), have also been exploited for ocular delivery as drug-loaded nanoformulations. Given that the surface of ocular tissues (e.g., the cornea and the conjunctiva) is negatively charged, the cationic colloidal nanoparticles are expected to confer better penetration potential through the ocular membranes and barriers. Of the polymers used for ocular delivery, a few polymers (CS, ERL, and ERS) grant positively charged nanoparticles (Bu *et al.*, 2007). Figure 2.8 (A) shows the chemical structures of some important polymers used in the preparation of nanoformulations. Of the biodegradable polymers, the PLGA copolymers (PLA, PGA, and PLGA) have been widely utilized as the most promising biodegradable materials (Fig. 2.8 B and C), which have also been reported to be the most safe polymers used *in vivo* successfully with no significant toxicity (Kobayashi *et al.*, 1992; Athanasiou *et al.*, 1996; Agnihotri and Vavia, 2009; Dong *et al.*, 2006).

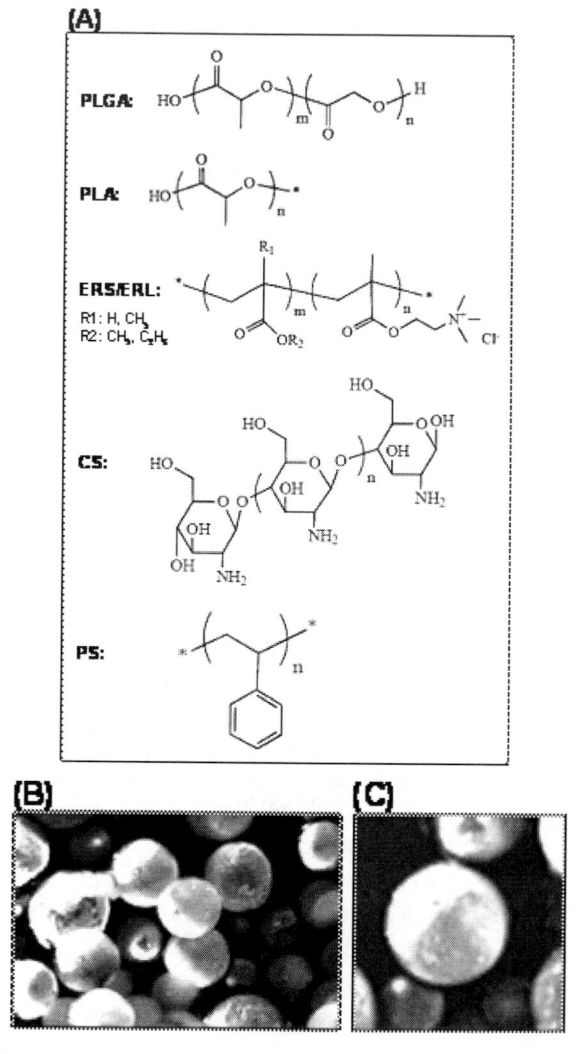

Figure 2.8 Chemical structures of some important polymers used in the preparation of nanoformulations (A) and scanning electron micrographs of PLGA microspheres — (B) and (C). Panels (B) and (C) show the magnified micrographs PLGA nanoparticles containing genomedicine (antisense against epidermal growth factor receptor). The images are from our unpublished work on genocompatibility of PLGA as a gene delivery system.

In a study, the neuroprotective effects of small pigment epithelium-derived factor (PEDF) peptides injected intravitreally as free peptides or delivered in PLGA nanospheres were tested in retinal ischemic injury in C57BL/6 mice. The injection of PEDF peptide (alone or as PLGA-based nanospheres) showed protective effects. However, the PLGA-PEDF nanospheres resulted in the longer-term protection of the retinal ganglion cell layer with no noticeable side effects at seven days, thus conferring higher clinical advantages for longer-term treatments of retinal diseases (Li *et al.*, 2006). Agnihotri and Vavia (2009) successfully loaded diclofenac sodium in PLGA nanosuspensions, which were applied to the rabbit eye and examined with a modified Draize test. These polymeric nanoparticles seemed to be devoid of any irritant effect on the cornea, the iris, and the conjunctiva. Further, a higher decrease of the sodium arachidonate–induced inflammation was obtained by means of PLGA nanoparticles incorporating flurbiprofen in the rabbit eye after topical instillation, indicating its usefulness for the inhibition of ocular inflammation (Vega *et al.*, 2006). Similarly, Dong and coworkers (2006) reported that the intravitreal implantation of the cyclosporin A (CyA)-loaded PLGA can effectively reduce intraocular inflammation in rabbits with no toxicity. Further, intravitreal injections of a suspension of PLA micro/nanospheres containing 1% adriamycin/doxorubicin was reported to provide sustained first-order release for approximately two weeks. Using microarray technology, we have examined the toxicogenomic potential of the PLGA-based nanoformulations using small arrays hosing 200 gene spots, as a result of which no significant gene expression changes were observed (our unpublished data).

CS, a deacetylated chitin, is biodegradable, biocompatible, and nontoxic polymer, whose nanoparticles have been demonstrated to effectively penetrate conjunctival and corneal epithelial cells. It is a promising ophthalmic vehicle because of its probable superior mucoadhesiviness caused by electrostatic interactions with the negative charges of the mucosal layers. In an interesting investigation, animals were treated with CyA–loaded CS nanoparticles, which resulted in significantly higher corneal and conjunctival drug levels than those treated with a suspension of CyA in a CS aqueous solution or in water (De Campos *et al.*, 2001). It has also been demonstrated that the amounts of fluorescent nanoparticles in the cornea and the conjunctiva were significantly higher than that of a control solution. These amounts were fairly constant for up to 24 hours. A higher retention of CS nanoparticles in the conjunctiva compared with in the cornea was observed (De Campos *et al.*, 2004).

2.5.5 Liposomal Nanomedicines

The vesicular lipid bilayers are basically defined as "liposomes," which can contain one or more aqueous compartments. Upon the number of bilayers, these lipid-based globular structures can be categorized into multilamellar and unilamellar vesicles. The unilamellar vesicles include small unilamellar vesicles (SUV) and large unilamellar vesicles (LUV). Drugs, based on their solubility characteristics, can be entrapped in the lipid bilayers or the aqueous compartment (Fenwick and Cullis, 2008).

Liposomal nanomedicines (LNM) were first developed to encapsulate small conventional therapeutic drugs, where the earliest attempts involved the passive entrapment of drugs resulted in the rapid production of stable, homogeneous populations of LUVs (~100 nm). Owing to the composition of LNMs, they are biodegradable and relatively nontoxic, which makes them interesting as drug-delivery systems. The cationic nanoliposomes have been evaluated for their genotoxicity potential in A431 and A549 cells, which resulted in significant gene expression changes mainly related to apoptosis signaling paths (Omidi *et al.*, 2005; Omidi *et al.*, 2003b).

Owing to the unique architecture of the nanoliposomes, when they are used as ocular DDS, the LNMs can come into intimate contact with corneal and conjunctival epithelial cells, facilitating drug absorption. The main goal of LNMs is to reduce side effects while maintaining or enhancing the efficacy of the administered medicament. It should be noticed that the LNMs are not usually taken up by healthy tissue as is the free drug because the normal tissues in corneal/noncorneal routes are continuous, nonfenestrated endothelium of the vasculature, with tight endothelial junctions (on the order of 5 nm) that prevent the extravasation of small liposomal carriers. The basal tissues also inhibit the extravasation of macromolecules. Based upon the disease/dugs used, the LNMs can be used to passively target the designated markers, at which drugs can preferentially selectively be accumulated at sites of disease (Fenwick and Cullis, 2008).

The impact of a single intravitreal injection of vasoactive intestinal peptide (VIP) loaded in rhodamine-conjugated liposomes (VIP-Rh-Lip) on experimental autoimmune uveoretinitis (EAU) has been investigated in Lewis rats. Clinical and histologic assessments showed that macrophages expressed transforming growth factor-beta2, low levels of major histocompatibility complex class II, and nitric oxide synthase-2 in VIP-Rh-Lip-treated eyes in which the intraocular levels of interleukin (IL)-2, interferon-gamma, IL-17, IL-4, GRO/KC, and CCL5 were reduced with increased IL-13. These findings clearly imply that the encapsulation of VIP within liposomes can effectively deliver VIP into the eye and prevent EAU (Camelo *et al.*, 2009). The elimination of liposomes from the vitreous occurs via a diffusional process through the anterior chamber, where SUVs and LUVs show half-life of 10 and 20 days, respectively (Barza *et al.*, 1987). Drug release from liposomal systems is dependent on the concentration of the drug in the liposome. Thus, in the case of long-term treatment, the high concentration of drugs encapsulated in liposomal carriers may raise problems associated with vitreous clouding; nevertheless these drawbacks may be acceptable in endophthalmiti. Besides, sometimes, liposome entrapment can decrease the efficacy of drugs as reported for amphotericin B in a rabbit model with fungal (Candida albicans) endophthalmitis (Barza *et al.*, 1987). Despite huge investigations, at this stage, the liposomal drugs approved by the FDA are liposomal daunorubicin (DaunoXome®, Gilead Sciences, Inc., approved in 1996), liposomal cytarabine (DepoCyt®, DepoTech Corporation, approved in 1999), liposomal Amphotericin B (AmBisone®, Fujisawa, approved in 1997), and liposomal doxorubicin HCl (Doxil®, ALZA Pharmaceuticals, approved in 2007). Still, nano-scaled formulations are under investigations for ocular use.

Of the lipid based nanoformulations, the cationic lipids (CLs) have been widely used as gene delivery systems. These structures were initially exploited by Felgner *et al.* (1987), who used liposomes consisting of N-[1-(2,3-dioleyloxy) propyl]-N,N,N-trimethylammonium chloride (DOTMA) and dioleoylphosphatidylethanolamine (DOPE) for DNA traverse across cell membranes and showed high-level expression of the encoded gene. A number of novel CLs have soon after been synthesized and shown to possess similar transfection activity within target cells. CLs possess either mono- or polycationic head groups. DOTMA, dimyristooxypropyl dimethyl hydroxyethyl ammonium bromide (DMRI), and dioleoyloxy-3-(trimet hylammonio)propane (DOTAP) are monocationic while dioctadecylamidoglicylspermin (DOGS), N-(1-(2,3-dioleyloxy)propyl)-N-2-(sperminecarboxamido)ethyl)-N,N-dimethyl-ammonium trifluoracetate (DOSPA), and 3-beta-(N-(N′,N′-dimethylaminoethane)-carbamoyl)cholesterol (DC-Chol) have polycationic head groups. DOGS (transfectam or lipofectin) and DOTMA are examples of most used CLs for transfection; the reader is directed to see Liu *et al.*, 2003, and Nicolazzi *et al.*, 2003. CL-based delivery systems possess positively charged surface, at which these lipid-based nanosystems can attach the cell surface that normally display negative charges. The cellular toxicity of CLs is deemed to be attributed with the surface charge potential of the CLs. It should be evoked that the lipid-DNA lipoplex is thought to enter cells via adsorptive endocytosis and, by mechanisms not fully understood as yet, release nucleic acids out of the endosomal/lysosomal compartments with the net effect of yielding high uptake and intracellular delivery of genes and oligonucleotides (Pedroso de Lima *et al.*, 2001).

2.5.6 Nanostructured Dendrimers

Tomalia *et al.* (1984) developed the first dendrimer, which was named the Starburst™ polyamidoamine (PAMAM) dendrimer due to its dendritic branches and controlled starburst growth. This macromolecule is built on an ammonia core with extending branches of alternating methyl acrylate and ethylene diamine molecules (Tomalia *et al.*, 1984). Dendrimers are composed of concentric, geometrically progressive layers created through radial amplification from a single, central initiator core molecule containing either three or four reactive sites such as ammonia or ethylene diamine. These nano-scale macromolecules are three-dimensional and highly branched monodispersed nanostructures that are obtained by an iterative sequence of reaction steps producing a precise, unique branching structure (Loutsch *et al.*, 2003). Figure 2.9 represents the chemical structures of polypropylenimine diaminobutane (DAB) dendrimers — that is, generation 2 (panel A) with 8 protonable surface amine groups and generation 3 (panel B) with 16 protonable surface amine groups. These nanostructures provide globular nanosystems of 1–100 nm depending on the molecular weight and number of generations. Its surface ultimately determines the structure's interactions with its environment, as a result of which drugs/genes can be incorporated with and released in a controlled manner (Vandervoort and Ludwig, 2007).

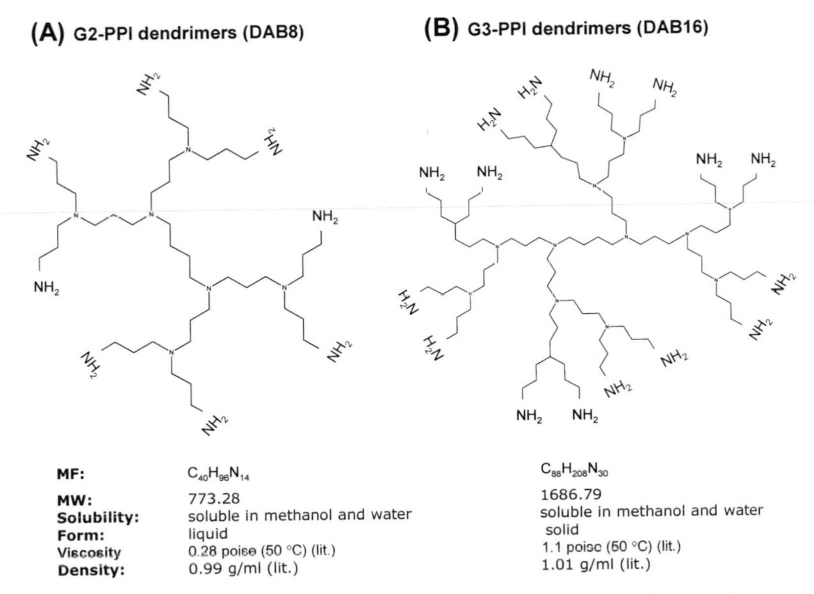

Figure 2.9 Chemical structures of polypropylenimine diaminobutane (DAB) dendrimers. Panel (A) shows the generation 2 (G2) PPI dendrimers (DAB8) with eight protonable surface amine groups. Panel (B) shows the generation 3 (G3) PPI dendrimers (DAB16) with 16 protonable surface amine groups. MF and MW represent molecular formula and molecular weight, respectively. The image was adapted from our work with permission (Omidi and Barar, 2009).

Interestingly, the influence of a controlled incremental increase in the size, molecular weight, and number of amine, carboxylate, and hydroxyl surface groups in several series of PAMAM dendrimers for controlled ocular drug delivery was investigated. The duration of residence time for various generations (1.5, 2–3.5, and 4) in the New Zealand albino rabbit resulted in longer residence time for the solutions containing dendrimers with carboxylic and hydroxyl surface groups, which was largely dependent on size and molecular weight (Vandamme and Brobeck, 2005). The modification of the dendrimer surface (e.g., the addition of functional groups) is achievable through the addition of either subnanoscopic (e.g., small molecules) or nanoscaled reactants (e.g., DNA, antibodies, and proteins). The latter appears to be the preferred approach. For example, in a study to inhibit laser-induced choroidal neovascularization (CNV), lipophilic amino-acid dendrimer was exploited to deliver an anti-VEGF oligonucleotide (ODN) into the eyes of rats and inhibit. Analysis of fluorescein angiograms of laser-photocoagulated eyes revealed that dendrimer plus ODN significantly inhibited the development of CNV for four to six months by up to 95% in the initial stages while ODN alone showed no significant difference (Marano *et al.*, 2005).

Interestingly, generation-2 polypropyleneimine octaamine dendrimers cross-linked with collagen were reported to support human corneal epithelial cell growth and adhesion, with no cell toxicity. Thus, these nanostructures might be suitable scaffolds for corneal tissue engineering (Duan and Sheardown, 2006). In ocular gene therapy, the control of gene transfection within the eye is merely an important issue, in particular when a light-induced delivery of DNA, drugs, or other biological factors is the main objective. In a study, Nishiyama *et al.* (2005) devised a ternary complex composed of a core containing DNA packaged with cationic peptides and enveloped in the anionic dendrimer phthalocyanine (with a photosensitizing action). They showed that the ternary complex was able to profoundly (hundredfold) enhance transgene expression *in vitro* with reduced photocytotoxicity, in which subconjuctival injection of the ternary complex followed by laser irradiation resulted in transgene expression only in the laser-irradiated site. This, surely, is a new biomedical application for dendrimeric nanostructures with successful results in the photochemical-internalization-mediated gene delivery *in vivo* (Nishiyama *et al.*, 2005).

2.6 Nanomedicines Paradigms in Ocular Diseases

In some diseases of the eye, such as diabetic retinopathy, central retinal vein occlusion, CNV, and intraocular solid tumors, angiogenesis plays a key role; thus, targeting the biomarkers within the ocular tissue is deemed to be an efficient treatment modality (Sahoo *et al.*, 2008). Further, explicitly, no lymph system is presented in the retina environment. Thus, in retinal diseases attributed with neovascularization (e.g., wet AMD), treatment modes could be similar to the strategies recruited against solid tumors, that is, displaying enhanced permeability and retention (EPR) effects. These facts further highlight the biological impacts on required pharmacotherapy to achieve enhanced drug permeation, controlled release of drugs, and targeted pharmacotherapy through specific targeting markers. The biological characteristics of the eye render this organ exquisitely impervious to the foreign substances; thus, for the attainment of an optimal concentration at the intended ocular tissue of action by circumventing the ocular barriers, colloidal nanoparticle drug carriers have been devoted a great deal of attention (Bu *et al.*, 2007).

The emergence of nano-scaled pharmaceuticals like nanosuspensions, solid–lipid nanoparticles, and liposomes appears to resolve the solubility-related problems of poorly soluble drugs such as piroxicam, dexamethasone, methylprednisolone, budenoside, and gancyclovir (Kayser *et al.*, 2005). Based upon the biological architecture of the eye together with the physicochemical characteristics of the nanostructured medicines (i.e., particle charge, surface properties, and relative hydrophobicity), these medications can be designed to successfully circumvent the BEB. Since the encapsulation of drugs can grant further protection as well as prolonged/controlled release, they confer better controlling tools for some chronic ocular diseases like chronic CMV retinitis, in which the intravitreal delivery of ganciclovir (GCV) seems to be the preferred strategy. Given its 13-hour half-life, frequent injections of GCV is necessary to maintain therapeutic levels; however, its use may be limited due to the consequential side effects such as cataract development, retinal detachment, and endophthalmitis (Jabs, 1995). Thus, to avoid repeated injections, intravitreal implants can be used to provide prolonged drug release drugs even though some drawbacks like astigmatism and vitreous hemorrhage as well as a couple of surgery requirements may limit its use too (Muccioli and Belfort, Jr., 2000). These difficulties can be overcome by using nanomedicines made up of various natural/biodegradable polymers like albumin and PLGA, because of their smaller size and controlled release properties (Sahoo *et al.*, 2008). Piloplex®, consisting of pilocarpine ionically bound to poly(methyl) methacrylate–co-acrylic acid, is a nano-scaled colloidal carrier system effectively used in glaucoma patients as twice-daily instillations. Multidimensional mechanisms appear to be involved for the pharmacologic action of ocular nanosystems, including extending the time of drug residency in the cornea/conjunctiva, sustaining drug release from its carrier, reducing the precorneal drug loss, and targeting the desired biomarker (Sahoo *et al.*, 2008; Bu *et al.*, 2007; Vandervoort and Ludwig, 2007). Thus, it is highly desirable to exploit bioadhesive materials for formulation of nanosystems to be retained in the cul-de-sac after topical administration. Various biodegradable and nonbiodegradable carriers have been used, for example. PLA, PLGA, CS, poly(isobutyl cyanoacrylate), and Eudragit RS100 or RL100 (Bu *et al.*, 2007). Erodible nanosystems are superior because the self-eroding process of the hydrolyzable polymer exerts less harm on tissue (Herrero-Vanrell and Refojo, 2001; Jose Alonso, 2004). For example, PLGA colloidal nanoparticles were exploited to deliver gene-based therapeutics to the retinal pigment epithelial cells (Bejjani *et al.*, 2005). The sustained-release nanosuspension of piroxicam and methylprednisolone acetate (MPA) was formulated using Eudragit to control the endotoxin-induced uveitis in rabbits (Adibkia *et al.*, 2007a; Adibkia *et al.*, 2007b). For the treatment of chronic ocular diseases (e.g., CMV retinitis), localized prolonged nanomedicines can be effective as a safer alternative of the frequent injections that may cause cataract development, retinal detachment, endophthalmitis, and vitreous hemorrhage (Sahoo *et al.*, 2008).

2.6.1 Nanosuspensions in Ocular Inflammation

The steroidal and nonsteroidal anti-inflammatory drugs (NSAIDs) are routinely used in ocular surgeries, even though they often impose some adverse reactions. These medications are the most studied drugs to be exploited as ocular nanomedicines. Accordingly, localized therapy of ocular inflammation by these pharmaceuticals needs to be optimized since most ocular diseases are classically treated with topical eyedrops, which usually require the frequent utilization of highly concentrated solutions. Enormous efforts, thus, have so far been devoted to maximize the localized delivery and targeting of desired pharmaceuticals using hydrogels, micro- and/ or nanoparticles, and liposomal formulations. We have previously reported that a nanosuspension of piroxicam can control endotoxin-induced uveitis (EU) in rabbits (Adibkia *et al.*, 2007b), where cationic polymer (i.e., Eudragit® RS100) was used to formulate nanosuspensions of piroxicam be means of the solvent evaporation/extraction technique (also called the single-emulsion technique); see Fig. 2.10.

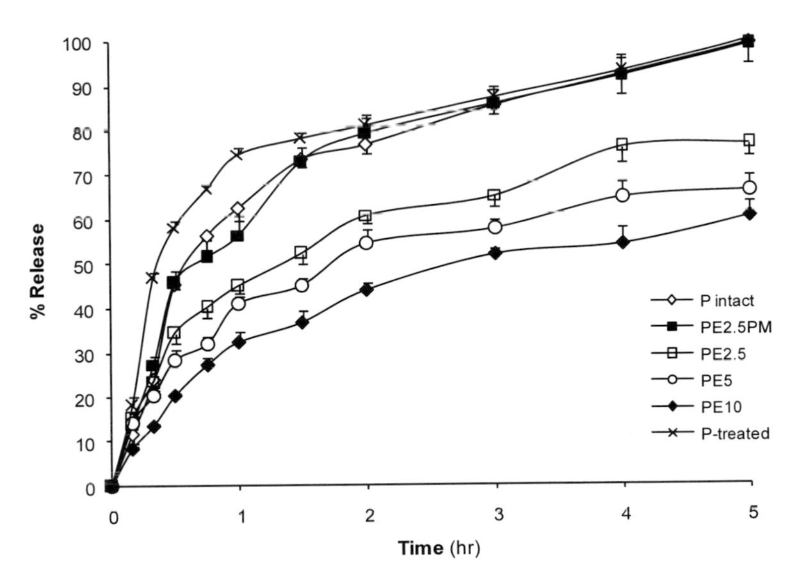

Figure 2.10 The release profile of piroxicam. P-intact: untreated intact piroxicam; P-treated: treated piroxicam; PE2.5: piroxicam: ERS nanoparticles (1:2.5 ratio); PM: physical mixture. The data represents the mean value of 4 replications ± standard error. ERS: Eudragit® RS100. The image was adapted from our work with permission (Adibkia *et al.*, 2007b).

Given that Eudragit® RS100 possesses an appropriate stability and size distribution characteristics together with its positive surface charge of about 30 mV, it is considered a suitable ocular DDS (Pignatello *et al.*, 2002a). The positively charged nanoformulations may interact with anionic mucins presented in the tear film and cause consequential prolongation of drug residency time on the corneal surface (Dillen *et al.*, 2006). Besides, the nanosuspensions may also ensure more comfort of and better acceptance by patients in comparison with the routine ophthalmic suspensions basically formulated in micrometer ranges and show poor characteristics (Zimmer and Kreuter, 1995). ERL nanoparticles containing cloricromene (a coumarine derivative with antithrombotic and anti-ischemic activities) with positive zeta potential values (+27.3 mV) and a particle size of 80 nm were topically applied to rabbit eyes and showed no sign of toxicity or irritation to ocular tissues. A sustained release was observed *in vitro* as well as *in vivo*, resulting in a doubled AUC compared with an aqueous solution (Bucolo *et al.*, 2004).

Overall, all nanoparticles showed a prolonged release profile without the burst effect (Fig. 2.4), in which the complete release of the drug after 24 hours (obeyed from Higuchi diffusion-controlled model kinetics) explicitly indicates that there exists a structural homogeneity of the polymeric matrix and also a more uniform distribution of the drug. Modeling of drug release from the nanoparticles of ciprofloxacin: Eudragit® has also been described by Dillen (2006), whose work showed that the release rate data fitted to the Higuchi's kinetic model. Based on our findings, treatment with piroxicam nanosuspensions significantly reduced observational symptoms of uveitis (based on Hogan's classification method) such as redness, presence of fibrin, photophobia, and lacrimation. We assume that the prolonged impacts of piroxicam nanosuspensions may be due to its interaction with local cellular components because of the positive surface charge of the nanoparticles in addition to the greater penetration and cellular uptake (Pignatello *et al.*, 2002a). Given the cellular responses to uveitis induced by the lipopolysaccharide (a component of gram-negative bacterial cell wall) (Koizumi *et al.*, 2003; Marie *et al.*, 1999), it can be assumed that the piroxicam nanosuspensions favor cellular recovery from EU by conferring a better therapeutic effect because of increased cellular uptake and enhanced inhibitory mechanism on the expression of the inflammatory mediators. Similarly, we formulated nanosuspensions of MPA using ERS to pursue their impacts on the inhibition of inflammatory symptoms in rabbits with EU. We found that the utilization of MPA-ERS nanosuspensions confers a controlled ocular delivery of MPA (Adibkia *et al.*, 2007a); see Fig. 2.11.

Although molecular biology aspects of such therapies for uveitis are yet to be mechanistically investigated, it appears that the application of these types of nanosuspensions as a noninvasive approach seems to be safer with controlled ocular delivery of anti-inflammation agents for the inhibition of the uveitis symptoms. Similar results have been reported for ibuprofen and flurbiprofen (Pignatello *et al.*, 2002a; Pignatello *et al.*, 2002b).

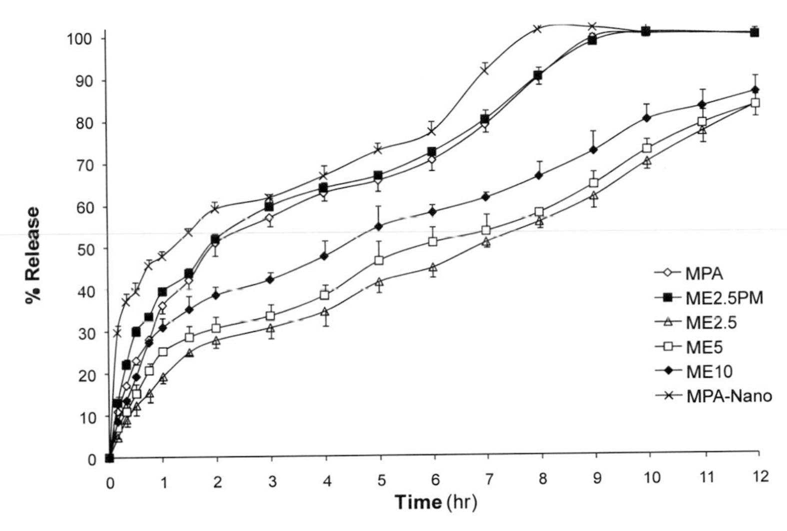

Figure 2.11 The release profile of methylprednisolone acetate. MPA: methylprednisolone acetate-intact powder; MPA-Nano: methylprednisolone acetate nanoparticles; ME2.5: MPA-ERS (1:2.5 ratio); ME5: MPA-ERS (1:5 ratio); ME10: MPA-ERS (1:10 ratio). The image was adapted from our work with permission (Adibkia *et al.*, 2007a).

Artificial vesicles such as liposomes, niosomes, and discomes have been successfully utilized as vehicles for ophthalmic drugs (e.g., oligonucleotides, acetazolamide, pilocarpine HCI, cyclopentolate, and timolol maleate) resulting in improved ocular bioavailability. Of these, positively charged nanostructures seem to be preferentially captured at the negatively charged corneal surface and slow down drug elimination by lacrimal flow (Sahoo *et al.*, 2008; Kaur *et al.*, 2004). Using laser-targeted delivery (LTD), it is now possible to release and activate the encapsulated drug within the heat-sensitive liposomes injected intravenously (Asrani *et al.*, 2006). By virtue of being encapsulated, the drug is confined into the liposomes and shielded from general metabolism, by which efficient pharmacological effects with minimal adverse reactions are expected.

2.6.2 Photodynamic Therapy: Implementation of Nanosystems

Photodynamic therapy (PDT) with verteporfin for CNV associated with RPE detachment AMD (Pece *et al.*, 2007) and the combination of PDT with aforementioned nanomedicines (Ju *et al.*, 2008; Lazic and Gabric, 2007) have revealed promising results. These medications are unable to completely cure AMD, but they significantly decelerate the progression of the lesion growth in a proportion of patients (El-Beik and Elligott, 2007). Ocular gene therapy has reached clinical trials (e.g., for inherited retinal degeneration), which possibly mark the culmination of decades of investigations (Bainbridge and Ali, 2008). The eye, as a valuable model system for gene therapy, is a unique highly compartmentalized organ for the efficient delivery of small volumes of viral (e.g., adeno/lenti-viral vectors) (Auricchio *et al.*, 2002; Auricchio, 2003; Hamilton *et al.*, 2006) or nonviral (e.g., PEGylated nanoliposomes and niosomes) (Sanders *et al.*, 2007; Bloquel *et al.*, 2006; Peeters *et al.*, 2005; Andrieu-Soler *et al.*, 2006) vectors. Among them, the PEGylated nonviral nucleic acid nanostructures prevent their interaction with undesired biomolecules and provide promising results (Sanders *et al.*, 2007). Besides, recent significant progresses in the mapping and cloning of retinal disease genes have provided great potential for gene therapy in the eye, for example, gene replacement in the inherited retinal degenerations (Leber's congenital amaurosis due to defects in the gene encoding the enzyme RPE65) (Le *et al.*, 2007; Bainbridge *et al.*, 2006). In 2005, Kataoka and his coworkers reported light-induced gene transfer from packaged DNA enveloped in a dendrimeric photosensitizer. For efficient transfection, the endosomal escape of the polyplexes is the main obstacle. This can be resolved by the use of polycationic systems that possess buffering capacity (the so-called proton sponge effect). Thus, to obtain efficient photochemical internalization (PCI), these researchers assumed that the control of the subcellular localization of photosensitizers may be a key to the PCI-mediated gene delivery with reduced cytotoxicity. At which, they developed a light-responsive gene carrier based on a ternary complex of pDNA, cationic peptides, and anionic dendrimer-based photosensitizers — dendrimer phthalocyanine (DPc). In their work, the core polyplex was formed from a quadruplicated cationic peptide (CP_4), where a peptide (CP_2: $C(YGRKKRRQRRRG)_2$) was dimerized through a disulphide linkage and pDNA was mixed with the CP_4 peptide at a molar ratio of cationic amino acids to a phosphate anion in DNA (i.e., N/P ratio of 2). Using a luciferase (Luc) reporter gene assay in HeLa cells, they showed the transfection efficiency and cytotoxicity of the pDNA/CP_4 polyplex and pDNA/CP_4/DPc ternary complexes with varying charge ratios of DPc after irradiation of the light with increasing fluence. For *in vivo* PCI-mediated gene delivery, they pursued the transfection of a reporter gene (a variant of yellow fluorescent proteins, Venus) to the conjunctival tissue in rat eyes on laser irradiation after subconjunctival injection of the ternary complex. The pDNA/CP_4/DPc ternary complex with a charge ratio of 1:2:1 achieved significant gene expression only at the laser-irradiated site in the conjunctiva two days after irradiation. This is a clear example of the emergence of nanosystems toward futuristic use in PDT.

2.6.3 Genonanomedicines, Monoclonal Antibodies, and Nanobodies

In September 2006, the global bionanotech company pSivida announced the initiation of a phase II clinical trial of Mifepristone as an eyedrop treatment for steroid-associated elevated intraocular pressure (see http://www.psivida.com/default.asp), for the formulation of which a nanocarrier has possibly been used. More recently, a branched PEGylated anti-VEGF aptamer (pegaptanib sodium marketed as Macugen®) was approved by the FDA for the treatment of neovascular AMD, which demonstrated the first ODN aptamer nanomedicine. It suppresses the pathological angiogenesis in the neovascular AMD by specifically targeting the extracellular VEGF, resulting in the inhibition of angiogenesis, reduction of permeability of the vascular bed, and diminution of inflammation (Bakri and Kaiser, 2006).

Further, ranibizumab is a recombinant humanized monoclonal antibody fragment (marketed as Lucentis®) that targets VEGF-A, an important mediator in the development of CNV, and reduces neovascularization and leakage in the wet AMD (Bakri and Kaiser, 2006). Ranibizumab (48 kDa) is a markedly smaller molecule than the RhuMAb VEGF (bevacizumab, Avastin®, 148 kDa) that is in early clinical testing for the treatment of CNV via the intravitreal route (Bakri and Kaiser, 2006). Unlike RhuMAb VEGF, ranibizumab is able to penetrate the retina and enter the subretinal space after intravitreal injection because of the notable size difference.

Heavy-chain antibodies (HCAbs) have recently been discovered in the blood of camelids. Because of their nano-scaled size (a diameter of ~2.5 nm and a height of ~4 nm), the antigen-binding units of these HCAbs comprise only a single Ig fold (see Fig. 2.12). Thus, they are called Nanobodies®. There several remarkable characteristics (i.e., being small, nonimmunogenic, very stable, highly soluble, and easy to produce in large quantities) make them ideal candidates as next-generation immunotherapies. Antigen-specific Nanobodies® can easily be derived from the V_{HH} of HCAbs that are circulating in the serum of immunized llamas or camels.

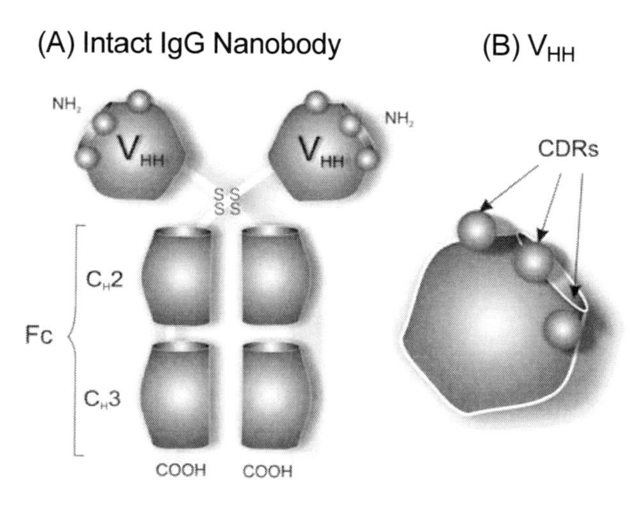

Figure 2.12 A graphical representation of the heavy-chain antibody. (A) A schematic structure of an intact IgG nanobody. (B) A schematic structure of V_{HH}.

Nanobodies® appear to be inherently soluble and stable. They usually do not aggregate and possess high homology with human V_H frameworks. Besides, they can be further humanized for use as therapeutics since these humanized nanostructured HCAbs are able to retain their characteristics and were shown to induce minimum immunogenicity (Muyldermans *et al.*, 2009). It should be evoked that Nanobodies® can also be derived from the V_H domains of conventional antibodies, at which humanized Nanobodies® (the process that is also called camelization) can be achieved through substitutions of specific amino acid to improve these unstable V_H domains so that they become more stabile with have higher solubility. In fact, the single-domain nature of HCAbs confers several unique features in comparison with conventional Abs, although the conventional Abs show various beneficial characteristics, including higher affinity and selectivity for a target. Nanobodies® display additional characteristics that make them superior as potential drug molecules. To our best knowledge, surprisingly, no studies have been conducted to use these unique structures for ocular targeting, but it is anticipated that they are not far from being put into practice.

2.7 Bioavailability of Ocular Nanomedicines

Within ocular tissues, a variety of drug delivery nanocarriers can be taken up by target cells through endocytic pathways. However, their characterization is limited to a qualitative basis only. The uptake percentage of the total dose nanoparticles and their contribution to overall ocular drug bioavailability remain unknown. In addition, an ophthalmic drug applied to the eye is subjected to metabolism when the drug penetrates across BEB into the site of action. In fact, there exist many research studies demonstrating the functional expression of various enzymes involved in a variety of stages of drug metabolism and detoxification (Duvvuri *et al.*, 2004; Rose and Bode, 1991). Some of these drug-metabolizing enzymes are oxidoreductases (e.g., aldehyde oxidase, ketone reductase, cyclooxygenase, monoamine oxidase, and P450), hydrolases (e.g., aminopeptidase, acetylcholinesterase, carboxylesterase, aryl sulfatase, and P-glucuronidase), and conjugating enzymes (e.g., arylamine acetyltransferase and glutathione S-transferase); to review, see Bu *et al.* (2007), Attar *et al.* (2005), and Duvvuri *et al.* (2004). These metabolizing machineries of the eye are primarily expressed in various tissues (e.g., the retina-choroid), which appear to play an important role in ocular homeostasis by preventing the entry of xenobiotics into, and/or eliminating xenobiotics from, the ocular tissues. Various cytochrome P450 (CYP) enzymes have been identified in ocular tissues, including CYPs 1A, 1B1, 2B, 2C, 2J, 3A, 4B1, 39A1, and NADPH reductase (Attar *et al.*, 2005). Ocular nanomedicines loom to optimize the ocular bioavailability. For example, a single topical instillation of acyclovir-PLA nanospheres in rabbits resulted in significantly higher drug levels compared to the free drug formulations and exhibited a sustained acyclovir release for up to 6 hours in aqueous humor (Giannavola *et al.*, 2003). Kassem *et al.* (2007) evaluated the effect of the particle size in the micro- and nanosize ranges as well as the effect of viscosity of the nanosuspension on the ocular bioavailability of glucocorticoid drugs (hydrocortisone, prednisolone, and dexamethasone) by measuring the intraocular pressure of normotensive albino rabbits. They showed that nanosuspensions always enhance the rate and extent of ophthalmic drug absorption as well as the intensity of drug action. This clearly highlights the higher bioavailability of nanosuspensions in comparison with micro-crystalline suspensions (Kassem *et al.*, 2007). Recently, to provide long-term extraocular drug delivery using CS polymer, CyA was formulated as nanoparticles by means of the ionic gelation technique. The CyA-CS nanoparticles yielded a mean size of 293 nm with a zeta potential of +37 mV. *In vitro* release studies revealed prolonged drug release for a 24-hour period. *In vivo* tests showed that, following the topical instillation of CyA-CS nanoparticles in rabbits, therapeutic concentration was obtained in the cornea and the conjunctiva for at least 48 hours, where the levels were significantly higher than those obtained following the instillation of a CS solution containing CyA and an aqueous CyA suspension (De Campos *et al.*, 2001). Very recently, to improve the precorneal residence time and the ocular bioavailability of IM, Badawi *et al.* (2008) deveoloped CS-based nanoparticles (280 nm) and nanoemulsion (220–690 nm) using ionic gelation and spontaneous emulsification techniques, respectively. *In vivo* studies on eyes of rabbits displayed clearer healing of the cornea by nanoemulsion, while CS nanocarriers were able to contact intimately with the cornea, providing slow gradual IM release with long-term drug levels, increasing delivery to both external and internal ocular tissues (Badawi *et al.*, 2008). These findings support similar previous results (Calvo *et al.*, 1996), in which suspensions of nanoparticles and nanocapsules made of poly-epsilon-caprolactone (PECL) yielded profound increased ocular bioavailability of IM in rabbit eyes. Similarly, enhanced bioavailability was reported for the topical use of nanoparticles of amikacin-poly(butyl cyanoacrylate) (PBCA), acyclovir-poly(ethyl cyanoacrylate), betaxolol-poly(isobutyl cyanoacrylate), cloricromene-ERL, cyclophosphamide-PBCA, hydrocortisone-BSA, ibuprofen-ERS/ERL, metipranolol-PIBCA/PCL, and progesterone-PBCA; for more details, readers should refer to Bu *et al.* (2007). All these animal model–based works are clear evidence for impacts of nano-scaled medicaments in ocular therapy despite the fact that their medical practices require clinical trials.

2.8 Future Prospective of Ocular Therapies

In recent years, for the treatment of many ocular disorders, there has been a profound shift toward the implementation of more efficient treatment paradigms. For example, the neurodegenerative disorder glaucoma, which is associated with elevated intraocular pressure, has impacted many patients' lives, while its treatment has fortunately moved from the management of intraocular pressure to the prevention of neurodegeneration and maintenance of retinal function. Artificial tears are no longer the main treatment for dry eye, which damages the ocular surface and is a common cause for patients to visit eye care specialists. It is now being controlled with Restasis® (CyA ophthalmic emulsion), which targeted the immune component of the disease (Attar *et al.*, 2005).

In ocular pharmacotherapy, the biggest challenges are the achievement of the preferred concentration at the intended ocular tissue. To tackle this issue, a variety of conventional ocular DDSs have been developed for the production of effective ophthalmic drug formulations. Most of these ophthalmic drugs are delivered to the eye via aqueous vehicles. Nonetheless, aqueous vehicles exhibit poor ocular bioavailability due to rapid drainage, lacrimation, and tear turnover, and if penetration occurs, only a short duration of action may be observed (Hillaireau *et al.*, 2006; Lang, 1995). Moreover, the application of many potentially active ophthalmic compounds is seriously limited because of their very low water solubility. They, accordingly, need to be administered either through alternative routes or by optimized the delivery system. Among various approaches for improving the ophthalmic delivery of lipophilic drugs, hydrogels, microparticles, nanoparticles, and liposomal formulations have been shown to favor topical targeting and improve drug bioavailability (Patravale *et al.*, 2004). Of these DDSs, nanoformulations have raised promising potential for efficient ocular delivery (Bucolo *et al.*, 2004). In fact, colloidal nanoparticle drug carriers emerge to be useful for ocular absorption enhancement through various mechanisms, including a prolonged drug residence time in the cornea and the conjunctiva, sustained drug release from the delivery system, and reduced precorneal drug loss (Bu *et al.*, 2007). Surprisingly, over the past two decades, nanoformulations of ophthalmic drugs have not yet been undertaken in clinical practice as fast as expected.

In ocular drug therapy, the need for the safe application of medications to the posterior segment is deemed to be even more important than the surface delivery. Treatment of intricate posterior segment diseases crucially necessitates safe drug delivery to the retina, the choroid, or the ciliary body. Systemic delivery and devices inserted into the vitreous are valuable strategies. So are the biodegradable/nonbiodegradable controlled-release implants inserted into both aqueous humor and vitreous humor. Moreover, in recent years, there has been a dramatic increase in the understanding of the pathobiology of ocular diseases at cellular/molecular level. There are now many drugs under development (Frank, 2003). For ocular drug therapy, this state of high flux resulted in a few advanced therapeutics such as Visudyne®, Macugen®, and the angiostatic anecortave acetate (Retaane®), which is administered as a periocular injection every six months (Hayek *et al.*, 2007; Bakri and Kaiser, 2006).

In close proximity, it is also predictable to perceive nano-scaled technologies in practice, providing a promising platform for improved noninvasive ocular drug delivery. However, further developments need to be accomplished to render the nanosystems more effective. The primary practical approach for providing nanomedicines with the necessary site adherence and site retention to achieve carrier and drug targeting in topical ocular therapy is to endow them with the ability to be a bioadhesive system, perhaps by the utilization of natural biopolymers such as hyaluronic acid. The mutual use of penetration enhancers along with nanomedicines without compromising the stability of the system could also provide higher ocular bioavailability. Bioadhesive nanosystems can maximize ocular drug absorption by prolonging the drug residence time in the cornea and the conjunctiva and minimize precorneal drug loss, resulting in increased patient compliance. For the development of ocular bioadhesive systems as localized sustained-release medications, nonbiodegradable systems appear to be adequate to treat perforations and ulcerations. Ideally, for long-term use, however, these systems should be nontoxic biodegradable adhesives with site specificity and minimal immunogenicity yet improving bioavailability by enhancing absorption (particularly for protein/peptide-based macromolecules) or inhibiting the metabolizing enzymes.

Because of its unique bioarchitecture, the eye is considered a perfect organ for gene therapy because the delivery vector can rarely escape to systemic sites. To date, ocular pathologies have been tackled with 17 trials (phase I/II) focused on different conditions, including retinitis pigmentosa, glaucoma, diabetic macular edema, and AMD, while 1,537 gene therapy clinical trials are in development; for more details, see the following website: http://www.wiley.co.uk/genmed/clinical. This website highlights the growing interest in the gene therapy of ocular diseases, for which futuristic genomedicines are deemed to become more effective therapeutics through the exploitation of molecular Trojan delivery systems for safe shuttling of genomedicines (e.g., antisense, ribozyme, and siRNA) and the targeting of the desired biomarkers (Janoria *et al.*, 2007; Maguire and Bennett, 2006). There is much excitement about the potential of the short interfering RNA (siRNA), which has remarkably rapidly moved toward applications. At this stage, nine clinical trials are being developed for its implementation and most of these trials are involved in the ocular disease: (1) a phase I trial on "Cand5 anti-VEGF RNAi evaluation," which was started in 2004 by Acuity Pharmaceuticals, (2) a phase II trial on "Cand5 anti-VEGF RNAi evaluation (CARE) trial," which was started in 2005 by Acuity Pharmaceuticals, (3) a phase II trial on "RNAi assessment of cand5 in diabetic macular edema (RACE) trial," which was started in 2006 by Acuity Pharmaceuticals, (4) a phase I trail on "Open-label, dose-escalation single dose trial with Ssrna-027 in patients with AMD," which was in 2005 by Allergan Inc., and (5) a phase II trial on "intravitreal injections of a siRNA in patients with AMD" targeting the vascular endothelial growth factor receptor-1 (Sirna-27), which was started in 2006 by Allergan Inc.

LTD and PDT seem to be promising methodologies to deliver and activate therapeutic and diagnostic agents to the retina and choroid. However, their successful applications largely depend on the appropriateness of the agent. Perhaps a combination of these techniques with gene therapy could benefit ocular diseases. Encapsulated cell technology (ECT) and cell therapy appear to grant treatment potentials for ocular diseases. ECT implants consist of living cells encapsulated within a semipermeable polymer membrane and supportive matrices, which are genetically engineered to produce a specific therapeutic substance to target a specific disease or condition. Once implanted, the implant allows the outward passage of the therapeutic product (Tao *et al.*, 2006). It is anticipated that the biological properties of the eye would undergo the desired alterations through the application of these technologies. However, for implementation of the cell therapy technology in human eyes, the validation of the technique will be a critical step. Besides, the cellular and subcellular/molecular aspects of the target tissues should be fully addressed and ocular disease–related biomarkers should be exclusively clarified. Possibly, high throughput screening technologies (e.g., DNA/protein array and phage display screening methodologies) would facilitate investigations toward specific targeting.

Finally, it should be stated that not all attempts to apply *de novo* nanotechnology approaches in biomedical sciences have met with the same success as those cited here in this review, and sometimes, these novel technologies tools provoke a great deal of challenges and hurdles. In fact, nanostructures appear not to function in the same predictive ways that routinely used small molecules act, although this field is experiencing a rapid growth period, with major advances in numerous diverse ways. Current preclinical investigations seem to provide new approaches to diagnose disease, to deliver specific therapy, and to monitor the biological impacts deeply. Although such fast inauguration methodological alterations will eventually literally convey new challenges in the regulatory processes, they will also grant a prolific platform from which many exciting, and yet unimagined, applications of biomedical nanotechnology will emerge.

References

1. Adibkia, K., Omidi, Y., Siahi, M.R., Javadzadeh, A.R., Barzegar-Jalali, M., Barar, J., Maleki, N., Mohammadi, G., and Nokhodchi, A. (2007a). Inhibition of endotoxin-induced uveitis by methylprednisolone acetate nanosuspension in rabbits. *J. Ocul. Pharmacol. Ther.*, **23**, pp. 421–432.
2. Adibkia, K., Siahi Shadbad, M.R., Nokhodchi, A., Javadzedeh, A., Barzegar-Jalali, M., Barar, J., Mohammadi, G., and Omidi, Y. (2007b).

Piroxicam nanoparticles for ocular delivery: physicochemical characterization and implementation in endotoxin-induced uveitis. *J. Drug Target*, **15**, pp. 407–416.

3. Agnihotri, S.M., and Vavia, P.R. (2009). Diclofenac-loaded biopolymeric nanosuspensions for ophthalmic application. *Nanomedicine*, **5**, pp. 90–95.
4. Ahmed, I. (2003). The noncorneal route in ocular drug delivery. In *Ophthalmic Drug Delivery Systems* (ed. A.K. Mitra), pp. 335–363. Marcel Dekker, New York.
5. Ambati, J., Canakis, C.S., Miller, J.W., Gragoudas, E.S., Edwards, A., Weissgold, D.J., Kim, I., Delori, F.C., and Adamis, A.P. (2000). Diffusion of high molecular weight compounds through sclera. *Invest. Ophthalmol. Vis. Sci.*, **41**, pp. 1181–1185.
6. Ashton, P. (2006). Retinal drug delivery. In *Intraocular Drug Delivery* (ed. G.J. Jaffe, P. Ashton, and P.A. Pearson), pp. 1–25. Taylor & Francis Group, LLC, New York.
7. Asrani, S., Goldberg, M.F., and Zeimer, R. (2006). Thermal-sensitive liposomes. In *Intraocular Drug Delivery* (ed. G.J. Jaffe, P. Ashton, and P.A. Pearson), pp. 143–156. Taylor & Francis Group, LLC, New York.
8. Athanasiou, K.A., Niederauer, G.G., and Agrawal, C.M. (1996). Sterilization, toxicity, biocompatibility and clinical applications of polylactic acid/polyglycolic acid copolymers. *Biomaterials*, **17**, pp. 93–102.
9. Atluri, H., Anand, B.S., Patel, J., and Mitra, A.K. (2004). Mechanism of a model dipeptide transport across blood-ocular barriers following systemic administration. *Exp. Eye Res.*, **78**, pp. 815–822.
10. Attama, A.A., Reichl, S., and Muller-Goymann, C.C. (2008). Diclofenac sodium delivery to the eye: *in vitro* evaluation of novel solid lipid nanoparticle formulation using human cornea construct. *Int. J. Pharm.*, **355**, pp. 307–313.
11. Attar, M., Shen, J., Ling, K.H., and Tang-Liu, D. (2005). Ophthalmic drug delivery considerations at the cellular level: drug-metabolising enzymes and transporters. *Expert Opin. Drug Deliv.*, **2**, pp. 891–908.
12. Auricchio, A. (2003). Pseudotyped AAV vectors for constitutive and regulated gene expression in the eye. *Vision Res.*, **43**, pp. 913–918.
13. Auricchio, A., Rivera, V.M., Clackson, T., O'Connor, E.E., Maguire, A.M., Tolentino, M.J., Bennett, J., and Wilson, J.M. (2002). Pharmacological regulation of protein expression from adeno-associated viral vectors in the eye. *Mol. Ther.*, **6**, pp. 238–242.

14. Badawi, A.A., El-Laithy, H.M., El Qidra, R.K., El, M.H., and El, d.M. (2008). Chitosan based nanocarriers for indomethacin ocular delivery. *Arch. Pharm. Res.*, **31**, pp. 1040–1049.

15. Bainbridge, J.W., and Ali, R.R. (2008). Ocular gene therapy trials due to report this year; keeping an eye on clinical trials in 2008. *Gene Ther.* (in press).

16. Bainbridge, J.W., Tan, M.H., and Ali, R.R. (2006). Gene therapy progress and prospects: the eye. *Gene Ther.*, **13**, pp. 1191–1197.

17. Bakri, S.J., and Kaiser, P.K. (2006). Antiangiogenic agents: intravitreal injection. In *Intraocular Drug Delivery* (ed. G.J. Jaffe, P. Ashton, and P.A. Pearson), pp. 71–84. Taylor & Francis Group, LLC, New York.

18. Barar, J., Javadzadeh, A.R., and Omidi, Y. (2008). Ocular novel drug delivery: impacts of membranes and barriers. *Expert. Opin. Drug Deliv.*, **5**, pp. 567–581.

19. Barza, M., Stuart, M., and Szoka, F., Jr. (1987). Effect of size and lipid composition on the pharmacokinetics of intravitreal liposomes. *Invest. Ophthalmol. Vis. Sci.*, **28**, pp. 893–900.

20. Baudouin, C. (1996). Side effects of antiglaucomatous drugs on the ocular surface. *Curr. Opin. Ophthalmol.*, **7**, pp. 80–86.

21. Bejjani, R.A., BenEzra, D., Cohen, H., Rieger, J., Andrieu, C., Jeanny, J.C., Gollomb, G., and Behar-Cohen, F.F. (2005). Nanoparticles for gene delivery to retinal pigment epithelial cells. *Mol. Vis.*, **11**, pp. 124–132.

22. Bill, A. (1986). The blood-aqueous barrier. *Trans. Ophthalmol. Soc. U.K.*, **105** (Pt 2), pp. 149–155.

23. Bloquel, C., Bourges, J.L., Touchard, E., Berdugo, M., BenEzra, D., and Behar-Cohen, F. (2006). Non-viral ocular gene therapy: potential ocular therapeutic avenues. *Adv. Drug Deliv. Rev.*, **58**, pp. 1224–1242.

24. Boado, R.J., Zhang, Y., Zhang, Y., Xia, C.F., Wang, Y., and Pardridge, W.M. (2008). Genetic engineering of a lysosomal enzyme fusion protein for targeted delivery across the human blood-brain barrier. *Biotechnol. Bioeng.*, **99**, pp. 475–484.

25. Bridges, C.C., El-Sherbeny, A., Roon, P., Ola, M.S., Kekuda, R., Ganapathy, V., Camero, R.S., Cameron, P.L., and Smith, S.B. (2001). A comparison of caveolae and caveolin-1 to folate receptor alpha in retina and retinal pigment epithelium. *Histochem. J.*, **33**, pp. 149–158.

26. Bu, H.Z., Gukasyan, H.J., Goulet, L., Lou, X.J., Xiang, C., and Koudriakova, T. (2007). Ocular disposition, pharmacokinetics, efficacy and safety of nanoparticle-formulated ophthalmic drugs. *Curr. Drug Metab.*, **8**, pp. 91–107.

27. Bucolo, C., Maltese, A., Maugeri, F., Busa, B., Puglisi, G., and Pignatello, R. (2004). Eudragit RL100 nanoparticle system for the ophthalmic delivery of cloricromene. *J. Pharm. Pharmacol.*, **56**, pp. 841–846.

28. Cai, X., Conley, S., and Naash, M. (2008). Nanoparticle applications in ocular gene therapy. *Vision Res.*, **48**, pp. 319–324.

29. Calvo, P., Alonso, M.J., Vila-Jato, J.L., and Robinson, J.R. (1996). Improved ocular bioavailability of indomethacin by novel ocular drug carriers. *J. Pharm. Pharmacol.*, **48**, pp. 1147–1152.

30. Camelo, S., Lajavardi, L., Bochot, A., Goldenberg, B., Naud, M.C., Brunel, N., Lescure, B., Klein, C., Fattal, E., Behar-Cohen, F., and De, K.Y. (2009). Protective effect of intravitreal injection of vasoactive intestinal peptide-loaded liposomes on experimental autoimmune uveoretinitis. *J. Ocul. Pharmacol. Ther.*, **25**, pp. 9–21.

31. Cantrill, H.L., Henry, K., Melroe, N.H., Knobloch, W.H., Ramsay, R.C., and Balfour, H.H., Jr. (1989). Treatment of cytomegalovirus retinitis with intravitreal ganciclovir. Long-term results. *Ophthalmology*, **96**, pp. 367–374.

32. Cao, Y., Zhang, C., Shen, W., Cheng, Z., Yu, L.L., and Ping, Q. (2007). Poly(N-isopropylacrylamide)-chitosan as thermosensitive *in situ* gel-forming system for ocular drug delivery. *J. Control Release*, **120**, pp. 186–194.

33. Chang, J.E., Basu, S.K., and Lee, V.H. (2000). Air-interface condition promotes the formation of tight corneal epithelial cell layers for drug transport studies. *Pharm. Res.*, **17**, pp. 670–676.

34. Chastain, J.E. (2003). General considerations in ocular drug delivery. In *Ophthalmic Drug Delivery Systems* (ed. A.K. Mitra), pp. 59–108. Marcel Dekker, New York.

35. Chiou, G.C., Shen, Z.F., and Zheng, Y.Q. (1991). Systemic absorption of oxytocin and vasopressin through eyes in rabbits. *J. Ocul. Pharmacol.*, **7**, pp. 351–359.

36. Choy, Y.B., Park, J.H., McCarey, B.E., Edelhauser, H.F., and Prausnitz, M.R. (2008). Mucoadhesive microdiscs engineered for ophthalmic drug delivery: effect of particle geometry and formulation on preocular residence time. *Invest. Ophthalmol. Vis. Sci.*, **49**, pp. 4808–4815.

37. Costabile, B.S. (1998). Treatment of cytomegalovirus retinitis with intraocular implants. *AORN J.*, **67**, pp. 356–368.

38. Dartt, D.A., Hodges, R.R., and Zoukhri, D. (2006). Tear and their secretion. In *The Biology of Eye* (ed. J. Fischbarg), pp. 21–82. Academic Press, New York.

39. Davis, A.A., Bernstein, P.S., Bok, D., Turner, J., Nachtigal, M., and Hunt, R.C. (1995). A human retinal pigment epithelial cell line that retains epithelial characteristics after prolonged culture. *Invest. Ophthalmol. Vis. Sci.*, **36**, pp. 955–964.

40. Davis, J.L., Gilger, B.C., and Robinson, M.R. (2004). Novel approaches to ocular drug delivery. *Curr. Opin. Mol. Ther.*, **6**, pp. 195–205.

41. De Campos, A.M., Diebold, Y., Carvalho, E.L., Sanchez, A., and Alonso, M.J. (2004). Chitosan nanoparticles as new ocular drug delivery systems: *in vitro* stability, *in vivo* fate, and cellular toxicity. *Pharm. Res.*, **21**, pp. 803–810.

42. De Campos, A.M., Sanchez, A., and Alonso, M.J. (2001). Chitosan nanoparticles: a new vehicle for the improvement of the delivery of drugs to the ocular surface. Application to cyclosporin A. *Int. J. Pharm.*, **224**, pp. 159–168.

43. Dey, S., and Mitra, A.K. (2005). Transporters and receptors in ocular drug delivery: opportunities and challenges. *Expert Opin. Drug Deliv.*, **2**, pp. 201–204.

44. Dey, S., Patel, J., Anand, B.S., Jain-Vakkalagadda, B., Kaliki, P., Pal, D., Ganapathy, V., and Mitra, A.K. (2003). Molecular evidence and functional expression of P-glycoprotein (MDR1) in human and rabbit cornea and corneal epithelial cell lines. *Invest. Ophthalmol. Vis. Sci.*, **44**, pp. 2909–2918.

45. Diebold, Y., Jarrin, M., Saez, V., Carvalho, E.L., Orea, M., Calonge, M., Seijo, B., and Alonso, M.J. (2007). Ocular drug delivery by liposome-chitosan nanoparticle complexes (LCS-NP). *Biomaterials*, **28**, pp. 1553–1564.

46. Dillen, K., Vandervoort, J., Van den Mooter, G., and Ludwig, A. (2006). Evaluation of ciprofloxacin-loaded Eudragit RS100 or RL100/PLGA nanoparticles. *Int. J. Pharm.*, **314**, pp. 72–82.

47. Dong, X., Shi, W., Yuan, G., Xie, L., Wang, S., and Lin, P. (2006). Intravitreal implantation of the biodegradable cyclosporin A drug delivery system for experimental chronic uveitis. *Graefes Arch. Clin. Exp. Ophthalmol.*, **244**, pp. 492–497.

48. Duan, X., and Sheardown, H. (2006). Dendrimer crosslinked collagen as a corneal tissue engineering scaffold: mechanical properties and corneal epithelial cell interactions. *Biomaterials*, **27**, pp. 4608–4617.

49. Dunn, K.C., Aotaki-Keen, A.E., Putkey, F.R., and Hjelmeland, L.M. (1996). ARPE-19, a human retinal pigment epithelial cell line with differentiated properties. *Exp. Eye Res.*, **62**, pp. 155–169.

50. Duvvuri, S., Majumdar, S., and Mitra, A.K. (2003). Drug delivery to the retina: challenges and opportunities. *Expert Opin. Biol. Ther.*, **3**, pp. 45–56.

51. Duvvuri, S., Majumdar, S., and Mitra, A.K. (2004). Role of metabolism in ocular drug delivery. *Curr. Drug Metab*, **5**, pp. 507–515.

52. Einmahl, S., Capancioni, S., Schwach-Abdellaoui, K., Moeller, M., Behar-Cohen, F., and Gurny, R. (2001). Therapeutic applications of viscous and injectable poly(ortho esters). *Adv. Drug Deliv. Rev.*, **53**, pp. 45–73.

53. El-Beik, S., and Elligott, R. (2007). Macular degeneration — Advances in treatment. *Hospital Pharmacist*, **14**, pp. 155–160.

54. Fenwick, B.W., and Cullis, P.R. (2008). Liposomal nanomedicines. *Expert. Opin. Drug Deliv.*, **5**, pp. 25–44.

55. Fischbarg, J. (2006a) *The Biology of the Eye*, 10th edn. Elsevier Science, Amsterdam.

56. Fischbarg, J. (2006b). The corneal endothelim. In *The Biology of Eye* (ed. J. Fischbarg), pp. 113–125. Academic Press, New York.

57. Fischbarg, J., Diecke, F.P., Iserovich, P., and Rubashkin, A. (2006). The role of the tight junction in paracellular fluid transport across corneal endothelium. electro-osmosis as a driving force. *J. Membr. Biol.*, **210**, pp. 117–130.

58. Frank, R.G. (2003). New estimates of drug development costs. *J. Health Econ.*, **22**, pp. 325–330.

59. Freddo, T.F. (2001). Shifting the paradigm of the blood-aqueous barrier. *Exp. Eye Res.*, **73**, pp. 581–592.

60. Fullard, R.J., and Tucker, D. (1994). Tear protein composition and the effects of stimulus. *Adv. Exp. Med. Biol.*, **350**, pp. 309–314.

61. Ganapathy, M.E., and Ganapathy, V. (2005). Amino Acid Transporter ATB^{0+} as a delivery system for drugs and prodrugs. *Curr. Drug Targets: Immune. Endocr. Metabol. Disord.*, **5**, pp. 357–364.

62. Gao, J., Sun, X., Yatsula, V., Wymore, R.S., and Mathias, R.T. (2000). Isoform-specific function and distribution of Na/K pumps in the frog lens epithelium. *J. Membr. Biol.*, **178**, pp. 89–101.

63. Gardner, T.W., Antonetti, D.A., Barber, A.J., Lieth, E., and Tarbell, J.A. (1999). The molecular structure and function of the inner blood–retinal barrier. Penn State Retina Research Group. *Doc. Ophthalmol.*, **97**, pp. 229–237.

64. Gaudana, R., Jwala, J., Boddu, S.H., and Mitra, A.K. (2009). Recent perspectives in ocular drug delivery. *Pharm. Res.*, **26**, pp. 1197–1216.

65. Gerhart, D.Z., Leino, R.L., and Drewes, L.R. (1999). Distribution of monocarboxylate transporters MCT1 and MCT2 in rat retina. *Neuroscience*, **92**, pp. 367–375.

66. Ghate, D., and Edelhauser, H.F. (2006). Ocular drug delivery. *Expert. Opin. Drug Deliv.*, **3**, pp. 275–287.

67. Giannavola, C., Bucolo, C., Maltese, A., Paolino, D., Vandelli, M.A., Puglisi, G., Lee, V.H., and Fresta, M. (2003). Influence of preparation conditions on acyclovir-loaded poly-d,l-lactic acid nanospheres and effect of PEG coating on ocular drug bioavailability. *Pharm. Res.*, **20**, pp. 584–590.

68. Gillies, M.C., Su, T., and Naidoo, D. (1995). Electrical resistance and macromolecular permeability of retinal capillary endothelial cells *in vitro*. *Curr. Eye Res.*, **14**, pp. 435–442.

69. Hamalainen, K.M., Kananen, K., Auriola, S., Kontturi, K., and Urtti, A. (1997). Characterization of paracellular and aqueous penetration routes in cornea, conjunctiva, and sclera. *Invest. Ophthalmol. Vis. Sci.*, **38**, pp. 627–634.

70. Hamann, S. (2002). Molecular mechanisms of water transport in the eye. *Int. Rev. Cytol.*, **215**, pp. 395–431.

71. Zeuthen, T., and Wilfred, D. (eds) *Molecular Mechanisms of Water Transport Across Biological Membranes*, vol. **215**, pp. 395–431. Academic Press.

72. Hamilton, M.M., Brough, D.E., McVey, D., Bruder, J.T., King, C.R., and Wei, L.L. (2006). Repeated administration of adenovector in the eye results in efficient gene delivery. *Invest. Ophthalmol. Vis. Sci.*, **47**, pp. 299–305.

73. Hayek, S., Scherrer, M., Barthelmes, D., Fleischhauer, J.C., Kurz-Levin, M.M., Menghini, M., Helbig, H., and Sutter, F.K. (2007). First clinical experience with anecortave acetate (Retaane). *Klin. Monatsbl. Augenheilkd.*, **224**, pp. 279–281.

74. Herrero-Vanrell, R., and Refojo, M.F. (2001). Biodegradable microspheres for vitreoretinal drug delivery. *Adv. Drug Deliv. Rev.*, **52**, pp. 5–16.

75. Hillaireau, H., Le, D.T., and Couvreur, P. (2006). Polymer-based nanoparticles for the delivery of nucleoside analogues. *J. Nanosci. Nanotechnol.*, **6**, pp. 2608–2617.

76. Holash, J.A., and Stewart, P.A. (1993). The relationship of astrocyte-like cells to the vessels that contribute to the blood-ocular barriers. *Brain Res.*, **629**, pp. 218–224.

77. Hornof, M., Toropainen, E., and Urtti, A. (2005). Cell culture models of the ocular barriers. *Eur. J. Pharm. Biopharm.*, **60**, pp. 207–225.

78. Hosoya, K., Horibe, Y., Kim, K.J., and Lee, V.H. (1998). Nucleoside transport mechanisms in the pigmented rabbit conjunctiva. *Invest. Ophthalmol. Vis. Sci.*, **39**, pp. 372–377.

79. Hosoya, K., Lee, V.H., and Kim, K.J. (2005). Roles of the conjunctiva in ocular drug delivery: a review of conjunctival transport mechanisms and their regulation. *Eur. J. Pharm. Biopharm.*, **60**, pp. 227–240.

80. Hosoya, K., Tomi, M., Ohtsuki, S., Takanaga, H., Ueda, M., Yanai, N., Obinata, M., and Terasaki, T. (2001). Conditionally immortalized retinal capillary endothelial cell lines (TR-iBRB) expressing differentiated endothelial cell functions derived from a transgenic rat. *Exp. Eye Res.*, **72**, pp. 163–172.

81. Huang, H.S., Schoenwald, R.D., and Lach, J.L. (1983a). Corneal penetration behavior of beta-blocking agents II: Assessment of barrier contributions. *J. Pharm. Sci.*, **72**, pp. 1272–1279.

82. Huang, H.S., Schoenwald, R.D., and Lach, J.L. (1983b). Corneal penetration behavior of beta-blocking agents III: *In vitro-in vivo* correlations. *J. Pharm. Sci.*, **72**, pp. 1279–1281.

83. Hunt, R.C., Dewey, A., and Davis, A.A. (1989). Transferrin receptors on the surfaces of retinal pigment epithelial cells are associated with the cytoskeleton. *J. Cell Sci.*, **92** (Pt 4), pp. 655–666.

84. Jabs, D.A. (1995). Controversies in the treatment of cytomegalovirus retinitis: foscarnet versus ganciclovir. *Infect. Agents Dis.*, **4**, pp. 131–142.

85. Janoria, K.G., Gunda, S., Boddu, S.H., and Mitra, A.K. (2007). Novel approaches to retinal drug delivery. *Expert Opin. Drug Deliv.*, **4**, pp. 371–388.

86. Jentsch, T.J., Keller, S.K., and Wiederholt, M. (1985). Ion transport mechanisms in cultured bovine corneal endothelial cells. *Curr. Eye Res.*, **4**, pp. 361–369.

87. Jose Alonso, M. (2004). Nanomedicines for overcoming biological barriers. *Biomed. Pharmacother.*, **58**, pp. 168–172.

88. Ju, M., Mailhos, C., Bradley, J., Dowie, T., Ganley, M., Cook, G., Calias, P., Lange, N., Adamis, A.P., Shima, D.T., and Robinson, G.S. (2008). Simultaneous but not prior inhibition of VEGF165 enhances the efficacy of photodynamic therapy in multiple models of ocular neovascularization. *Invest. Ophthalmol. Vis. Sci.*, **49**, pp. 662–670.

89. Karla, P.K., Pal, D., Quinn, T., and Mitra, A.K. (2007). Molecular evidence and functional expression of a novel drug efflux pump (ABCC2) in human corneal epithelium and rabbit cornea and its role in ocular drug efflux. *Int J. Pharm.*, **336**, pp. 12–21.

90. Kassem, M.A., Abdel Rahman, A.A., Ghorab, M.M., Ahmed, M.B., and Khalil, R.M. (2007). Nanosuspension as an ophthalmic delivery system for certain glucocorticoid drugs. *Int. J. Pharm.*, **340**, pp. 126–133.

91. Kaur, I.P., Garg, A., Singla, A.K., and Aggarwal, D. (2004). Vesicular systems in ocular drug delivery: an overview. *Int. J. Pharm.*, **269**, pp. 1–14.

92. Kayser, O., Lemke, A., and Hernandez-Trejo, N. (2005). The impact of nanobiotechnology on the development of new drug delivery systems. *Curr. Pharm. Biotechnol.*, **6**, pp. 3–5.

93. Kim, S.H., Lutz, R.J., Wang, N.S., and Robinson, M.R. (2007). Transport barriers in transscleral drug delivery for retinal diseases. *Ophthalmic Res.*, **39**, pp. 244–254.

94. Kimura, H., and Ogura, Y. (2001). Biodegradable polymers for ocular drug delivery. *Ophthalmologica*, **215**, pp. 143–155.

95. Klyce, S.D., and Crosson, C.E. (1985). Transport processes across the rabbit corneal epithelium: a review. *Curr. Eye Res.*, **4**, pp. 323–331.

96. Kobayashi, H., Shiraki, K., and Ikada, Y. (1992). Toxicity test of biodegradable polymers by implantation in rabbit cornea. *J. Biomed. Mater. Res.*, **26**, pp. 1463–1476.

97. Koizumi, K., Poulaki, V., Doehmen, S., Welsandt, G., Radetzky, S., Lappas, A., Kociok, N., Kirchhof, B., and Joussen, A.M. (2003). Contribution of TNF-alpha to leukocyte adhesion, vascular leakage, and apoptotic cell death in endotoxin-induced uveitis *in vivo*. *Invest. Ophthalmol. Vis. Sci.*, **44**, pp. 2184–2191.

98. Kompella, U.B., Sundaram, S., Raghava, S., and Escobar, E.R. (2006). Luteinizing hormone-releasing hormone agonist and transferrin functionalizations enhance nanoparticle delivery in a novel bovine *ex vivo* eye model. *Mol. Vis.*, **12**, pp. 1185–1198.

99. Kothuri, M.K., Pinnamaneni, S., Das, N.G., and Das, S.K. (2003). Microparticles and nanoparticles in ocular drug delivery. In *Ophthalmic Drug Delivery Systems* (ed. A.K. Mitra), pp. 437–466. Marcel Dekker, New York.

100. Kuang, K., Li, Y., Yiming, M., Sanchez, J.M., Iserovich, P., Cragoe, E.J., Diecke, F.P., and Fischbarg, J. (2004). Intracellular [Na^+], Na^+ pathways, and fluid transport in cultured bovine corneal endothelial cells. *Exp. Eye Res.*, **79**, pp. 93–103.

101. Kurz, D., and Ciulla, T.A. (2002). Novel approaches for retinal drug delivery. *Ophthalmol. Clin. North Am.*, **15**, pp. 405–410.

102. Kyyronen, K., and Urtti, A. (1990). Improved ocular: systemic absorption ratio of timolol by viscous vehicle and phenylephrine. *Invest. Ophthalmol. Vis. Sci.*, **31**, pp. 1827–1833.

103. la Cour, M., and Ehinger, B. (2006). The retina. In *The Biology of Eye* (ed. J. Fischbarg), pp. 195–252. Academic Press, New York.

104. Lang, J.C. (1995). Ocular drug delivery conventional ocular formulation. *Adv. Drug Deliv. Rev.*, **16**, pp. 39–43.

105. Lazic, R., and Gabric, N. (2007). Verteporfin therapy and intravitreal bevacizumab combined and alone in choroidal neovascularization due to age-related macular degeneration. *Ophthalmology*, **114**, pp. 1179–1185.

106. Le, M.G., Stieger, K., Smith, A.J., Weber, M., Deschamps, J.Y., Nivard, D., Mendes-Madeira, A., Provost, N., Pereon, Y., Cherel, Y., Ali, R.R., Hamel, C., Moullier, P., and Rolling, F. (2007). Restoration of vision in RPE65-deficient Briard dogs using an AAV serotype 4 vector that specifically targets the retinal pigmented epithelium. *Gene Ther.*, **14**, pp. 292–303.

107. Lee, B., Litt, M., and Buchsbaum, G. (1992). Rheology of the vitreous body: part 1: Viscoelasticity of human vitreous. *Biorheology*, **29**, pp. 521–533.

108. Lee, B., Litt, M., and Buchsbaum, G. (1994a). Rheology of the vitreous body: part 2. Viscoelasticity of bovine and porcine vitreous. *Biorheology*, **31**, pp. 327–338.

109. Lee, B., Litt, M., and Buchsbaum, G. (1994b). Rheology of the vitreous body: part 3. Concentration of electrolytes, collagen and hyaluronic acid. *Biorheology*, **31**, pp. 339–351.

110. Lee, T.W., and Robinson, J.R. (2004). Drug delivery to the posterior segment of the eye III: the effect of parallel elimination pathway on the vitreous drug level after subconjunctival injection. *J. Ocul. Pharmacol. Ther.*, **20**, pp. 55–64.

111. Lee, V.H. (1990). New directions in the optimization of ocular drug delivery. *J. Ocul. Pharmacol.*, **6**, pp. 157–164.

112. Lee, V.H., Carson, L.W., Kashi, S.D., and Stratford, R.E., Jr. (1986). Metabolic and permeation barriers to the ocular absorption of topically applied enkephalins in albino rabbits. *J. Ocul. Pharmacol.*, **2**, pp. 345–352.

113. Leeming, J.P. (1999). Treatment of ocular infections with topical antibacterials. *Clin. Pharmacokinet.*, **37**, pp. 351–360.

114. Lehr, C.M., Lee, Y.H., and Lee, V.H. (1994). Improved ocular penetration of gentamicin by mucoadhesive polymer polycarbophil in the pigmented rabbit. *Invest. Ophthalmol. Vis. Sci.*, **35**, pp. 2809–2814.

115. Li, H., Tran, V.V., Hu, Y., Mark, S.W., Barns, C.J., and Tombran-Tink, J. (2006). A PEDF N-terminal peptide protects the retina from ischemic injury when delivered in PLGA nanospheres. *Exp. Eye Res.*, **83**, pp. 824–833.

116. Liaw, J., Chang, S.F., and Hsiao, F.C. (2001). *In vivo* gene delivery into ocular tissues by eye drops of poly(ethylene oxide)-poly(propylene oxide)-poly(ethylene oxide) (PEO-PPO-PEO) polymeric micelles. *Gene Ther.*, **8**, pp. 999–1004.

117. Lin, H., Kenyon, E., and Miller, S.S. (1992). Na-dependent pHi regulatory mechanisms in native human retinal pigment epithelium. *Invest. Ophthalmol. Vis. Sci.*, **33**, pp. 3528–3538.

118. Liu, D., Ren, T., and Gao, X. (2003). Cationic transfection lipids. *Curr. Med. Chem.*, **10**, pp. 1307–1315.

119. Lo, W.K., Mills, A., Zhang, W., and Zhu, H. (1991). Polarized distribution of coated pits and coated vesicles in the rat lens: an electron microscopy and WGA-HRP tracer study. *Curr. Eye Res.*, **10**, pp. 1151–1163.

120. Lo, W.K., Zhou, C.J., and Reddan, J. (2004). Identification of caveolae and their signature proteins caveolin 1 and 2 in the lens. *Exp. Eye Res.*, **79**, pp. 487–498.

121. Lopez-Cortes, L.F., Pastor-Ramos, M.T., Ruiz-Valderas, R., Cordero, E., Uceda-Montanes, A., Claro-Cala, C.M., and Lucero-Munoz, M.J. (2001). Intravitreal pharmacokinetics and retinal concentrations of ganciclovir and foscarnet after intravitreal administration in rabbits. *Invest. Ophthalmol. Vis. Sci.*, **42**, pp. 1024–1028.

122. Loutsch, J.M., Ong, D., and Hill, J.M. (2003). Dendrimers: an innovative and enhanced ocular drug delivery system. In *Ophthalmic Drug Delivery Systems* (ed. A.K. Mitra), pp. 467–492. Marcel Dekker, New York.

123. Ludwig, A. (2005). The use of mucoadhesive polymers in ocular drug delivery. *Adv. Drug Delivery Rev.*, **57**, pp. 1595–1639.

124. Macha, S., and Mitra, A.K. (2003). Overview of ocular drug delivery. In *Ophthalmic Drug Delivery Systems* (ed. A.K. Mitra), pp. 1–12. Marcel Dekker, New York.

125. Maguire, A.M., and Bennett, J. (2006). Gene therapy for retinal disease. In *Intraocular Drug Delivery* (ed. G.J. Jaffe, P. Ashton, and P.A. Pearson), pp. 157–173. Taylor & Francis Group, LLC, New York.

126. Mannermaa, E., Vellonen, K.S., and Urtti, A. (2006). Drug transport in corneal epithelium and blood–retina barrier: emerging role of transporters in ocular pharmacokinetics. *Adv. Drug Deliv. Rev.*, **58**, pp. 1136–1163.

127. Marano, R.J., Toth, I., Wimmer, N., Brankov, M., and Rakoczy, P.E. (2005). Dendrimer delivery of an anti-VEGF oligonucleotide into the eye: a long-term study into inhibition of laser-induced CNV, distribution, uptake and toxicity. *Gene Ther.*, **12**, pp. 1544–1550.

128. Marie, O., Thillaye-Goldenberg, B., Naud, M.C., and de Kozak, Y. (1999). Inhibition of endotoxin-induced uveitis and potentiation of local TNF-alpha and interleukin-6 mRNA expression by interleukin-13. *Invest. Ophthalmol. Vis. Sci.*, **40**, pp. 2275–2282.

129. McLaughlin, B.J., Caldwell, R.B., Sasaki, Y., and Wood, T.O. (1985). Freeze-fracture quantitative comparison of rabbit corneal epithelial and endothelial membranes. *Curr. Eye Res.*, **4**, pp. 951–961.

130. Mitra, A.K., Anand, B.S., and Duvvuri, S. (2006). Drug delivery to the eye. In *The Biology of Eye* (ed. J. Fischbarg), pp. 307–351. Academic Press, New York.

131. Mo, Y., Barnett, M.E., Takemoto, D., Davidson, H., and Kompella, U.B. (2007). Human serum albumin nanoparticles for efficient delivery of Cu, Zn superoxide dismutase gene. *Mol. Vis.*, **13**, pp. 746–757.

132. Muccioli, C., and Belfort, R., Jr. (2000). Treatment of cytomegalovirus retinitis with an intraocular sustained-release ganciclovir implant. *Braz. J. Med. Biol. Res.*, **33**, pp. 779–789.

133. Muyldermans, S., Baral, T.N., Retamozzo, V.C., De, B.P., De, G.E., Kinne, J., Leonhardt, H., Magez, S., Nguyen, V.K., Revets, H., Rothbauer, U., Stijlemans, B., Tillib, S., Wernery, U., Wyns, L., Hassanzadeh-Ghassabeh, G., and Saerens, D. (2009). Camelid immunoglobulins and nanobody technology. *Vet. Immunol. Immunopathol.*, **128**, pp. 178–183.

134. Myles, M.E., Neumann, D.M., and Hill, J.M. (2005). Recent progress in ocular drug delivery for posterior segment disease: emphasis on transscleral iontophoresis. *Adv. Drug Deliv. Rev.*, **57**, pp. 2063–2079.

135. Andrieu-Soler, C., Bejjani, R.A., de Bizemont, T., Normand, N., BenEzra, D., and Behar-Cohen, F. (2006). Ocular gene therapy: a review of nonviral strategies. *Mol. Vis.*, **12**, pp. 1334–1347.

136. Nicolazzi, C., Garinot, M., Mignet, N., Scherman, D., and Bessodes, M. (2003). Cationic lipids for transfection. *Curr. Med. Chem.*, **10**, pp. 1263–1277.

137. Nishiyama, N., Iriyama, A., Jang, W.D., Miyata, K., Itaka, K., Inoue, Y., Takahashi, H., Yanagi, Y., Tamaki, Y., Koyama, H., and Kataoka, K. (2005). Light-induced gene transfer from packaged DNA enveloped in a dendrimeric photosensitizer. *Nat. Mater.*, **4**, pp. 934–941.

138. Omidi, Y., Barar, J., Ahmadian, S., Heidari, H.R., and Gumbleton, M. (2008). Characterization and astrocytic modulation of system L transporters in brain microvasculature endothelial cells. *Cell Biochem. Funct.* (in press).

139. Omidi, Y., Barar, J., and Akhtar, S. (2005). Toxicogenomics of cationic lipid-based vectors for gene therapy: impact of microarray technology. *Curr. Drug Deliv.*, **2**, pp. 429–441.

140. Omidi, Y., Campbell, L., Barar, J., Connell, D., Akhtar, S., and Gumbleton, M. (2003a). Evaluation of the immortalised mouse brain capillary endothelial cell line, b.End3, as an in vitro blood-brain barrier model for drug uptake and transport studies. *Brain Res.*, **990**, pp. 95–112.

141. Omidi, Y., and Gumbleton, M. (2005). Biological membranes and barriers. In *Biomaterials for Delivery and Targeting of Proteins Nucleic Acids* (ed. R.I. Mahato), pp. 232–274. CRC Press, New York.

142. Omidi, Y., Hollins, A.J., Benboubetra, M., Drayton, R., Benter, I.F., and Akhtar, S. (2003b). Toxicogenomics of non-viral vectors for gene therapy: a microarray study of lipofectin- and oligofectamine-induced gene expression changes in human epithelial cells. *J. Drug Target*, **11**, pp. 311–323.

143. Palmgren, J.J., Toropainen, E., Auriola, S., and Urtti, A. (2002). Liquid chromatographic-electrospray ionization mass spectrometric analysis of neutral and charged polyethylene glycols. *J. Chromatogr. A*, **976**, pp. 165–170.

144. Parascandola, J. (1991). The development of the Draize test for eye toxicity. *Pharm. Hist*, **33**, pp. 111–117.

145. Pardridge, W.M. (2007). Blood-brain barrier delivery of protein and non-viral gene therapeutics with molecular Trojan horses. *J. Control Release*, **122**, pp. 345–348.

146. Patravale, V.B., Date, A.A., and Kulkarni, R.M. (2004). Nanosuspensions: a promising drug delivery strategy. *J. Pharm. Pharmacol.*, **56**, pp. 827–840.

147. Pece, A., Isola, V., Vadala, M., and Calori, G. (2007). Photodynamic therapy with verteporfin for choroidal neovascularization associated with retinal pigment epithelial detachment in age-related macular degeneration. *Retina*, **27**, pp. 342–348.

148. Pedroso de Lima, M.C., Simoes, S., Pires, P., Faneca, H., and Duzgunes, N. (2001). Cationic lipid-DNA complexes in gene delivery: from biophysics to biological applications. *Adv. Drug Deliv. Rev.*, **47**, pp. 277–294.

149. Peeters, L., Sanders, N.N., Braeckmans, K., Boussery, K., de Voorde, V., d., De Smedt, S.C., and Demeester, J. (2005). Vitreous: a barrier to nonviral ocular gene therapy. *Invest. Ophthalmol. Vis. Sci.*, **46**, pp. 3553–3561.

150. Pignatello, R., Bucolo, C., Ferrara, P., Maltese, A., Puleo, A., and Puglisi, G. (2002a). Eudragit RS100 nanosuspensions for the ophthalmic controlled delivery of ibuprofen. *Eur. J. Pharm. Sci.*, **16**, pp. 53–61.

151. Pignatello, R., Bucolo, C., Spedalieri, G., Maltese, A., and Puglisi, G. (2002b). Flurbiprofen-loaded acrylate polymer nanosuspensions for ophthalmic application. *Biomaterials*, **23**, pp. 3247–3255.

152. Prausnitz, M.R., and Noonan, J.S. (1998). Permeability of cornea, sclera, and conjunctiva: a literature analysis for drug delivery to the eye. *J. Pharm. Sci.*, **87**, pp. 1479–1488.

153. Qaddoumi, M.G., Gukasyan, H.J., Davda, J., Labhasetwar, V., Kim, K.J., and Lee, V.H. (2003). Clathrin and caveolin-1 expression in primary pigmented rabbit conjunctival epithelial cells: role in PLGA nanoparticle endocytosis. *Mol. Vis.*, **9**, pp. 559–568.

154. Quinn, R.H., and Miller, S.S. (1992). Ion transport mechanisms in native human retinal pigment epithelium. *Invest. Ophthalmol. Vis. Sci.*, **33**, pp. 3513–3527.

155. Raghava, S., Hammond, M., and Kompella, U.B. (2004). Periocular routes for retinal drug delivery. *Expert Opin. Drug Deliv.*, **1**, pp. 99–114.

156. Rana, Z.A., and Pearson, P.A. (2006). Pharmacologic treatment in diabetic macular edema. In *Intraocular Drug Delivery* (ed. G.J. Jaffe, P. Ashton, and P.A. Pearson), pp. 291–300. Taylor & Francis Group, LLC, New York.

157. Robinson, M.R., Lee, S.S., Kim, H., Kim, S., Lutz, R.J., Galban, C., Bungay, P.M., Yuan, P., Wang, N.S., Kim, J., and Csaky, K.G. (2006). A rabbit model for assessing the ocular barriers to the transscleral delivery of triamcinolone acetonide. *Exp. Eye Res.*, **82**, pp. 479–487.

158. Rocha, E.M., Cunha, D.A., Carneiro, E.M., Boschero, A.C., Saad, M.J., and Velloso, L.A. (2002). Identification of insulin in the tear film and insulin receptor and IGF-1 receptor on the human ocular surface. *Invest. Ophthalmol. Vis. Sci.*, **43**, pp. 963–967.

159. Rose, R.C., and Bode, A.M. (1991). Ocular ascorbate transport and metabolism. *Comp. Biochem. Physiol. A: Physiol.*, **100**, pp. 273–285.

160. Sabah, J.R., Schultz, B.D., Brown, Z.W., Nguyen, A.T., Reddan, J., and Takemoto, L.J. (2007). Transcytotic passage of albumin through lens epithelial cells. *Invest. Ophthalmol. Vis. Sci.*, **48**, pp. 1237–1244.

161. Saha, P., Kim, K.J., and Lee, V.H. (1996). A primary culture model of rabbit conjunctival epithelial cells exhibiting tight barrier properties. *Curr. Eye Res.*, **15**, pp. 1163–1169.

162. Saha, P., Yang, J.J., and Lee, V.H. (1998). Existence of a p-glycoprotein drug efflux pump in cultured rabbit conjunctival epithelial cells. *Invest. Ophthalmol. Vis. Sci.*, **39**, pp. 1221–1226.

163. Sahoo, S.K., Dilnawaz, F., and Krishnakumar, S. (2008). Nanotechnology in ocular drug delivery. *Drug Discov. Today*, **13**, pp. 144–151.

164. Sanders, N.N., Peeters, L., Lentacker, I., Demeester, J., and De Smedt, S.C. (2007). Wanted and unwanted properties of surface PEGylated nucleic acid nanoparticles in ocular gene transfer. *J. Control Release*, **122**, pp. 226–235.

165. Sasaki, H., Yamamura, K., Tei, C., Nishida, K., and Nakamura, J. (1995). Ocular permeability of FITC-dextran with absorption promoter for ocular delivery of peptide drug. *J. Drug Target*, **3**, pp. 129–135.

166. Schlingemann, R.O., Hofman, P., Klooster, J., Blaauwgeers, H.G., van der, G.R., and Vrensen, G.F. (1998). Ciliary muscle capillaries have blood-tissue barrier characteristics. *Exp. Eye Res.*, **66**, pp. 747–754.

167. Schoenwald, R.D., and Huang, H.S. (1983). Corneal penetration behavior of beta-blocking agents I: physiochemical factors. *J. Pharm. Sci.*, **72**, pp. 1266–1272.

168. Schorderet, D.F., Manzi, V., Canola, K., Bonny, C., Arsenijevic, Y., Munier, F.L., and Maurer, F. (2005). D-TAT transporter as an ocular peptide delivery system. *Clin. Experiment. Ophthalmol.*, **33**, pp. 628–635.

169. Selvin, B.L. (1983). Systemic effects of topical ophthalmic medications. *South. Med. J.*, **76**, pp. 349–358.

170. Shedden, A.H., Laurence, J., Barrish, A., and Olah, T.V. (2001). Plasma timolol concentrations of timolol maleate: timolol gel-forming solution (TIMOPTIC-XE) once daily versus timolol maleate ophthalmic solution twice daily. *Doc. Ophthalmol.*, **103**, pp. 73–79.

171. Shen, J., Cross, S.T., Tang-Liu, D.D., and Welty, D.F. (2003). Evaluation of an immortalized retinal endothelial cell line as an *in vitro* model for drug transport studies across the blood–retinal barrier. *Pharm. Res.*, **20**, pp. 1357–1363.

172. Shen, J., Samul, R., Silva, R.L., Akiyama, H., Liu, H., Saishin, Y., Hackett, S.F., Zinnen, S., Kossen, K., Fosnaugh, K., Vargeese, C., Gomez, A., Bouhana,

K., Aitchison, R., Pavco, P., and Campochiaro, P.A. (2006). Suppression of ocular neovascularization with siRNA targeting VEGF receptor 1. *Gene Ther.*, **13**, pp. 225–234.

173. Shimoyama, Y., Akihara, Y., Kirat, D., Iwano, H., Hirayama, K., Kagawa, Y., Ohmachi, T., Matsuda, K., Okamoto, M., Kadosawa, T., Yokota, H., and Taniyama, H. (2007). Expression of monocarboxylate transporter 1 in oral and ocular canine melanocytic tumors. *Vet. Pathol.*, **44**, pp. 449–457.

174. Smith, M., Omidi, Y., and Gumbleton, M. (2007). Primary porcine brain microvascular endothelial cells: biochemical and functional characterisation as a model for drug transport and targeting. *J. Drug Target*, **15**, pp. 253–268.

175. Stewart, P.A., and Tuor, U.I. (1994). Blood-eye barriers in the rat: correlation of ultrastructure with function. *J. Comp Neurol.*, **340**, pp. 566–576.

176. Stone, T.W., and Jaffe, G.J. (2000). Reversible bull's-eye maculopathy associated with intravitreal fomivirsen therapy for cytomegalovirus retinitis. *Am. J. Ophthalmol.*, **130**, pp. 242–243.

177. Sun, X.C., Bonanno, J.A., Jelamskii, S., and Xie, Q. (2000). Expression and localization of Na^+-HCO_3^- cotransporter in bovine corneal endothelium. *Am. J. Physiol. Cell Physiol.*, **279**, pp. C1648–C1655.

178. Sunkara, G., and Kompella, U.B. (2003). Membrane transport processes in the eye. In *Ophthalmic Drug Delivery Systems* (ed. A.K. Mitra), pp. 13–58. Marcel Dekker, New York.

179. Tao, W., Wen, R., Laties, A., and Aguirre, G.D. (2006). Cell-based delivery systems: development of encapsulated cell technology for ophthalmic applications. In *Intraocular Drug Delivery* (ed. G.J. Jaffe, P. Ashton, and P.A. Pearson), pp. 111–128. Taylor & Francis Group, LLC, New York.

180. Tomalia, D.A., Baker, H., Dewald, J., Hall, M., Kallos, G., Martin, S., Roeck, J., Ryder, J., and Smith, P. (1984). A new class of polymers: starburst-dendritic macromolecules. *Polymer J.*, **17**, pp. 117–132.

181. Toropainen, E., Ranta, V.P., Talvitie, A., Suhonen, P., and Urtti, A. (2001). Culture model of human corneal epithelium for prediction of ocular drug absorption. *Invest. Ophthalmol. Vis. Sci.*, **42**, pp. 2942–2948.

182. Urtti, A. (2006). Challenges and obstacles of ocular pharmacokinetics and drug delivery. *Adv. Drug Deliv. Rev.*, **58**, pp. 1131–1135.

183. Urtti, A., Rouhiainen, H., Kaila, T., and Saano, V. (1994). Controlled ocular timolol delivery: systemic absorption and intraocular pressure effects in humans. *Pharm. Res.*, **11**, pp. 1278–1282.

184. Urtti, A., and Salminen, L. (1993a). Animal pharmacokinetic studies. In *Ophthalmic Drug Delivery Systems* (ed. A.K. Mitra), pp. 121–136. Marcel Dekker, New York.

185. Urtti, A., and Salminen, L. (1993b). Minimizing systemic absorption of topically administered ophthalmic drugs. *Surv. Ophthalmol.*, **37**, pp. 435–456.

186. Vandamme, T.F., and Brobeck, L. (2005). Poly(amidoamine) dendrimers as ophthalmic vehicles for ocular delivery of pilocarpine nitrate and tropicamide. *J. Control Release*, **102**, pp. 23–38.

187. Vandervoort, J., and Ludwig, A. (2007). Ocular drug delivery: nanomedicine applications. *Nanomedicine*, **2**, pp. 11–21.

188. Vega, E., Egea, M.A., Valls, O., Espina, M., and Garcia, M.L. (2006). Flurbiprofen loaded biodegradable nanoparticles for ophtalmic administration. *J. Pharm. Sci.*, **95**, pp. 2393–2405.

189. Visor, G.C. (1994). Drug design strategies for ocular therapeutics. *Adv. Drug Delivery Rev.*, **14**, pp. 269–279.

190. Wood, T.O., McLaughlin, B.J., and Boykins, L.G. (1985). Electron microscopy of corneal surface microdiathermy. *Curr. Eye Res.*, **4**, pp. 885–895.

191. Wu, J., Zhang, J.J., Koppel, H., and Jacob, T.J. (1996). P-glycoprotein regulates a volume-activated chloride current in bovine non-pigmented ciliary epithelial cells. *J. Physiol.*, **491** (Pt 3), pp. 743–755.

192. Yang, J.J., Ann, D.K., Kannan, R., and Lee, V.H. (2007). Multidrug resistance protein 1 (MRP1) in rabbit conjunctival epithelial cells: its effect on drug efflux and its regulation by adenoviral infection. *Pharm. Res.*, **24**, pp. 1490–1500.

193. Zimmer, A., and Kreuter, J. (1995). Microspheres and nanoparticles used in ocular delivery systems. *Adv. Drug Deliv. Rev.*, **16**, pp. 61–73.

Chapter 3

Immunonanosystems to CNS Pathologies: State of the Art

G. Tosi, B. Ruozi, L. Badiali, L. Bondioli, D. Belletti, F. Forni, and M. A. Vandelli

Department of Pharmaceutical Sciences, University of Modena and Reggio Emilia, Via Campi 183, 41100, Modena, Italy

gtosi@unimore.it

3.1 Introduction

The delivery of pharmacologically active substances, such as synthetic drugs, natural compounds, gene material, and many other pharmaceutical products, has been widely studied and investigated over the last half century. In fact, scientists working in the field of pharmacological active substances easily understood that the main problem of such molecules is represented by their wide and nonspecific biodistribution once administered in the human body. This reflects, without any doubt, in an increase in toxicity and contemporaneously in both a decreased patient compliance and decreased benefit-risk ratio.

On the other hand, it is also true that a number of specific diseases are considered "difficult to treat" due to the presence of pathogen-defensive systems, which protect against the progression

Nanotechnology in Health Care
Edited by Sanjeeb K. Sahoo

ISBN 978-981-4267-21-2 (Hardcover), 978-981-4267-35-9 (eBook)
www.panstanford.com

of the pathology (e.g., leukemia and viral infection). Moreover the presence of natural barriers would hinder the entrance/invasion of pathogens into the tissue to be protected, but contemporaneously also the effectiveness of drugs once the infection or the pathologies grow.

In this view, the development of drug delivery systems, able to improve the pharmacokinetic profile of drugs, thus protecting the body from the exposure of a great amount of drugs and decreasing the circulating doses, is surely one of the most innovative improvements of the last decade of pharmaceutical research. New drug delivery systems have been prepared mainly from biodegradable and biocompatible starting materials (polymers, lipids, proteins, etc.), obtaining direct application on the pharmaceutical market and reaching valuable results (Bawa, 2008) against a wide spectrum of pathologies.

The step forward, nowadays strongly necessary, is to increase the selectivity of drugs and thus the selectivity of therapies. In fact, in order to maximize the therapeutic effect, the new "smart" drug delivery systems need to be further engineered to obtain "ultraselective" carriers able to deliver drugs (which could be loaded into or bound to the systems) to the correct sites of action.

This specialized therapy is now going in the same direction as the so-called personalized medicine. In fact, the new age of pharmacoproteomic and pharmacogenomic invading medicine has created the need for obtaining a more selective therapeutic protocol of treatments. These approaches are mainly based on the differences among patients in terms of hematochemical parameters, metabolisms, elimination, and drug biodistribution.

If personalized medicine is a way to increase the selectivity of a chosen drug and to maximize the pharmacological effect, the other way is to use systems (such as drug delivery systems) that are able to both decrease the adverse effects and to be much more selective than the free drugs or unmodified drug carriers or conventional formulations.

The main advance of the drug delivery systems, in comparison with personalized medicine, is surely represented by the costs. Even if polymers and preparation protocols for nanoparticulate formulations are not cheap, the genomic and proteomic analysis needed to be applied to every patient in order to reach the personalized-medicine goal represents a nonsustainable cost for public sanity. On the contrary, a drug delivery system should be able to hit specifically a target tissue, diseased and pathological, characterized by common features (e.g., surface antigens [Ags], histological characteristics, different pH environment, or variation in the temperature) and so relatively easily targeted.

In fact, drug targeting and personalized medicine represent parallel approaches because both strategies have the common aim to improve the current therapies but they follow completely different (or maybe complementary) methodologies. In fact, drug targeting considers pathologies as the final objective of the therapy while personalized medicine considers the patient as the subject of the pathology to be intimately studied for the obtainment of the best therapy.

Regarding the pathologies that are nowadays commonly considered as "difficult to treat," it is possible to cite several diseases, mostly aiming brain diseases. The main reason for this difficulty is the presence of the most important homeostatic defensive mechanism of the human body, the blood–brain barrier (BBB).

3.1.1 BBB Features

The BBB is the most important physiological barrier of the CNS, and it represents the unique protective system for the life and equilibrium of the cerebral environment.

The BBB consists of walls formed by capillaries that separate the brain from the circulating blood; its low permeability is due to its anatomical structure, expression of efflux transporters, and low level of enzyme activity. Unlike the rest the body, capillaries within the CNS lack intercellular clefts and fenestra while showing tight junctions and low pinocytotic activity (Weiss *et al.*, 2009). Thus, due to the difficulty for drugs to enter the brain when the BBB is in a healthy state, there has been in-depth study of and progress in drug delivery strategies to cross the BBB.

As many authors describe, the BBB represents a strong defensive barrier, pivotal to life and working as an artificial dam.

In fact, if in the past, the BBB was thought to be a very static membrane, impermeable to hydrophilic substances and permeable only to lipophilic ones, nowadays, the BBB is radically thought to be a very dynamic interface, mediating the passage of nutrients and substances by using different pathways. The movement of substances *from the blood to the brain* is mainly mediated by the so-called *influx systems*, such as the paracellular aqueous pathway (transporting water-soluble agents), the transcellular lipophilic pathways (transporting lipid-soluble agents), the transport protein pathways (for glucose, amino acids, and purines), and the more complex transport mechanisms such as specific-receptor-mediated endocytosis (insulin or Tf) or adsorptive endocytosis (for albumin and other plasma proteins).

The movement of substances or pathogens from the *brain to the blood* is instead mediated by efflux systems, such as P-glycoprotein (P-gp), multidrug resistance proteins (MRP), and organic anion transporter (OAT) efflux pumps. These systems really represent the brain's defensive mechanism, preventing the passage of a number of molecules potentially damaging the brain life.

Unfortunately, the efflux system often represents the most important cause of the failure of the treatment of brain pathologies. In fact, it is estimated that over 98% of drugs able to treat brain disease (from anticancer to antiretroviral drugs or antibiotics) are not able to enter the brain due to the presence of P-gp and other efflux systems or to the fact that these drugs do not have specific active transport influx systems. Firstly, a deep study of the anatomy and pathophysiology of the BBB must be at the basis of all the studies and approaches for the CNS drug delivery, because it is true that certain pathologies do affect BBB integrity.

In these cases, drug delivery to the CNS must not be thought of as delivery across the BBB but as delivery to target pathologies. In fact, the protective role of the BBB is totally lost in the BBB-disrupting diseases (de Vries *et al.*, 1997) and the delivery of drugs may be facilitated; this is the case shown for hypertension or seizures or during cerebral inflammation such as multiple sclerosis, experimental allergic encephalomyelitis, bacterial meningitis (Afonso *et al.*, 2008) and some cerebral tumors such as glioblastoma (Schneider *et al.*, 2004; Plate *et al.*, 1992).

Totally different is the case of those pathologies in which BBB integrity is completely maintained, rendering the treatment much more difficult and hampered both by the complexity of BBB-crossing mechanisms and the difficulty of reaching the correct target site, cells, or parenchyma.

3.1.2 BBB Strategies for Drug Delivery

Considering the complexity of the BBB, it is clear how the therapies against brain diseases represent a huge challenge for physicians and scientists — the inability of the drugs to reach the target site.

To date, in clinical treatments, the most widely used approach is based on invasive techniques of neurosurgery (intracerebral infusions or implants) (Bobo *et al.*, 1994; Kroll *et al.*, 1996) with direct drug delivery to the target site. This approach shows advantages in terms of increased efficacy, since the drug is directly placed into the brain; however, on the other hand, neurosurgical costs and the risks of infections rapidly increase. Most of all, it is fundamental to seriously consider patient compliance, which radically decreases when invasive techniques are applied.

Alongside this approach, a temporary chemical or physical disruption of the BBB, produced by some biochemical and immunological changes or by an osmotic shift (Siegal *et al.*, 2000; Doolittle *et al.*, 1998), could be used to allow the drug to cross the BBB.

Although this approach could really improve drug access to the CNS district, increasing drug efficacy, it is important to remember that this temporary disruption could create physiological stress or a transient increase in the intracranial pressure, exposing the brain to infections and damages from toxins.

For many reasons — firstly to enhance patient compliance and in order to improve drug delivery to the brain — noninvasive techniques have been investigated (the medicinal chemistry approach or the nanotechnological approach).

In fact, the medicinal chemistry approach based on the modification of the physicochemical properties of drugs (Anderson, 1996; Ricci *et al.*, 2006) has been demonstrated to be efficacious for CNS treatment along with a biological approach based on the conjugation of molecules with Abs or ligands targeting the BBB (Pardridge, 2002; Gaillard *et al.*, 2005).

The nanotechnological approach consists of the use of nanosystems (colloidal carriers) that could be made from polymer-based (NPs), solid-lipid (SLNPs), and lipid-based (LPs) materials.

Generally, the use of colloidal systems in the field of drug delivery has a long-time background (Soppimath *et al.*, 2001; Hans *et al.*, 2002), while the concept of an ideal carrier able to target the drugs to specific regions, organs, or cells is certainly more recent (Emerich, 2005; Fahr *et al.*, 2007; Torchilin, 2006; Fahmy *et al.*, 2005; Sachdeva, 1998), being connected to the development of pharmaceutical technology.

3.2 Nanoparticulate Systems: Brain Disease Nanomedicine and Nanotoxicology

In recent years, the application of nanotechnology to the field of medicine represented the most innovative strategy to cope with diseases — named *nanomedicine*, it is applied to difficult-to-treat diseases.

As previously said, in this field of research, the most important goal to be reached is an increase in selectivity and specificity of drug action. Several results with stimulating findings in preclinical or clinical phases have been reached by using nanocarriers, delivering agents to targeted pathologies (Bawa, 2008).

But besides this aspect, a new field of research has been developed by toxicologists and it concerns the possible toxicity of nanoparticulate matters for the human health. In fact, it has been shown how nanoparticulate matters could be reasonably thought as a possible cause of damages, tumors, and other invasive pathologies when inhalated or accidently injected.

This new field of research, called *nanotoxicology*, mainly dealing with environmental damages due to nanoparticulate matters, is now looking to nano-drug delivery systems, showing possible damages and adverse effect due to the nanoparticulate approach.

It has to be clarified that even if a deep study is needed on the toxicity of drug delivery systems once administered in the human body, in line with the first aim of not creating toxicity, a nanoparticulate approach could be useful in the treatment of those pathologies that are now not treatable or at least for those pathologies in which a therapeutic intervention, even if not totally safe, is the last possibility of life. Furthermore, nano-drug delivery systems have to be planned starting from Food and Drug Administration (FDA)-approved polymers, featured by high-purity-grade, biodegradable, biocompatible, a-toxic, and nontumorogenic materials.

Thus, the design of nanosystems that are able to achieve drug targeting must consider some fundamental properties not yet fully optimized, such as their drug-loading capacities and *in vivo* fate, the interaction of these systems with the body and with its mechanisms of defense (that is, the non-self properties of these carriers), and the possible defensive reaction of the body's immune system.

At the same time, researchers have to cope with the overall cost, the scale-up production, the stability, and finally the acute and chronic toxicity.

3.2.1 Polymeric NPs

Generally talking, polymeric NPs are solid colloid matrix-like particles 1 to 1,000 nm in size made of polymers (Soppiamath *et al.*, 2001) of a different nature and encapsulate drugs during the preparation process, which could be chosen by using different approaches depending on both the polymers and the drug to be delivered.

Usually, small quantities of organic solvents are used in order to render much more ecocompatible the process of preparation and purification of these systems. In some cases, when the drug to be loaded into the NP possesses certain chemicophysical parameters (e.g., lipophilicity), the use of organic solvent is required, but suitable purification processes are always applied.

There are several natural or synthetic polymers often mixed during the preparation of NPs. Considering the stringent request of FDA guidelines in terms of biodegradability and biocompatibility for *in vivo* administration, the list of polymers that could be used to prepare NP systems is very short, with few polymers available for drug delivery systems preparation and approved for systemic administration.

In particular, it is a common opinion that the toxicology of a nanodevice should be related both to morphological and structural parameters of the systems (size, surface charge, shape) and the polymers used.

3.2.1.1 Polymers

In the field of brain delivery by using polymeric NPs, considering the synthetic polymers, poly-lactide (PLA), poly-lactide-co-glycolide

(PLGA), and polyalkylcyanoacrylate (PACA) are the most widely used polymers. In particular, PACA (Vauthier *et al.*, 2007) is at present not approved by the FDA for intravenous (IV) administration, although some of these polymers have been described to be devoid of toxicity (Müller *et al.*, 1990; Müller *et al.*, 1992; Lukowski *et al.*, 1992; Lherm *et al.*, 1992; Kante *et al.*, 1982; Kattan, 1992).

On the other hand, PACA NPs have been considered for the treatment of several resistant tumors (lung, brain, and liver) (Vauthier *et al.*, 2003). Phase I studies with PACA NPs loaded with the antitumoral drug doxorubicin (Kattan *et al.*, 1992) have shown good tolerance. At present, these NPs have reached Phase II clinical trials for the treatment of resistant cancer (Vauthier *et al.*, 2003).

Generally talking, poly-butyl-cyanoacrylate (PBCA) NPs have been widely studied and applied to a large number of therapeutic applications and with different drugs (Calvo *et al.*, 2001a; Ramge *et al.*, 2000; Gelperina *et al.*, 2002; Soma *et al.*, 2000; Kreuter, 2002a). Along with different *in vivo* and *in vitro* experiments regarding the proof-of-concept of drug delivery mediated by these kinds of NPs, several works have been performed regarding the safety on PBCA NP coated with polysorbate 80 for the drug delivery of doxorubicin to glioblastoma-bearing rats.

In these studies, the acute toxicity of doxorubicine associated with polysorbate 80-PBCA NP in healthy rats, along with the establishment of the therapeutic dose range against glioblastoma intracranially implanted in rats, was evaluated (Gelperina *et al.*, 2002), demonstrating the relative safety (no mortality and no differences in the weights of the internal organs) of the formulation.

In another work (Pereverzeva *et al.*, 2007), a toxicological study was performed after IV injection of polysorbate 80–coated PBCA NPs loaded with doxorubicin at the therapeutic doses, with the animals followed up for 15 and 30 days, demonstrating a considerably reduced cardio and testicular toxicity as compared with the free drug.

Finally, a very recent work (Pereverzeva *et al.*, 2008) demonstrated, after two–three months of single- or multiple-dose treatment, a maintenance of basal parameters (body weight, hematological features, blood biochemical parameters, urinalysis) without any damages, confirmed by pathomorphological (macroscopic and microscopic assays) and histological evaluation.

It must be considered that polysorbate 80, usually employed in these kinds of research, covering the surface of NPs with a non-covalent or covalent linkage, has been found to be toxic and disrupting for the BBB. In fact, it has been proved that a dose of polysorbate 80 of 3–30 mg/kg will cause BBB disruption in mice (Pardridge *et al.*, 2005; Azmin *et al.*, 1985; Sakane *et al.*, 1989). This fact is currently debated in the scientific community, with other authors routinely using polysorbate 80 as the delivery force (Petri *et al.*, 2007).

PLGA and PLA are FDA approved and, therefore, represent two of the most promising polymers for the preparation of NPs. PLA or PLGA degradation occurs by an autocatalytic cleavage of the ester bonds, through spontaneous hydrolysis into oligomers and monomers of lactic and glycolic acids, which are substrates of the Krebs' cycle (Li *et al.*, 1999). It is remarkable that, depending on their molecular weights (MW) and their conjugation with other polymers (such as polyethylene glycol, or PEG), these biodegradable polymers show different times of elimination from the body (Li *et al.*, 1999; Bazile *et al.*, 1992).

3.2.1.2 NP fate

When polymeric NPs are planned along with the choice of the polymers, it is pivotal to have strong knowledge of the fate of the NPs once administered in the body. In literature, there are a number of papers and reviews dealing with this aspect, which is determinant in understanding the potential and the limits of these systems.

The activation of defensive systems such as the reticulo-endothelial system (RES, mainly in the liver, spleen, and lung) is strictly connected with the surface characteristics of the NPs (charge, functional groups, etc.) and the system's geometry and size.

Considering the surface properties, NPs with a hydrophobic surface and negative charges promote protein adsorption and activate the complement system (Moghimi *et al.*, 2001).

Considering PLA/PLGA NPs, it has been shown that these NPs undergo a sudden removal when injected into the peripheral circulation (Bazile *et al.*, 1992; Von Burkersroda *et al.*, 1997; Stolnik *et al.*, 1994), with a blood half-life of around two–three minutes (Verrecchia *et al.*, 1995; Le Ray *et al.*, 1994; Li *et al.*, 2001). The same NP fate has been demonstrated for a variety of polymeric NPs, such as PBCA NPs (Beck *et al.*, 1997; Grislain *et al.*, 1983; Douglas *et al.*, 1986; Waser *et al.*, 1987; Simeonova *et al.*, 1988; Verdun *et al.*, 1990; Lobenberg *et al.*, 1998), that, lacking stealth properties when administered intravenously, are rapidly cleared from the bloodstream by the monuclear phagocyte system (MPS) and mainly accumulate in the liver and the spleen.

The final size of NPs is another important parameter that partially determines their biological fate upon administration (Moghimi *et al.*, 2001). Particles under 10 nm are rapidly removed after an extensive extravasation and renal clearance, whereas NPs of over 200 nm are rapidly filtrated by the spleen and removed by the RES cells. On the contrary, NPs with a size smaller than 100 nm have a lower possibility of being uptaken by macrophages or recognized by opsonins. On the other hand, a small diameter of the NP corresponds to a large relative surface area, which could promote their aggregation.

Once this first issue of CNS delivery — choosing and accurately preparing NPs — is addressed, it is important to remember that these systems, if not engineered, are totally unable to cross the BBB in its healthy state.

Thus, a further improvement in the drug delivery has been reached by using the so-called *targeted system technology*. This technology is well known, especially in the field of tumor-targeting, and its development is connected to the need to obtain increased specificity and selectivity in drug therapies.

Considering the brain as a protected artificial dam barrier, the role of NP surface engineering represents the milestone for a promising future application in *difficult-to-treat* brain pathologies.

Thus, NPs can be engineered with specific ligands or, more generally, substances able to increase their ability to cross the BBB by means of specific mechanisms, such as absorptive-mediated transcytosis or receptor-mediated endocytosis. Since specific receptors have been identified on the brain capillaries for Tf, insulin, and insulin-like growth factor (Tusij *et al.*, 2000, Brasnjevic *et al.*, 2009), attempts were made to link these ligands to the NP surface in order to realize a BBB targeting.

As reported below, there are several approaches (Tosi *et al.*, 2008) to be used for increasing drug delivery to the brain by applying NP surface modifications:

- *Magnetic-NP approach* (based on magnetic fields that drive the nanocarriers to the target site) (Pankhurst *et al.*, 2003; Alexiou *et al.*, 2000; Mornet *et al.*, 2006; Ito *et al.*, 2005; Lübbe *et al.*, 1996; Kopelman *et al.*, 2005; Chertok *et al.*, 2008; Hassan *et al.*, 1993; Pulfer *et al.*, 1998; Pulfer *et al.*, 1999; Yellen *et al.*, 2005)

- *Surface charge–based approach* (based on the adsorptive-mediated transcytosis of surface-charged NPs) (Koziara *et al.*, 2003; Lockman *et al.*, 2003a; Lockman *et al.*, 2003b; Koziara *et al.*, 2004)
- *Surfactant-based approach* (based on surfactant-coated or surfactant-linked NPs) (Tröester *et al.*, 1992; Kreuter *et al.*, 1997; Alyautdin *et al.*, 1997; Ambruosi *et al.*, 2003; Ambruosi *et al.*, 2006; Steiniger *et al.*, 2004; Friese *et al.*, 2000; Kreuter *et al.*, 1995; Calvo *et al.*, 2001; Kreuter, 2001; Kreuter *et al.*, 2002b; Gessner *et al.*, 2001; Anderberg, 1992; Nerurkar *et al.*, 1997; Yamazaki *et al.*, 2000; Woodcock, 1992; Raub, 1992; Olivier *et al.*, 1999; Kreuter *et al.*, 2003; Sun *et al.*, 2004)
- *PEG-approach* (based polyethylene glycols–conjugated long-circulating NPs) (Harris *et al.*, 2003; Torchilin, 1998; Gref *et al.*, 1995; Stolink *et al.*, 2001; Moghimi *et al.*, 2003; Gref *et al.*, 2000; Calvo *et al.*, 2001a; Brigger *et al.*, 2002; Garcia-Garcia *et al.*, 2005a; Garcia-Garcia *et al.*, 2005b; Kim *et al.*, 2007a; Kim *et al.*, 2007b; Kim *et al.*, 2007c; Dams *et al.*, 2000; Laverman *et al.*, 2001a; Laverman *et al.*, 2001b; Ishida *et al.*, 2002; Ishida *et al.*, 2003a; Ishida *et al.*, 2003b; Ishida *et al.*, 2004; Ishida *et al.*, 2005; Ishida *et al.*, 2006a; Ishida *et al.*, 2006b)
- *Ligand-based approach* (based on the conjugation of NPs with specific ligands able to increase or promote BBB crossing)

Considering the surface charge–based approach as an example, interesting studies have been carried out using PEG-PLA NPs conjugated with cationic bovine serum albumin (CBSA) (Lu *et al.*, 2005), showing some NP amount in the brain coming from *in vitro* and *in vivo* experiments. These studies were also confirmed by using a plasmid (pORF-hTRAIL) localized in both brain and tumor microvasculature and with a decreased tumor growth after repeated treatments.

Considering the PEG approach, *in vivo* studies (Calvo *et al.*, 2001b) on pegylated ^{14}C-PHDCA NPs described an enhanced penetration into the brain, demonstrating the ability of NPs to cross the BBB owing to their long-circulating characteristics. Another confirmation of this approach has been assessed by the accumulation of these NPs into the brain after *in vivo* studies on rats infected by allergic encephalomyelitis (Calvo *et al.*, 2002) and on rats bearing a gliosarcoma (Brigger *et al.*, 2002).

In order to increase the selectivity for brain targeting by colloidal systems, the ligand-based strategy is one of the most interesting and promising approaches. Its rationale of use is based on the presence of specific receptors on brain capillaries, such as receptors for insulin, insulin-like growth factors, angiotensin II, atrial natriuretic peptide, brain natriuretic peptide, interleukin 1, and Tf; thus these molecules, related peptides, or Abs, could be conjugated with the particles in order to access the brain parenchyma via receptor-mediated transport systems (Bickel *et al.*, 2001). Following the interaction with the receptor, the ligands are internalized by means of receptor-mediated endocytosis or transcytosis (see section 3.3 of this chapter, "Rationale of a Ligand-Based Approach").

3.2.2 SLNPs

Recently, if an important step toward the evolution and application of polymeric NP in medicine has been reached with the evidence of a number of advantages (drug delivery and drug targeting, accessibility to difficult-to-reach sites of action, etc.), a number of critical issues related to this approach have also been shown. Possible residual contamination from the production process (organic solvents) polymerization initiation, large polymer aggregates, toxic monomers, or degradation products should be in fact strongly taken into account. The most important limits of polymeric NPs are represented by the possible toxicity, and, most of all, their stability over time.

In association with this technological problem, the uptake and deactivation of the NPs (meaning metabolism and degradation) by RES systems must be considered.

In this view, SLNPs (addressed by a number of researchers) represent a possibility in order to overcome these limits. These kinds of particles, consisting of spherical nanometric solid-lipid carriers, dispersed in water or in an aqueous surfactant solution, show generally a solid hydrophobic core, having a monolayer of phospholipid coating. Several authors corroborate the hypothesis of a number of advantages of SLNP use over polymeric NP use, such as the ideal decreased activation of RES system, controlled release over time (several weeks), stability in the formulation and feasibility of incorporating both hydrophilic and hydrophobic drugs, and finally the avoidance of toxic organic solvents during the preparation, leading to the possibility of obtaining easy and not-expensive scale-up procedures (Blasi *et al.*, 2007).

It is interesting to note that the same strategies of surface conjugation/engineering for specific targeting applied for polymeric NPs have been utilized for SLNPs and, in particular, the ligand-based approach.

One of the first studies on modified SLNPs for brain delivery has been developed by using stealth and nonstealth SLNPs of doxorubicin using PEG 2000 at various concentrations (Zara *et al.*, 2002), administered intravenously, increasing transport across the BBB tenfold. Other researchers applied the surfactant-based approach (polysorbate coating) to SLNP carriers (Goppert *et al.*, 2005), stabilizing the SLNPs and confirming the adsorption of apolipoprotein (Apo) C1 and Apo CII, thus inhibiting the receptor-mediated binding of Apo E to low-density lipoprotein (LDL) receptors after oral administration.

Another example of SLNPs for brain delivery could be recognized in the Poloxamer 188–stabilized stearic acid camptothecin-loaded SLNP targeted to the brain after both oral and IV administration in mice (Yang *et al.*, 1999a; Yang *et al.*, 1999b).

Positively and negatively charged tripalmitin SLNPs were loaded with labeled etoposide, and their organ biodistribution was compared to that of free-labeled drugs in mice after IV administration. Positively charged SLNPs showed higher brain accumulation compared with both negatively charged SLNPs and free-labeled drugs. The etoposide concentration, achieved using positively charged SLNPs, was more than tenfold higher with respect to the negatively charged SLNPs. Even though the overall concentration was not as high, some preferential BBB uptake could be hypothesized (Reddy *et al.*, 2004).

Finally, Peira and colleagues proposed a BBB-diagnostic application of SLNPs by using superparamagnetic iron oxide–loaded SLNPs as a new type of nuclear magnetic resonance contrast agent (Peira *et al.*, 2003). After IV injection in rats, SLNPs were able to cross the BBB and accumulate in the brain parenchyma.

One of the most recent examples of SLNP-mediated delivery to the brain is represented by the application of ligands (such as Abs) to

SLNPs, thus creating immunonanosystems (Beduneau *et al.*, 2008), confirmed to be effective in increasing brain delivery or brain cell adhesion.

The field of pharmaceutical technology dealing with SLNPs is certainly new, and it needs, as happened in the past for NPs and LPs, to be much more developed, with greater understanding of the real potential of SLNPs in CNS drug delivery but more generally in nanomedicine.

If it is true that SLNPs represent a "middle course" between polymeric NPs and LPs, with great advantages in formulative and technological aspect, it is true that the body's response to these new kinds of nanosystems must be comprehensively investigated in the near future.

3.2.3 LPs

LPs are the most studied and old *smart* systems, applied in different field of medicine research, representing the first innovative approach for the treatment of challenging pathologies, like cancer, HIV, strokes, and many other diseases that require selective therapies.

As described for NPs, LPs need a surface modification in order to promote specific delivery and targeting of the embedded drugs.

Generally speaking, it is surprising that good *in vitro* results do not reflect *in vivo* confirmations, leading to a very low applicability of the LP approach in the treatment protocols. Some problems connected with *in vivo* delivery (very quick elimination and degradation when injected into the bloodstream, along with the type and properties of phospholipids that are constituents of the LPs) have been addressed using different strategies such as using stabilizers or modification of preparation procedures.

Particularly, conjugation with molecules able to protect the LPs from degradation (GM1, poloamine, polaxamer, and PEG) or able to induce an increased affinity to the diseased cells represented one of the most applied strategies. In fact, the principal objectives of surface conjugation are similar to those illustrated for NPs — stealth property, biostability, and specificity improvements.

The pegylation technology offers a potential resolution to the problem of LPs' biostability, connected to the liposomal intravenous administration.

In fact, pegylation prevents binding with opsonins and, therefore, prevents recognition by phagocytic cells, strongly influencing the pharmacokinetics and distribution parameters. In the case of a simple pegylation, a passive targeting, facilitated by the environment of the solid-state tumor, is the only possible mechanism. On the contrary, in order to increase the minimal affinity to the diseased cells and to avoid the toxic effect on nondiseased tissues, an active targeting due to functionalization of the surface of the LP is hardly needed.

In fact, different coupling strategies could be applied, all of them with the scope of attaching proteins to phospholipids or PEG-phospholipids in order to preserve biological functionality.

Among the different coupling strategies, covalent coupling represents one of the best choices as it is based on the conjugation of molecules to the phospholipid headgroups on the LP surface, by making use of amide or disulfide bonds.

As previously shown, it is also possible to use pegylated lipids to prepare LPs and to modify their biodistribution and pharmacokinetics. In this case, it is important to remember that the most important limitation is the shielding effect of PEG chains to the attached molecules, preventing interaction between ligands and receptors. To overcome this restriction, the coupling procedure could be applied by utilizing the terminus of the PEG chains, making the PEG a spacer and giving to the conjugation architecture more flexibility and, therefore, accessibility. A particular consideration has to be done when coupling proteins to pegylated phospholipids; in reality, the first choice has to be evaluated in relation with the will of obtaining a cleavable or stable bond, respectively represented by a disulfide bond and a thioether, amide, or imide bond. The following choices must consider the coupling efficiency, the maintenance of the antigenicity, and a possible control of the orientation of the Ab fragments, which relates with the accessibility to the receptors.

Several LP-based approaches were proposed to improve the systemic delivery of active agents to the brain. Naoi and Yagi used LPs composed of phospatidilcholine (PC), cholesterol (CHOL) and sulphatides to deliver enzymes (glucose oxidase, horseradish peroxidise) across the BBB into the rat brain tissue (Naoi *et al.*, 1980) as evidenced by the presence of peroxidase in brain cells, proved by histochemical analysis (Yagi *et al.*, 1982).

Conventional LPs prepared using egg yolk PC, CHOL, and dipalmitoylphosphatidic acid (DPPA) were found to successfully deliver 9-amino-1,2,3,4-tetrahydroacridine (THA), although the accumulation of THA in the spleen and kidney was observed (Kobayashi *et al.*, 1996).

To treat malignant glioma patients, Kakinuma and coworkers, along with Aoki and coworkers, proposed a targeting chemotherapy using local hyperthermia and thermosensitive LPs. It was found that drugs concentrations in the tumors were significantly higher following treatment with liposomal drugs than with free drugs; this finding demonstrated that thermosensitive LPs, releasing their contents in response to mild hyperthermia, have a greater therapeutic efficacy for malignant brain tumors (Kakinuma *et al.*, 1996; Aoki *et al.*, 2004).

The use of conventional and pegylated LPs to accumulate drugs in brain when the BBB is compromised was evaluated in a number of publications. LPs prepared with natural phospholipids and cholesterol more efficiently delivered the entrapped adenosine-3′-5′-cyclic monophosphate to the mouse brain after disruption of the BBB with iperosmolar mannitol (Gomes *et al.*, 2004). Conventional and PEG-LPs were also used to deliver glucocorticosteroids to the inflamed CNS in experimental autoimmune encephalomyelitis (EAE) (Schmidt *et al.*, 2003; Linker *et al.*, 2008). Probably, the mechanism of brain accumulation in disease may involve enhanced permeability and retention effect (EPR) of LPs at sites of pathology-induced compromised BBB.

As previously introduced, it is remarkable that, notwithstanding the fact that the application of Ab-mediated delivery of nanocarriers results in a specificity of action when applied to brain tumor, this approach must be intended as tumor delivery and not as brain delivery.

Another important approach hypothesized that negatively charged LPs enter efficaciously the brain of animals via the activation of monocytes as the transport mechanism. Afergan and colleagues, studying the uptake in monocytes and neutrophils *in vitro* and *in vivo* (rabbits and rats), demonstrated that large conventional LPs encapsulating serotonin are phagocyted by these immune system cells, prolonging the circulation time of LPs and promoting the drug brain uptake (Afergan *et al.*, 2008).

3.3 Rationale of the Ligand-Based Approach

The ligand-based approach has become an interesting choice for a more specific and selective drug delivery to the CNS district. This approach is based on the covalent linkage of ligands to the polymers/lipids or to the nanosystems in order to promote direct interaction with transport systems (Vyas *et al.*, 2001; Newton, 2006).

The ligands that could be used in CNS drug delivery have to be chosen with appropriate characteristics in order to take advantage or receptor-mediated trancytosis or receptor-mediated endocytosis. Possible ligands could be natural substrates or targeting moieties (such as Tf, insulin, and thiamine) but also synthetic or natural peptides and Abs.

3.3.1 Natural Substrates and Targeting Moieties as Ligands

Several examples of engineered NP with ligands have been proved to be efficacious drug delivery systems, able to enter the brain and carry a suitable drug (not generally able to cross the BBB) into the cerebral parenchyma.

To better understand the rationale of this approach, it is important to consider that these applications of peptides able to mediate drug delivery to the brain are also known as "chimeric peptide technology." This approach is based on the observation that peptide receptors are present on the brain capillary endothelium and that some of them mediate the transcytosis of the circulating peptide through the BBB.

A chimeric peptide is formed when a nontransportable drug is conjugated to a brain drug delivery vector. The latter may be an endogenous peptide, a modified protein, or a peptidomimetic monoclonal antibody (MAb) that undergoes *in vivo* receptor-mediated or absorptive-mediated transcytosis through the BBB on one of the endogenous transport systems. This approach has been used to deliver both neurodiagnostic (Wu *et al.*, 1997; Kurihara *et al.*, 1999) and neurotherapeutic molecules (Wu *et al.*, 1996; Wu *et al.*, 1999) across the rodent or primate BBB.

As another example, a new strategy for NP brain targeting by using PLGA derivatized with peptides (Tosi *et al.*, 2007; Costantino *et al.*, 2005) was recently demonstrated to be efficacious. In fact, some categories of opioid peptides have been shown to penetrate the BBB (Egleton *et al.*, 2005) and they have demonstrated the ability to cross the BBB to a higher extent when glycosilated (Polt, 2005; Polt *et al.*, 1994; Kihlberg *et al.*, 1995; Negri *et al.*, 1998; Dhanasekaran *et al.*, 2005).

Starting from an opioid peptide able to enter the brain via the biousian mechanism (Polt *et al.*, 2001), a newly simil-opioid peptide was synthetized, glycosylated, and conjugated to the PLGA polymer in order to obtain, by means of a nanoprecipitation procedure, engineered NPs able to enter the brain (Costantino *et al.*, 2005; Costantino *et al.*, 2006). These NPs, showing on the surface the ligands for CNS targeting (Tosi *et al.*, 2007), were loaded with loperamide, an opioid not able to cross the BBB, and administered through rat tail vein. The evidence of loperamide delivery in the brain was achieved by the hotplate test (nociception assay), with the recognition of a high antinociceptive activity four hours after IV administration, with the analgesic effect lasting over eight hours.

More recent studies (Vergoni *et al.*, 2009) demonstrated the effectiveness of this carrier for brain targeting, comparing the effect of the administration of loperamide-loaded NP with the effect of an intracerebroventricular administration of the drug (with at least 13% of the injected dose active in the CNS).

Moreover, the biodistribution of these NPs showed localization into the CNS in a quantity about two orders of magnitude (at least 15% of the injected dose) greater than that found with the other known NP drug carriers.

Another approach has been developed recently by Hu and colleagues with the preparation of lactoferrin (Lf)-conjugated PEG-PLA NPs as potential brain delivery vectors (Hu *et al.*, 2009).

Lf receptors have in fact been proved to exist on BBB and involved in Lf transport across the BBB *in vitro* and *in vivo*. In order to assess Lf presence on Lf-NP surface, a Lf-ELISA has been performed, suggesting an average number of 55 Lf molecules conjugated on each NP.

To evaluate the brain delivery properties of the Lf-NP, a fluorescent probe, coumarin-6, has been encapsulated and its uptake evaluated *in vitro* through a mouse brain endothelial line (bEnd-3), demonstrating fluorescence values at 1 h after incubation threefold higher with respect to fluorescent NP without any surface modification.

Furthermore, coumarin-6-loaded Lf-NP have been intravenously administrated *in vivo* to mice, pointing out about a threefold increase of dye accumulation within brain tissues carried by Lf-NP compared to that granted by unmodified NPs, thus suggesting Lf-NP as a new promising brain drug delivery system.

Another interesting ligand family conjugated with NP is the Apo proteins: in this case, the colloidal carriers functionalized with Apos mimic lipoprotein particles. These NPs were recognized by receptors on the brain endothelial cells of the BBB and act as Trojan horses. In reality, Apos A1 and E are the principal cholesterol-carrying molecules in the brain (Dietschy *et al.*, 2001; Yamauchi *et al.*, 1999); in fact, Apo E plays an important role in the brain transport of lipoproteins, which bind to and are internalized by the LDL-receptor and the LDL-receptor-related protein. The LDL-receptor is specifically upregulated on the surface of the endothelium that forms the BBB (Dehouck *et al.*, 1997).

HSA-NPs covalently linked to Apo E were able to deliver to the brain the drug loperamide (Michaelis *et al.*, 2006); the same effect was obtained with HSA NPs covalently linked to Apo A-I and B100 (Kreuter *et al.*, 2007): in this case, the delivery to brain can be mediated by the interaction with the scavenger receptor class B type I (SR-BI) expressed by the brain vessels' endothelial cells.

The same effect is also shared by functionalized LPs (Sauer *et al.*, 2005); the highly cationic tandem dimer of Apo E residues was coupled covalently onto PEG-derivatized LPs, and the membrane binding and cellular uptake was monitored qualitatively by confocal-laser-scanning microscopy as well as quantitatively using a fluorescence assay. The results demonstrated that the peptide mediated an efficient, energy-dependent translocation of LPs across the membrane of brain capillary endothelial cells.

In another work, Apo E peptide properties were confirmed to be relevant for peptide-LP complexes to initiate an endocytotic cellular uptake. In fact, efficient internalization of LPs bearing about 180 peptide derivatives on the surface into brain capillary endothelial cells was monitored by confocal laser scanning microscopy (Sauer *et al.*, 2006).

Moreover, considering the affinity for the GLUT1, the nutrient transporter that promotes the passage of glucose from the blood to the brain through the BBB, mannose-LPs (prepared incorporating mannose derivatives on the surface of LPs) seem to be able to cross the BBB, but only using a mouse model (Umezawa *et al.*, 1988). In fact, rat brain accumulation was not enhanced compared with conventional formulation (Mora *et al.*, 2002).

More recently, Madhankumar and coworkers proposed interleukin 13 (IL-13)-conjugated LPs as drug carriers in brain tumors (Madhankumar *et al.*, 2009). The receptors for interleukin 13 is a tumor-specific receptor overexpressed in glioblastoma multiform (Husain *et al.*, 2003) and consequently the IL-13 is attractive as a targeting moiety for LPs. This study demonstrated the potential therapeutic efficacy of IL-13-targeted LPs to deliver doxorubicin to a subcutaneous glioma tumor model in mice.

Several studies have been performed also using ligands such as arginine-glycine-aspartic acid (RGD) and RMP-7 for the brain delivery of LPs: for example, RMP-7, a ligand to the B2 receptor on brain microvascular endothelial cells (BMVEC), known to be able to increase the permeability of the BBB tumor barrier, was combined with 1,2-dioleoyl-sn-glycero-3-phosphoethanolamine-n-[poly(ethylenegly-col)]-hydroxy succinimide (DSPE-PEG-NHS) to obtain DSPE-PEG-RMP-7.

The DSPE-PEG-RMP-7 incorporated into the LP surface targeted sterically stabilized LPs (SSL-T) to the brain, and at the same time, a reduction of toxicity brought by RMP-7's BBB opening has been also observed. This approach was used to transport the exogenous nerve growth factor as a possible drug for treating Alzheimer's disease (Xie *et al.*, 2005) and amphotericine for serious inflammation (Zhang *et al.*, 2003). In another study, Jain and coworkers (Jain *et al.*, 2003) optimized the condition for the preparation of magnetic LPs in order to develop an effective biophysically modulated cellular-mediated coordinated targeting strategy. To this end, RGD peptide was covalently coupled to negatively charged LPs composed of phospatidylcoline, cholesterol, phosphatidylserine, and phosphatidylethanolamine. These targeted systems were used to transport the anti-inflammatory drug to the brain under inflammatory condition.

In fact, RGD selectively binds the integrin receptors expressing on the surface of monocytes and neutrophils, optimizing the cell uptake of drug. These cells rapidly migrate to inflammatory sites under the guidance of the external magnetic field, thus targeting the active substance to any poorly accessible inflammatory site, that is, the brain. Moreover, the data obtained after the *in vivo* administration of magnetic-RGD-coated LPs suggested that the liver uptake was significantly bypassed and high brain levels of drug were quantified.

Several approaches have been investigated by both *in vivo* and *in vitro* experiments by using natural substrates of brain endothelial cell receptors or overexpressed in diseased brain parenchyma as targeting moieties, such as folic acid or Tf, and they will be reviewed in the next chapters.

Considering the attempt for SLNP application, the ligand-based approach has been applied mainly using Brje 78, emulsifying wax, and thiamine ligand (Th).

In the very first studies, the authors tested labeled Th-coated SLNPs to evaluate *in vivo* brain uptake after an "*in situ* brain perfusion" in comparison with blank SLNPs (Lockman *et al.*, 2003), with results describing a nonlinear, delayed brain uptake after 45 seconds. Prolonging the time up to 120 seconds, the brain uptake was linear for both coated and uncoated SLNPs with a transfer rate for Th-coated SLNPs greater than the control. The administration of free Th produced the inhibition of the uptake of Th-coated SLNPs, suggesting that Th-coating of SLNPs can be a successful technology to enhance brain delivery of SLNPs due to a specific mediated transport across the BBB.

Another work based on this kind of SLNP loaded with paclitaxel demonstrated that the entrapment of paclitaxel in SLNPs significantly increased the drug brain uptake and its toxicity toward P-gp-expressing tumor cells. It was hypothesized that this SLNP could mask paclitaxel characteristics, limiting its binding to P-gp, leading to higher brain and tumor cell uptake of the otherwise effluxed drug (Koziara *et al.*, 2004). A further improvement of this approach with Th is still going on, confirmed by a preclinical study performed in the United States (Muthu *et al.*, 2009).

3.3.2 Ligand-Based Approach and Immunonanosystems

Among the possible ligands utilized to actively direct the nanosystems against a diseased tissue or cell population, the use of polyclonal or monoclonal Ab represents an interesting and efficacious approach due to the high selectivity of the recognition reaction with the proper Ag. In fact, this approach has been applied in the targeting aim on several pathologies (Wang *et al.*, 2008; Dimitrov *et al.*, 2008) such as cancer (Cho *et al.*, 2008).

The high selectivity of the nanovectors engineered with Ab is the most important feature of the immune-mediated drug delivery. Nonetheless, some important characteristics of both carriers and pathologies have to be strongly considered.

Regarding the pathology and choice of the Ab, it is essential that the pathology (or the diseased cells) possess a distinctive Ag pattern; those pathologies characterized by cells with a unique (or at least overexpressed) pattern of Ags are optimal candidates for drug delivery via Ab-mediated reaction.

On the contrary, those diseases expressing a low level of specific Ags or not exposing any signal of the disease are really not targetable. Moreover, it is important to study in depth the reactivity of the chosen Ab, and, if possible, it is better to work with monoclonal Ab, recognizing only a determinate and specific stadium of the target pathology.

Regarding the carriers, their stability and the possibility of avoiding the macrophage attack are essential properties. This fact could seem obvious, but, considering the wide literature dealing with "stealth" carriers (Moghimi *et al.*, 2001), it clearly appears that a shield of hydrophilic substances (e.g., PEG) is needed to obtain long-circulating systems. This shield obviously creates a sort of coverage of the surface of the carriers, and thus the possible recognition of Ab-Ag could be decreased or radically impeded.

This approach, which could be called *immune-nanomedicine*, when applied to brain pathology is based on the conjugation of the carriers with antibodies, able to bind to the brain microvessels and to make use of the transcytosis mechanism for passage through the BBB (Miller *et al.*, 1994; Shin *et al.*, 1995; Banks *et al.*, 1997, Fig. 3.1).

If considering this kind of transport, some features and obliged actions have to be underlined as well as planned accurately before the experiments. It is pivotal, in fact, to remember that this process requires a specific interaction of the Ab (or a portion of it) with moieties expressed at the luminal surface of endothelial cells, which triggers internalization of the Ab-conjugate (drug, polymer, or nanodevices) into endocytic vesicles as well as their movement through the endothelial cytoplasm and exocytosis at the abluminal side.

Once the correct Ag to be targeted is recognized, it is also important to consider the unicity of the Ag pattern, which means a unique possibility to achieve transport across the BBB, avoiding possible different body/tissue/organ distribution of the Ab-conjugate.

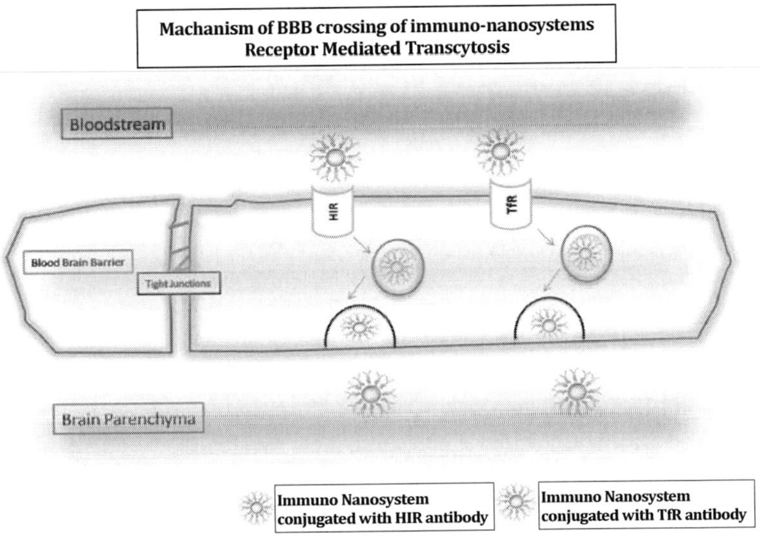

Figure 3.1 The mechanism of the entrance of immunonanosystems. Examples of HIR-Ab- and TfR-modified nanosystems. See also Color Insert.

As previously evidenced, the "chimeric peptide technology" was applied by using a peptidomimetic MAb that undergoes receptor-mediated or absorptive-mediated transcytosis through the BBB *in vivo* as a brain drug delivery vector. Thus, in order to make this approach useful for BBB drug targeting in humans, the peptidomimetic MAb transport vector should be genetically engineered to remove the immunodominant murine sequences that would produce immune reactions in humans. Human/mouse chimeric MAbs are genetically engineered Abs wherein approximately 85% of the sequence is human and 15% is murine.

In fact, more recently (Boado *et al.*, 2009), Pardridge and colleagues have investigated the possibility of delivering protein therapeutics across the BBB by genetic fusion to a BBB molecular Trojan horse, which is an endogenous peptide or a peptidomimetic MAb against a BBB receptor, such as the human insulin receptor (HIR) or the transferrin receptor (TfR).

Fusion proteins have been engineered with the MAb against the HIR and, in particular, the cloning and sequencing of the variable region of the heavy chain (VH) and light chain (VL) of the rat 8D3 TfRMAb were analyzed in order to produce a new chimeric TfRMAb. The affinity of the chimeric TfRMAb for the murine TfR was found to be equal to the 8D3 MAb using a radio-receptor assay and mouse fibroblasts and when the radiolabeled chimeric TfRMAb was injected into mice for a pharmacokinetics study of the clearance of the chimeric TfRMAb, a sudden uptake of the chimeric TfRMAb at a level comparable to the rat 8D3 MAb was demonstrated.

3.4 Abs Used in Brain Targeting

3.4.1 TfR

Tf is an Fe-binding protein, and its receptor (TfR) is heterogeneously distributed into the brain (de Boer *et al.*, 2003).

The unusually high expression of TfRs on the surface of the normal BBB provides a potential advantage for the delivery of drugs into the brain. In fact, various therapeutic agents have been chemically linked to Tf in order to deliver it to brain (Quian *et al.*, 2002) with Tf mediating the transport of iron to the brain by means of its interaction with TfR (Jefferies *et al.*, 1984). Moreover, TfR undergoes receptor-mediated trancytosis and it is highly expressed by brain capillaries (Pardridge *et al.*, 1987).

It should however be remembered that Tf itself is limited as a brain drug transport vector since the TfRs are almost saturated under physiological conditions due to the high endogenous plasma concentration of Tf.

In fact, the use of Tf itself as a drug delivery vector is also prevented by the large concentration of Tf in the plasma, which is about 25 μM, a level that is 3 log orders of magnitude in excess of the dissociation constant (KD) governing the BBB Tf receptor (Tf-R)/Tf binding reaction (Pardridge, 1995a).

Tf-coupled LPs were used to enhance the delivery of 5-fluorouracil to the brain (Soni *et al.*, 2005; Soni *et al.*, 2008).

Significantly increased gliomal doxorubicin uptake was achieved by drug encapsulation within Tf-coupled LPs compared to encapsulation within noncoupled LPs (Eavarone *et al.*, 2000). Tf-coupled LPs encapsulating horseradish peroxidase (HRP) were found to be able to translocate across the BBB in *in vitro* experiments (Visser *et al.*, 2005) (brain capillary endothelial cells culture, BCEC).

Another study (Mishra *et al.*, 2006), in which the Tf ligand-based approach has been applied, concerns engineered pegylated albumin NPs encapsulating azidothymidine (AZT), a water-soluble antiviral drug. The surface of these NPs was modified by anchoring Tf, and *in vivo* studies (fluorescence microscopy) demonstrated an enhancement in NP accumulation within the brain tissues.

This approach was also applied to NanoGel (Vinogradov *et al.*, 2004). In order to target the NanoGel to the CNS district, the use the PEG technology coupled with the avidin-biotin method has been applied for the attachment of Tf or insulin. In particular, the biotin-modified NanoGel was loaded with oligonucleotides (ODN) and the formed ODN-loaded biotin-NanoGel complex was reacted with the preformed complex of avidin and biotinylated Tf or insulin. This study was built on *in vitro* experiments on bovine brain microvessel endothelial cells (BBMEC) and *in vivo* tests on mice. The mechanisms of Rhodamine-labeled NanoGel's transport in endothelial cells, the toxicity of NanoGel and ^{3}H-NanoGel, and ^{3}H-ODN biodistribution in different organs (including the brain) have been investigated. The *in vitro* and *in vivo* results suggested that insulin- or Tf-modificated NanoGels were non-toxic. Furthermore, the permeability increased twelvefold compared to free ODNs; thus, NanoGel carriers can protect ODNs from rapid clearance by peripheral tissues and increase ODN transport to the brain.

3.4.1.1 OX26 Ab to TfR

If it clearly appears that the use of Tf as a ligand is hampered by endogenous competition, the Abs that bind to the TfR have been shown to selectively target the BBB endothelium due to the high levels of TfR expressed by these cells (Quian *et al.*, 2002).

One of the best studied and applied ligands for CNS drug delivery is the Ab OX26, a monoclonal Ab to the rat TfR (Friden *et al.*, 1991). In fact, it was found that there was no *in vivo* competition of the colloidal carriers with endogenous Tf (Huwlyer *et al.*, 1996), demonstrating that OX26 recognized a binding site different from the natural ligand Tf (Huwlyer *et al.*, 1997; Pardridge, 1995a).

The mechanism by which OX26 gains access to the CNS remains unresolved. In liver cells, the internalization of OX26 is thought to follow the generally accepted mechanism for the uptake of iron-containing Tf, which involves receptor-mediated endocytosis and transport to the endosomal compartment (Trinder *et al.*, 1988; Wu *et al.*, 1998). In terms of uptake of iron–Tf by bovine endothelial cells (BCECs), quantitative studies performed on the transport of iron–Tf strongly indicate that this is the principal mechanism for the uptake of iron–Tf at the BBB.

However, the fractional appearance of iron transported into the brain is much higher than that of Tf, which implies that only the iron is transported into the brain parenchyma, whereas most of the Tf recycles to the plasma (Taylor *et al.*, 1991; Morris, 1992; Ueda *et al.*, 1993). Nonetheless, it is claimed that the immunoglobulin OX26 undergoes receptor-mediated transcytosis through the BBB, resulting in a higher transport than is achieved with nonimmune immunoglobulins (Friden *et al.*, 1991; Pardridge *et al.*, 1991; Lee *et al.*, 2000). There is also emerging evidence for iron transport across the blood-cerebrospinal fluid barriers (Lee *et al.*, 2000), which makes it possible that the transport of OX26 through the choroid plexuses may account for OX26 in the brain.

3.4.1.2 8D3 MAb and R17-217 to TfR

8D3 MAb and R17-217 are another monoclonal Ab to the mouse TfR, active as BBB transport vector in mice and rats.

In fact, a study based on a comparison between OX26 and other two rat monoclonal Abs, 8D3 and RI7-217, showing comparable permeability-surface area products at the mouse BBB *in vivo* demonstrated that the mouse brain uptake of the 8D3 Ab was higher when compared with the brain uptake of the RI7 Ab. Moreover, the mouse brain uptake of the OX26 Ab, which does not recognize the mouse TF-R, was negligible. The brain uptake of the 8D3 Ab was saturable, consistent with a receptor-mediated transport process (Lee *et al.*, 2000).

3.4.2 Insulin

Over the past few years, it has become clear that insulin has also profound effects in the CNS, where it regulates key processes such as energy homeostasis, reproductive endocrinology, and neuronal survival. The actions of insulin are mediated via the INS-R, which belongs to the family of tyrosine kinase receptors and consists of two α-subunits and two β-subunits forming an α2β2 heterotetramer.

Binding by insulin leads to rapid autophosphorylation of the receptor, followed by the tyrosine phosphorylation of INS-R substrate (INS-R-S) proteins, which induce the activation of downstream pathways such as the PI3K and the mitogen-activated protein kinase (MAPK) cascades (White, 2003). The conformation change takes place, allowing tyrosine kinase activity and subsequent receptor internalization (Ullrich *et al.*, 1985).

An INS-R like the TfR is found on the luminal membrane of brain capillary endothelial cells (Havrankova *et al.*, 1981; Smith *et al.*, 2006) and it can undergo receptor-mediated transcytosis across the BBB endothelium (Duffy *et al.*, 1987).

Insulin is not produced in the brain, but it is present in the brain and arises from the blood via transport across the BBB in the endothelial INS-R. (Duffy *et al.*, 1987). The major limitation in this approach is the fact that the use of insulin, per se, as a vector would be problematical because the administration of the drug/insulin conjugate would cause hypoglycemia owing to the activation of INS-R in peripheral tissues.

As evidenced before in the chapter on Tf-R, considering NanoGel, the attachment of insulin to the NanoGel produced an increase in the ODN transport to the brain (Vinogradov *et al.*, 2004)

3.4.2.1 83-14 MAb to HINS-R

83-14 MAb is the murine monoclonal Ab to the HINS-R (HINS-R-MAb). The HINS-R is expressed at both the BBB interface with human brain gliomas and at the plasma membrane of human glioma cells.

83-14 murine MAb is a 150 kDa insulin peptidomimetic MAb that binds an exofacial epitope of the α-subunit of the HINS-R (Prignet *et al.*, 1990). This MAb generally undergoes receptor-mediated transcytosis through the BBB *in vivo* in Old World primates such as the rhesus monkey, but not New World primates such as the squirrel monkey (Pardridge *et al.*, 1995b). This observation is consistent with the greater genetic similarity between humans and Old World primates compared with New World primates (Swindler *et al.*, 1986). The 83-14 HIR MAb has a very high affinity for the human or Old World primate INS-R and is both an endocytosing Ab in isolated human brain capillaries and a BBB-transcytosing Ab in anesthetized rhesus monkeys.

The 83-14 MAb to the HINS-R is the most potent brain drug delivery vector known to date and has a BBB permeability-surface area product in the primate that is ninefold greater than murine MAbs to the human TfR (Wu *et al.*, 1997).

For this reason, in gene targeting in humans, the HIR MAb is preferred over the TfRMAb. Firstly, OX26 MAb (targeting rat TfR) and 8D3 Ab (targeting mouse TfR) are generally active in mice and rats but not in humans and primates.

Then, it was proved that the MAb directed at the HINS-R is transported across the primate BBB nearly ten times faster than the MAb directed at the human TfR (Pardridge, 2001).

3.4.3 Folic Acid

Folate receptors (FR) mediate via potocytosis the uptake of various serum folates (F), which serve as carbon donors for purine and thymidine synthesis. Distinct FR isoforms that exhibit greater than 70% homology have been identified in humans (FR-a, FR-b, and FR-g) and in mice (FR-a and FR-b) (Brigle *et al.*, 1991; Shen *et al.*, 1994).

The affinity of FRs for F is of the order of 1 nM KD. The exact role of the high affinity FR remains unclear. Interestingly, while FR is not necessary to meet the metabolic requirements of tumor cells *in vitro*, neoplastic cells transfected with FRs are capable of increased F acquisition and enhanced cell growth. Moreover, FRs are overexpressed in a large number of tumors, such as carcinoma and brain tumors (Weitman *et al.*, 1992).

The targeting of the FR has been shown considerably promising in mediating uptake of variety of drugs. Several experiments show that there is a significant difference in uptake by folate-targeted LPs between cells with overexpression and those with absence of expression of FR (Lee *et al.*, 1995; Wang *et al.*, 1995; Anderson *et al.*, 2001). In fact, folate-targeted drug delivery emerged as an alternative therapy for the treatment and imaging of many cancers and inflammatory diseases.

Due to the small molecular size and high binding affinity for cell surface FR, folate conjugates display the ability to deliver a variety of molecular complexes to pathologic cells without causing harm to normal tissues.

To date, complexes that have been successfully delivered to FR-expressing cells include protein, toxins, immune stimulants, chemotherapeutic agents, LPs, NPs, and imaging agents.

As another example, commercially available doxorubicin-loaded long-circulating LPs, modified with the monoclonal nucleosome (NS)-specific 2C5 antibody (MAb 2C5), which recognizes a broad variety of tumors via the tumor cell surface-bound NSs, have been tested *in vitro*, demonstrating the ability to kill various tumor cells *in vitro* with efficiency higher than nontargeted doxorubicin-loaded LPs (Lukyanov *et al.*, 2004).

It must be considered that folate-receptor-mediated delivery represents a huge chance to treat brain tumors, but it represents a delivery to the tumor and not real brain delivery of ligand-modified molecules or carriers. In fact, in the major percentage of brain tumors, the BBB is not able to preserve its integrity, facilitating the passage of molecules, macromolecules, and carriers.

As an example, LPs have been specifically delivered to FR-bearing cells via chemical conjugation to folic acid (Lee, 1995) and Saul and colleagues (Saul *et al.*, 2003) demonstrated that it is possible to target doxorubicin to the C6 rat glioma cells using folic acid–coupled LPs, minimizing nonspecific uptake in normal cells by means of optimization of the number of targeting ligand on the liposomal surface.

3.5 Immuno-NPs

3.5.1 TfR Abs (OX26, R17-217) as Ligands

One the most relevant works on the synthesis of NPs conjugated with Abs is the recent preparation of peglyated immunonanoparticles (Olivier *et al.*, 2002; Pardridge *et al.*, 2005), made by PEG-PLA and coupled with OX26 MAb; moreover, polymers different from PLA were also used.

For example, chitosan nanospheres conjugated with PEG-bearing OX26 monoclonal Ab were shown to enhance BBB transport (Aktaş *et al.*, 2005). After *in vivo* administration (mice), the authors established the presence of fluorescently labeled NP in the brain areas, outside the intravascular compartments. This technology was applied to the transport of a caspase inhibitor (peptide Z-DEVD-FMK), which is able to significantly reduce the death of the neuronal cell after an ischemic attack.

Another example of a semipolymeric NP conjugated to OX26 was based on PEG-polycaprolactone polymersomes (self-assembled vesicles of amphiphilic block copolymers with thicker and tougher membranes than lipids) (Pang *et al.*, 2008). In this case, a model peptide was incorporated into these particles (100 nm diameter) and its pharmacological activity assessed in rats: the peptide NC-1900 was able to improve scopolamine-induced learning and memory impairments via IV administration.

In a recent study (Ulbrich *et al.*, 2009), Kreuter and colleagues prepared human serum albumin (HSA) NPs by desolvation to which Tf or Tf-R monoclonal Abs (OX26 or R17217) were covalently coupled using the NHS-PEG-MAL-5000 cross-linker.

Loperamide was used as a model drug since it normally does not cross the BBB and it was bound to the NPs by adsorption. Loperamide-adsorbed HSA NPs with covalently bound Tf or the OX26 or R17217 Ab-induced significant antinociceptive effects in the tail-flick test mice after intravenous injection, demonstrating that Tf or these Ab covalently coupled to HSA NPs are able to transport loperamide and possibly other drugs across the BBB.

In this study, above the *in vivo* proof of brain delivery mediated by Tf or Ab action, a deep investigation into the measurement of unbound free Tf and free Ab was performed, showing a high percentage of the bound Tf or Ab to the NPs compared to the total ligand amount (from 45% to 90%), strongly dependent on time and excess of 2-iminothiolane used for the covalent conjugation.

3.5.2 INS-R Abs (83-14 MAb) as Ligands

In planning ligand-based approach, the use of insulin as an endogenous ligand is not suitable due to of its rapid degradation in the bloodstream (serum half-life of only 10 minutes) and the possible interference with the natural insulin balance (Bickel *et al.*, 1993). However, like the TfR, Abs recognizing the INS-R have been used as BBB-targeting vectors.

Extensive research using the 83–14 mouse MAb against the human INS-R as a receptor-mediated transport delivery vector has been performed, mainly in primates (rhesus monkey) (Pardridge *et al.*, 1995b).

Unfortunately, to date, no examples of polymeric NPs have been conjugated with 83-14 MAb.

3.6 Immuno-SLNPs

Considering SLN application to immune-nanomediated delivery to the CNS, one of the unique literature evidence is the work of Benoit and colleagues (Beduneau *et al.*, 2008). In fact, considering the relative novelty of the use of SLN for brain targeting, a deep study of the features of such novel carriers is strongly required.

3.6.1 TfR Ab (OX26) as Ligand

In this work, Benoit and colleagues prepared a novel generation of targeted SL nanocapsules and created very specialized systems by engineering these SLNPs with monoclonal Abs (OX26) to improve accumulation in the brain parenchyma (immunonanocapsules).

In a previous work, Benoit and colleagues deeply studied the chemical, physical, and morphological properties of these systems in order to obtain an engineered carrier able to target the brain. (Béduneau *et al.*, 2007).

Along with this modification, the authors were interested in evaluating the potential of Fab' fragments conjugated with SLNPs (to obtain Fab'-immunonanocapsules) in decreasing the uptake and recognition of immune-SLNs by RES systems (mechanism that appears to be connected to the Fc receptor) (Maruyama *et al.*, 1997).

In this work, both *in vitro* and *in vivo* studies were applied to understand the capability of adhesion of immuno-SLNPs to rat brain endothelial cells and SLNP biodistribution in healthy rats, respectively.

It is remarkable that these SLNPs have been prepared using Solutol ™HS15, a substance conferring to SLNP shell "stealth" properties but inhibiting the P-gp efflux pump (Buckingham *et al.*, 1995). It is clear that this property of SLNP composition would reflect in an inhibition of P-gp activity and, thus, in an increase in drug delivery efficacy of substance which undergo to P-gp efflux.

During SLNP preparation, the authors deeply studied the number of Abs linked by means of the postinsertion technique to the SLNP surface (30–40 molecules of whole OX26 or Fab' fragments) along with the encapsulation efficiency of radionucleotide ^{188}Re. The *in vitro* results based on flow cytometry analysis showed that immuno-SLNs with the whole OX26 created a much more effective cell association, confirmed by an increase in the fluorescence intensity with respect to the Fab' fragment conjugated to SLNPs. The authors hypothesized that the Fc portion of the Ab played the role of a spacer between the SLNP surface and the recognition site, promoting an improvement in cell adhesion.

After *in vivo* experiments, biodistribution studies on healthy rats showed a number of interesting results; in the blood, all kinds of SLNPs (OX26, Fab', unconjugated) were rapidly eliminated over three hours, with only less than 10% of the injected dose remaining in the bloodstream. Moreover, the longer circulation time of SLNPs conjugated with the Fab' fragments compared with whole OX26 was confirmed by an increased AUC considering the period of 0–24 hours.

Considering the liver uptake, a higher percentage of OX26-SLNP was recognized by macrophages and opsonins (60% after 30 minutes and 1 hour) compared with Fab' fragment-SLNP (40% considering the same experimental times).

It is interesting to note that SLN functionalized with the spacer but not bearing any Abs or fragments displayed a similar liver uptake level (45% after 30 minutes and 1 hour).

It is also surprising that, notwithstanding the presence of Solutol, described to be able to create a stealth surface of SLNP, all kinds of SLNPs were immediately recognized as non-self entities when injected into the bloodstream, thus allowing to reconsider the potential of Solutol as a stealth property–conferring molecule.

Considering the accumulation in the brain parenchyma after 30 minutes, OX26-SLNPs were found in a 0.05% of the injected dose (with a decrease to 0.02% after 24 hours), Fab' fragment-SLNP with 0.04% (with a decrease to 0.01% after 24 hours), and nonimmuno-SLNP with 0.02% (with a decrease to 0.01% after 24 hours).

It is clear that OX26 as the entire Ab, when conjugated to the surface of SLNPs, allows the obtainment of targeted systems, able to enter the brain to an increased extent, with respect to Fab' fragment–conjugated SLNPs and nonimmuno SLNPs. It is important to note that these values are not high enough to be considered as therapy, above all if considering the very high rate of elimination from the body, but it is remarkable the success of the application of Ab-surface engineering to SLNP.

3.7 Immuno-LP

There are several applications of LP technology to the CNS drug delivery, and the aim of this chapter is to underline the choices regarding the kind of ligands, the methodology of coupling, and the efficacy of the treatment with reliable *in vivo/in vitro* confirmation.

3.7.1 TfR Abs (OX26 and 8-D3) as Ligands

In one of the first evidence works on pegylated immunoliposomes as brain drug delivery vehicles, Huwlyer and colleagues (Huwlyer *et al.*, 1996), before encapsulating daunomycin, prepared LPs starting from distearoylphosphatidylcholine, cholesterol, and DSPE dissolved in chloroform/methanol. For the preparation of PEG-LPs and immunoliposomes, DSPE was substituted by DSPE-PEG. A lipid film was prepared by vacuum evaporation followed by hydration of the dried lipid films. Lipids were subjected to freeze-thaw cycles followed by extrusion through a 100-nm pore size polycarbonate membrane. Making use of maleimide linker, thiolated OX26 (by using Traut's reagent) was conjugated, obtaining stabilized immunoliposomes loaded with daunomycin. The results demonstrated important brain localization, and several evaluations concerning the saturation of receptors have been discussed.

Moreover, the optimal Ab density was investigated, suggesting that 30 Ab per LP was the best ratio and conjecturing that an increase of the ratio (plus that 30 Ab/LP) leads to an increase of steric stabilization of PEG and a poor targeting efficiency.

The coupling technology applied in this approach is based on the use of *neutral lipids*. The choice of using neutral lipids rather than cationic ones is based on the evidence that cationic lipids, producing unilamellar LPs of 80–100 nm, demonstrated rapid aggregation when in contact with different pH environments.

Besides, cationic LPs showed a preferential deposition in the lungs due to an aggregation and a deposit in the lung microvasculature after the pulmonary circulation. This localization, which renders the cationic LPs unable to perform brain targeting, could be due to their specific binding to heparin proteoglycans on the pulmonary endothelial surfaces. On the contrary, neutral pegylated lipids allow the obtainment of LPs with a prolonged plasma residence along with an ideal anchoring set, but, mostly, they do not accumulate in the lung.

Alternatively, Shi and Pardridge (Shi *et al.*, 2000) investigated noninvasive gene targeting to the brain, mixing anionic and neutral lipids such as 1-palymotyl-2-oleolyl-sn-glycerol-3-phosphocholine (POPC), DPSE-PEG_{2000}, and DSPE-PEG_{2000}-maleimide with a cationic lipid bromide (DDAB). Immuno-LPs were prepared dissolving the lipids in organic solvents, evaporated from the solvent, and dispersed in TRIS buffer. After sonication (10 minutes), the DNA (luciferase or B-galactosidase plasmids) was added and then the solution was evaporated to the final concentration. Then, freeze-thaw cycles and an extrusion filtration with polycarbonate membranes were applied to give homogenous size distribution population of LPs. The excess of plasmid and the plasmid adsorbed onto the LP were eliminated by using nuclease digestion. Then, the coupling procedure with the OX26 MAb via preliminar thiolation of the Ab with 2-imino-thiolane (Traut's reagent) was achieved by conjugating the thiolated groups with the maleimide moiety.

The efficacy of the brain targeting was confirmed evaluating Luciferase gene expression and β-galactosidase gene expression in the CNS district, after IV administration of the liposomal formulations into rats.

In another paper, Shi and Pardridge (Shi *et al.*, 2001a) investigated something through this technology to confirm gene delivery to the brain with an *in vivo* test. The experiments were carried out by using LPs in which 1% of the neutral LPs surface, showing PEG strands, were engineered with OX26 MAb, targeting the TfR.

The results clearly showed a prolonged (six days) widespread expression of β-galactosidase gene not only in the brain but also in liver and spleen parenchyma. The major concern regarding the off-target expressions of gene in the spleen and the liver is not to be ascribed to RES activation since it is well known that in the case of pegylated carriers, it is not relevant, confirmed by the lack of expression when a generic IgG was conjugated on behalf of OX26 MAb.

In this case, liver and spleen localization is due to the presence of Tf-Rs not only at the BBB level but also in the splenic and hepatic parenchyma, representing one of the most important limitations of the active specific targeting by using OX26 MAb as a ligand. (Schnyder *et al.*, 2005).

Biotinylated LPs created starting from cholesterol, DSPC, PEG-DSPE, and biotinylated PEG-DSPE were loaded with daunomycin using a pH gradient method. Biotin molecules at the distal end of PEG chains were noncovalently conjugated with OX26 MAb using a 1:1 molar ratio of biotinylated-PEG-DSPE:OX26-streptavidin-linked.

In vitro studies were performed on a multidrug-resistant cell line (RBE4) revealing an increased cellular uptake when daunomycin was loaded to immunoliposomes.

Pharmacokinetic parameters and tissues distribution of different liposomal formulations of daunomycin were determined in rat after IV injections, demonstrating that daunomycin-loaded LPs produced a significant increase in plasma clearance compared to free drugs even though OX26 immunoliposomes are more quickly removed than stealth systems. Moreover, it is important to note that the noncovalent binding of OX26 MAb produced a significantly higher brain accumulation as compared to control immunoliposomes.

In a recent work, Zhang and Pardridge (Zhang *et al.*, 2008) proposed the use of pegylated OX26 LPs loaded with glial-derived neurotrophic factor (GDNF) plasmid DNA as a possible therapy for Parkinson's disease. The GDNF plasmid was encapsulated in LPs made of POPC, DDAB, DSPE-PEG$_{2000}$, and DSPE-PEG$_{2000}$-maleimide (29% encapsulation efficiency). These authors suggested the use of both OX26 Ab and a rat tyrosine hydroxylase promoter in order to restrict GDNF expression to catecholaminergic cells within the brain. Rats were treated with three-weekly injections of LP formulation, and a strong (87%) reduction of aphomorphine-induced rotation was observed with a GDNF brain expression confined to substantia nigra that expresses the Th gene.

To overcome Tf-off target expression, researchers have introduced an important step forward — a more fine and engineered technology. Starting from the criticism that there was an invalidating abundance of TfR in different tissues (liver and spleen), the authors chose a solution based on the association of the pegylated immunoliposome gene targeting technology with a brain-specific promoter.

Particularly, the authors targeted the plasmid DNA to the brain by the conjugation of PEG-LPs with 8D3-MAb directed to mouse Tf-R and drove the expression of plasmids by two promoters — a general promoter (SV 40, simian virus) (Segovia *et al.*, 1998) and a brain-specific promoter (the human glial fibrillary acidic protein promoter) (GFAP) (Shi *et al.*, 2001b). The transgene was expressed in both brain and peripheral tissues when the simian virus 40 promoter was used, but the expression of the exogenous gene was confined to the brain when the transgene is under the influence of the brain-specific GFAP promoter. This study indicated that the following are possible: (1) a specific expression of the gene in the brain tissues, without any effect on different tissues (spleen, liver, and heart), (2) a prolonged expression over four days, and (3) no evidence of expression in the lungs, thus improving the specificity of the pegylated immunoliposomes.

Ko *et al.* (2009) described the use of anionic LPs to encapsulate a PEI/ODN complex. A dried anionic lipid film, consisting of a mixture of POPC, POPG, DSPE-PEG$_{2000}$, and biotinylated DSPE-PEG$_{2000}$ was mixed with a positively charged PEI/ODN complex for over four hours at room temperature with intermittent mixing and finally extruded through a polycarbonate membrane of 100 nm pore size. Immuno-LPs were obtained by the addition of 8D3 MAb conjugated with streptavidin to preformed biotinylated LPs. 8D3-LPs have been found to be efficiently internalized by brain-derived endothelial cells and to induce a relevant decrease of VCAM-1 expression under the stimulation of NFkB pathway with TNF-α when the specific transcription factor decoy ODN to NFkB was delivered.

In vivo pharmacokinetic parameters and biodistribution studies were performed to elucidate the different organ accumulations of 8D3-LPs compared to PEG-biotinylated systems. One hour after administration, a tenfold greater brain uptake was observed as compared to nontarget biotinylated LPs, indicating that the action was mediated by the targeting Ab.

3.7.2 INS-R Ab (83-14 MAb) as Ligand

A further improvement of Ab technology was obtained considering that OX26 MAb (targeting rat TfR) and 8D3 Ab (targeting mouse TfR) are generally active in mice and rats, but they are not active in humans and primates. The idea was to substitute these Abs with a murine 83-14 MAb active to the HINS-R (HINS-R-MAb).

Zhang and coworkers well described the use of pegylated immunoliposomes derivatized with the 83-14 murine MAb to target an EGFR antisense gene, driven by the SV40 to U87 human glioma cells. This targeting resulted in a 70–80% inhibition in cancer cell growth (Zhang *et al.*, 2002a). Moreover, the HIR-MAb-pegylated immunoliposomes showing an anionic superficial charge produced levels of gene expression comparable to those observed with a cationic and toxic lipid (lipofectamine).

Recently, the same research team added a promoter (SV 40) in order to perform a better and higher brain expression of β-galactosidase gene in primate brain (Zhang *et al.*, 2003a). The formulation of LPs has been planned on the basis of the previous works and briefly was composed of cationic lipids (DDAB) and of anionic or neutral ones (POPC, DSPE-PEG, and DPSE-PEG-Maleimide). This composition leads to a total negative surface charge; in order to compare the different targeting efficacy, 83-14 HIR MAb and OX26 TfRMAb were used. The results on monkeys after IV administration demonstrated a high expression of β-galactosidase gene in the brain; there was also evidence of peripheral gene expression in particular in those tissues with permeable vasculature (liver and spleen), expressing INS-Rs. In this case, the addition of a brain-specific promoter eliminated the off-target expression. Moreover, no expression in peripheral tissues with a continue vasculature and endothelium (heart, skeletal, muscles, and kidney) was recovered. Finally, comparing the efficiency of gene expression, the use of HIR MAb created a fiftyfold higher expression than TfRMAb-pegylated immunoliposomes. The authors of this work concluded that SV40, which is proper for simians, could easily be replaced with a human brain–specific promoter (e.g., GFAP), minimizing the expression in other tissues and possible immunoreactions, therefore improving brain-specific delivery and targeting.

Very recent works (Zhang *et al.*, 2003b; Zhang *et al.*, 2004) applied the pegylated-immunoliposomal technology to treat Parkinson's disease. In this work, the aim was to normalize striatal tyrosine hydroxylase (TH) activity in rats representing a PD model (lesionated in 6-OH-dopamine). The contemporaneous use of brain-specific promoter (GFAP), compared with generic promoter (SV-40), and of MAb for TfR (OX26) and for HIR (83-14 MAb) was evaluated after an IV injection of pegylated immuno (1–2% MAb conjugated with PEG strains) LPs. The results showed a high reduction of the effect of PD, reversing the induce motor impairment, and that the couple OX26 MAb and SV-40 led to an expression not only in the brain but also in the liver. On the contrary, the couple OX26 MAb and GFAP avoided the expression in the liver, only confining the gene expression to neurons with no expression in astrocytes.

In conclusion, it was possible to obtain a transduction of the entire striatum with nonviral exposure due to the possibility of the engineered LP to cross the BBB via a transvascular route.

3.7.3 Coupled Ab Technology: 8D3 MAb (to TfR) and 83-14 MAb (to HIR)

An important improvement was obtained considering the possibility to decorate LPs with two different peptidomimetic Ab. In this case, the idea was to merge two different finalities by making use of two different Abs. In particular, one Ab should be responsible for the brain tissue targeting and the second one should have the role of inducing cellular uptake or incrementing cellular transport.

Zhang and colleagues (Zhang *et al.*, 2002b), with the aim of delivering mRNA specifically to the brain, applied coupled conjugation technology. They used 8D3 MAb to TfR, ideally making use of transport across the tumor vasculature and exploiting receptor-mediated transcytosis across the tumor BBB and 83-14 MAb to human INS-R, improving the transport across the plasma membranes and nuclear membrane of human brain cancer cells. The tests were carried out on rats bearing human glioma cells (intracerebral injection of U87 tumor cell lines). The LPs composition was mainly of neutral lipids (POPC), with slight percentages of both cationic lipids (DDAB), anionic pegylated lipids (DPSE-PEG_{2000}), and activated anionic pegylated lipids (DPSE-PEG_{2000}-maleimide). The procedure of preparation of LP was the same as previously explained, and the Abs were preliminarily thiolated by using 2-imino-thiolane.

The results clearly showed that without dual targeting, it is not possible for the gene to reach deep localization because the cancer cells lay distal from the microvasculature barrier. On the contrary, using this coupled technology, the *in vivo* experiments showed a 100% survival after weekly administrations.

The same approach was recently used in gene therapy using RNA interference (RNAi) toward oncogenic gene such as EGFR (Zhang *et al.*, 2004). In this study, the authors joined the new form of antisense gene therapy, wherein an expression plasmid encodes for a short hairpin RNA (shRNA) with a nonviral targeting technology based on the creation of a doubly conjugated immunoliposomes. The delivery of RNAi, causing interference of EGFR gene expression-encapsulated immunoliposomes (83-14 MAb/8D3 MAb pegylated immunoliposomes) in cultured glioma cells, resulted in a 95% suppression of gene function and in an 88% increase in survival time of mice with advanced intracranial brain cancer after IV administration.

3.7.4 Others

Another attempt of brain targeting by using different ligands was made by Kabanov and coworkers to formulate micelles of poly(oxyethylene)-poly(oxypropylene) block copolymers (pluronic) surface modified with an Ab (Ab, anti-α_2-GP) to brain glial cells α_2-glycoprotein (Kabanov *et al.*, 1992).

These micelles have been alternatively loaded with fluorescein isothiocyanate (FITC) (a fluorescent probe) or haloperidol (a neuroleptic), intravenously administered to mice.

Qualitative distribution data has pointed out increased fluorescence in mice brain after treatment with FITC-loaded Ab-pluronic P85 micelles compared with FITC unmodified micelles.

Similarly, behavioral tests evaluating neuroleptic effects have demonstrated that haloperidol-loaded Ab-P85 dramatically decreases mouse mobility and grooming (which are typical central effects) in comparison with P85 haloperidol micelles.

Nonetheless, it is worth noting that α_2-GP-antigens, located in brain glial cells, can interact with Abs only after micelles cross the BBB: the authors expect anti-α_2-GP-Abs to be polyclonal Abs being able to bind first to Ags located in the external side of the BBB, and after passed the barrier, to recognize the proper glial target.

Chekhonin and coworkers carried out a remarkable series of collateral experiments using pegylated immunoliposomes conjugated with thiolated MAb directed against human gliofibrillary acidic proteins (GFAP) (Chekhonin *et al.*, 2008; Chekhonin *et al.*, 2009; Chekhonin *et al.*, 2005).

In these works, the coupling strategy was based once again on the reaction of thiolated Abs with maleimide derivatives of phosphatidylethanolamine of LP membranes.

The lipids used in the preparation of the LPs were PC, Chol, Maleimide-PE, and DSPE-PEG_{2000} (respectively in the ratio of 23:16:1:1.6:0.4). The thiolation of the Ab was conducted with Traut's reagent for 1 hour at room temperature and then conjugation was carried out for one day at 4°C under argon and in the dark. The *in vitro* experiments showed the preservation of the immune-chemical properties of the Abs and the specific and competitive binding of stealth immunoliposomes (directed against human gliofibrillary acidic protein) to embryonic rat brain astrocytes. This finding demonstrated that these immunoliposomes may be useful in delivering drugs to glial brain tumors or the other pathological loci in the brain with a partially disintegrated BBB (Chekhonin *et al.*, 2005).

Another interesting approach deals with the use of anti-amyloid Ab as a ligand conjugated to NPs for the treatment of Alzheimer's disease. In fact, Agyare prepared a chitosan polymeric core NP coated with polyamine-modified Fab' fragment of IgG4.1, an anti-amyloid Ab, to target cerebrovascular amyloid deposits, a typical feature of Alzheimer's disease (Agyare *et al.*, 2008).

Considering the preparation, the obtainment of optimal pH values (adjusted to 6.5 to reduce cationic repulsion) has been found to be pivotal in enhancing Fab' fragment adsorption. The polyamine-modified fragment Ab maintains excellent permeability at the BBB, when compared to the whole Ab and the unmodified Fab' fragment, without compromising the Ag-binding activity. This moiety was also labeled with I125 and Alexa Fluor 647 for *in vitro* and *in vivo* tests.

In vitro studies were performed on both bovine brain microvascular cell and on Transwell® filter–coated wildtype 1 rat tail collagen and bovine fibronectin (simulating the BBB). The uptake of FITC-BSA loaded into NP systems demonstrated that Fab' fragment-coated NPs exhibit greater fluorescence than the control NPs; moreover, the passage across the BBB have been registered only using NPs coated with the fragment.

For the *in vivo* studies performed on female mice at 16 weeks, after IV administration, modified NPs were administered intravenously and at the end of each experiment the brains were removed, dissected into various anatomical regions, and analyzed for I125 radioactivity. Modified NPs were found to be present in each brain region to a greater extent than unmodified NPs.

References

1. Afergan E., Epstein H., Dahan R., Koroukhov N., Rohekar K., Danenberg H. D., and Golomb G. (2008). Delivery of serotonin to the brain by monocytes following phagocytosis of liposomes, *J. Control. Re*lease, **132**, pp. 84–90.
2. Afonso P. V., Ozden S., Cumont M. C., Seilhean D., Cartier L., Rezaie P., Mason S., Lambert S., Huerre M., Gessain A., Couraud P. O., Pique C., Ceccaldi P. E., and Romero I. A. (2008). Alteration of blood–brain barrier integrity by retroviral infection, *Plos. Pathog.*, **4**, e1000205, pp. 2–11.
3. Agyare E. K., Curran G. L., Ramakrishnan M., Yu C. C., Poduslo J. F., and Kandimalla K. K. (2008). Development of a smart nano-vehicle to target cerebrovascular amyloid deposits and brain parenchymal plaques observed in alzheimer's disease and cerebral amyloid angiopathy, *Pharm. Res.*, **25**, pp. 2674–2684.
4. Aktaş Y., Yemisci M., Andrieux K., Gürsoy R. N., Alonso M. J., Fernandez-Megia E., Novoa-Carballal R., Quiñoá E., Riguera R., Sargon M. F., Celik H. H., Demir A. S., Hincal A. A., Dalkara T., Capan Y., and Couvreur P. (2005). Development and brain delivery of chitosan-PEG nanoparticles functionalized with monoclonal antibody OX26, *Bioconjugate Chem.*, **16**, pp. 1503–1511.
5. Alexiou C., Arnold W., Klein R. J., Parak F. G., Hulin P., Bergemann C., Erhardt W., Wagenpfeil S., and Lübbe A. S. (2000). Locoregional cancer treatment with magnetic drug targeting, *Cancer Res.*, **60**, pp. 6641–6648.
6. Alyautdin R. N., Petrov V. E., Langer K., Berthold A., Kharkevich D. A., and Kreuter J. (1997). Delivery of loperamide across the blood-brain barrier with polysorbate 80-coated polybutylcyanoacrylate nanoparticles. *Pharm. Res.*, **14**, pp. 325–328.
7. Ambruosi A., Yamamoto H., and Kreuter J. (2003). Body distribution of polysorbate-80 and doxorubicin-loaded [14C]-poly(butyl cyanoacrylate) nanoparticles after i.v. administration in rats, *J. Drug Targeting*, **13**, pp. 535–542.
8. Ambruosi A., Khalansky A. S., Yamamoto H., Gelperina S. E., Begley D. J., and Kreuter J. (2006). Biodistribution of polysorbate 80-coated doxorubicin-loaded [14C]-poly(butyl cyanoacrylate) nanoparticles after intravenous administration to glioblastoma-bearing rats, *J. Drug Targeting*, **14**, pp. 97–105.

9. Anderberg E. K., Nyström C., and Artursson P. (1992). Epithelial transport of drugs in cell culture.VII: effects of pharmaceutical surfactant excipients and bile acids on transepithelial permeability in monolayers of human intestinal epithelial (Caco-2) cells, *J. Pharm. Sci.*, **81**, pp. 879–887.

10. Anderson B. D. (1996). Prodrugs for improved CNS delivery, *Adv. Drug Del. Rev.*, **19**, pp. 171–202.

11. Anderson K. E., Eliot L. A., Stevenson B. R., and Rogers J. A. (2001). Formulation and evaluation of a folic acid receptor targeted oral vancomycin liposomal dosage form, *Pharm. Res.*, **18**, pp. 316–322.

12. Aoki H., Kakinuma K., Morita K., Kato M., Uzuka T., Igor G., Takahashi H., and Tanaka R. (2004). Therapeutic efficacy of targeting chemotherapy using local hyperthermia and thermosensitive liposome: evaluation of drug distribution in a rat glioma model, *Int. J. Hyperther.*, **20**, pp. 595 – 605.

13. Azmin M. N., Stuart J. F., and Florence A. T. (1985). The distribution and elimination of methotrexate in mouse blood and brain after concurrent administration of polysorbate 80, *Cancer Chem. Pharmacol.*, **14**, pp. 238–242.

14. Banks W. A., Jaspan J. B., and Kastin A. J. (1997). Selective, physiological transport of insulin across the blood-brain barrier: novel demonstration by species-specific radioimmunoassay, *Peptides*, **18**, pp. 1257–1262.

15. Bawa R. (2008). Nanoparticles-based therapeutics in humans: a survey, *Nanotech. Law & Business*, **5**, pp. 135–155.

16. Bazile D. V., Ropert C., Huve P., Verrecchia T., Marlard M., Frydman A., Veillard M., and Spenlehauer G. (1992). Body distribution of fully biodegradable [14C]-poly(lactic acid) nanoparticles coated with albumin after parenteral administration to rats, *Biomaterials*, **13**, pp. 1093–1102.

17. Beck R. P., Fichtner I., Hentschel M., Richter J., and Kreuter J. (1997). Body distribution of free, liposomal and nanoparticle-associated mitoxantrone in b16-melanoma-bearing mice, *JPET*, **280**, pp. 232–237.

18. Béduneau A., Saulnier P., Hindrè F., Clavreul A., Leroux J. C., and Benoit J. F. (2007). Design of targeted lipid nanocapsules by conjugation of whole antibodies and antibody Fab' fragments, *Biomaterials*, **28**, pp. 4978–4990.

19. Béduneau A., Hindrè F., Clavreul A., Leroux J. C., Saulnier P., and Benoit J. P. (2008). Brain targeting using novel lipid nanovectors, *J. Control. Release*, **126**, pp. 44–49.

20. Bickel U., Yoshikawa T., and Pardridge W. M. (1993). Delivery of peptides and proteins through the blood-brain barrier, *Adv. Drug Deliv. Rev.*, **10**, pp. 205–245.

21. Bickel U., Yoshikawa T., and Pardridge W. M. (2001). Delivery of peptides through the blood brain barrier, *Adv. Drug Del. Rev.*, **46**, pp. 247–279.

22. Blasi P., Giovagnoli S., Schoubben A., Ricci M., and Rossi C. (2007). Solid lipid nanoparticles for targeted brain drug delivery, *Adv. Drug Del. Rev.*, **59**, pp. 454–477

23. Boado R. J., Zhang Y., Wang Y., and Pardridge W. M. (2009). Engineering and expression of a chimeric transferring receptor monoclonal antibody for blood brain barrier delivery in the mouse, *Biotechnol. Bioeng.*, **102**, pp. 1251–1258.

24. Bobo R. H., Laske D. W., Akbasak A., Morrison P. F., Dedrick R. L., and Oldfield E. H. (1994). Convection-enhanced delivery of macromolecules in the brain, *Proc. Natl. Acad. Sci.*, **91**, pp. 2076–2080.

25. Brasnjevic I., Steinbusch H. W. M., Schmitz C., and Martinez-Martinez P. (2009). Delivery of peptide and protein drugs over the blood–brain barrier, *Progr. Neurobiol.*, **87**, pp. 212–251.

26. Brigger I., Morizet J., Aubert G., Chacun H., Terrier-Lacombe M. J., Couvreur P., and Vassal G. (2002). Poly(ethylene glycol)-coated hexadecylcyanoacrilate nanospheres display a combined effect for brain tumor targeting, *J. Pharm. Exp. Ther.*, **303**, pp. 928–936.

27. Brigle K. E., Westin E. H., Houghton M. T., and Goldman I. D. (1991). Characterization of two cDNAs encoding folate-binding proteins from L1210 murine leukemia cells. Increased expression associated with a genomic rearrangement, *J. Biol. Chem.*, **266**, pp. 17243–17249.

28. Buckingham L. E., Balasubramanian M., Emanuele R. M., Clodfelter K. E., and Coon J. S. (1995). Comparison of Solutol HS 15, Cremophor EL and novel ethoxylated fatty acid surfactans as multidrug resistance modification agents, *Int. J. Cancer*, **62**, pp. 436–442.

29. Calvo J. P., Gouritin B., and Villarroya H. (2002). Quantification and localization of PEGylated polycyanoacrylate nanoparticles in brain and spinal cord during experimental allergic encephalomyelitis in rats, *Eur. J. Neurosci.*, **15**, pp. 1317–1326.

30. Calvo P., Gouritin B., Chacun H., Desmaële D., D'Angelo J., Noel J. P., Georgin D., Fattal E., Andreux J. P., and Couvreur P. (2001a). Long-circulating PEGylated polycyanoacrylate nanoparticles as new drug carrier for brain delivery, *Pharm. Res.*, **18**, pp. 1157–1166.

31. Calvo P., Gouritin B., Brigger I., Lasmezas C., Deslys J., Williams A., Andreux J. P., Dormont D., and Couvreur P. (2001b). PEGylated polycyanoacrylate nanoparticles as vectors for drug delivery in prion diseases, *J. Neurosci. Met.*, **111**, pp. 151–155.

32. Chekhonin V. P., Zhirkov Y. A., Gurina O. I., Ryabukhin I. A., Lebedev S. V., Kashparov I. A., and Dmitriyeva T. B. (2005). PEGylated immunoliposomes directed against brain astrocytes, *Drug Deliv.*, **12**, pp. 1–6.

33. Chekhonin V. P., Gurina O. I., Ykhova O. V., Ryabinina A. E., Tsibulkina E. A., and Zhirkov Y. A. (2008). Polyethylene glycol-conjugated immunoliposomes specific for olfactory ensheathing glial cells, *Bull. Exp. Biol. Med.*, **145**, pp. 449–451.

34. Chekhonin V. P., Baklaushev V. P., Yusubalieva G. M., and Gurina O. I. (2009). Targeted transport of 125I-labeled antibody to GFAP and AMVB1 in an experimental rat model of C6 glioma, *J. Neuroimmune Pharmacol.*, **4**, pp. 28–34.

35. Chertok B., Moffat B. A., David A. E., Yu F., Bergemann C., Ross B. D., and Yang V. C. (2008). Iron oxide nanoparticles as a drug delivery vehicle for MRI monitored magnetic targeting of brain tumors, *Biomaterials*, **29**, pp. 487–496.

36. Cho K., Wang X., Nie S., Chen Z., and Shin D. M. (2008). Therapeutic nanoparticles for drug delivery in cancer, *Clin. Cancer Res.*, **14**, pp. 1310–1316.

37. Costantino L., Gandolfi F., Tosi G., Rivasi F., Vandelli M. A., and Forni F. (2005). Peptide-derivatized biodegradable nanoparticles able to cross the blood-brain barrier, *J. Control. Re*lease, **108**, pp. 84–96.

38. Costantino L., Gandolfi F., Bossy-Nobsb L., Tosi G., Gurny R., Rivasi F., Vandelli M. A., and Forni F. (2006). Nanoparticulate drug carriers based on hybrid poly (d,l-lactide-co-glycolide)-dendron structures, *Biomaterials*, **27**, pp. 4635–4645.

39. Dams E. T. M., Laverman P., Oyen W. J. G., Storm G., Scherphof G. L., van der Meer J. W. M., Corstens F. H. M., and Boerman O. C. (2000). Accelerated blood clearance and altered biodistribution of repeated injections of sterically stabilized liposomes, *J. Pharmacol. Exp. Ther.*, **292**, pp. 1071–1079.

40. de Boer A. G., van der Sandt I. C. J., and Gaillard P. J. (2003). The role of drug transporters at the blood-brain barrier, *Annu. Rev. Pharmacol. Toxicol.*, **43**, pp. 629–656.

41. de Vries H. E., Kuiper J., de Boer A. G., Van Berkel T. J. C., and Breimer D. D. (1997). The blood-brain barrier in neuroinflammatory diseases, *Pharmacol. Rev.*, **49**, pp. 143–156.

42. Dehouck B., Fenart L., Dehouck M. P., Pierce A., Torpier G., and Cecchelli R. (1997). A new function for the LDL receptor: transcytosis of LDL across the blood-brain barrier, *J. Cell Biol.*, **138**, pp. 877–889.

43. Dhanasekaran M. and Polt R. (2005). New prospects for glycopeptide based analgesia: glycoside-induced penetration of the blood brain barrier, *Curr. Drug Del.*, **2**, pp. 59–73.

44. Dietschy J. M. and Turley S. D. (2001). Cholesterol metabolism in the brain, *Curr. Opin. Lipidol.*, **12**, pp. 105–112.

45. Dimitrov D. S., Feng Y., and Prabakaran P. (2008). Antibody-guided nanoparticles, *J. Comput. Theor. Nanosci.*, **5**, pp. 751–759.

46. Doolittle N. D., Petrillo A., Bell S., Cummings P., and Eriksen S. (1998). Blood-brain barrier disruption for the treatment of malignant brain tumors: the National Program, *J. Neurosci. Nurs.*, **30**, pp. 81–90.

47. Douglas S. J., Davis S. S., and Illum L. (1986). Biodistribution of poly(butyl 2-cyanoacrylate) nanoparticles in rabbits, *Int. J. Pharm.*, **34**, pp. 145–152.

48. Duffy K. R. and Pardridge W. M. (1987). Blood-brain barrier transcytosis of insulin in developing rabbits, *Brain Res.*, **420**, pp. 32–38.

49. Eavarone D. A., Yu X., and Bellamkonda R. V. (2000). Targeted drug delivery to C6 glioma by transferring-coupled liposomes, *J. Biomed. Mat. Res.*, **51**, pp. 10–14.

50. Egleton R. D. and Davis T. P. (2005). Development of neuropeptide drugs that cross the blood brain barrier, *NeuroRx*, **2**, pp. 44–53.

51. Emerich D. F. (2005). Nanomedicine-prospective therapeutic and diagnostic applications, *Exp. Opin. Biol. Ther.*, **5**, pp. 1–5.

52. Fahmy T. M., Fong P. M., and Goyal A., Saltzman W. M. (2005). Targeted for drug delivery, *Nanotoday*, **8**, pp. 18–26.

53. Fahr A. and Liu X. (2007). Drug delivery strategies for poorly water-soluble drugs, *Exp. Opin. Drug Del.*, **4**, pp. 403–416.

54. Friden P. M., Walus L. R., Musso G. F., Taylor M. A., Malfroy B., and Starzyk R. M. (1991). Anti-transferrin receptor antibody and antibody–drug conjugates cross the blood–brain barrier, *Proc. Natl Acad. Sci.*, **88**, pp. 4771–4775.

55. Friese A., Seiller E., Quack G., Lorenz B., and Kreuter J. (2000). Increase of the duration of the anticonvulsive activity of a novel NMDA receptor antagonist using poly(butylcyanoacrylate) nanoparticles as a parenteral controlled release system, *Eur. J. Pharm. Biopharm.*, **49**, pp. 103–109.

56. Gaillard P. J., Visser C. C., and de Boer A. G. (2005). Targeted delivery across the blood-brain barrier, *Exp. Opin. Drug Deliv.*, **2**, pp. 299–309.

57. Garcia-Garcia E., Andrieux K., Gil S., Kim H. R., Le Doan T., Desmaele D., d'Angelo J., Taran F., Georgin D., and Couvreur P. (2005a). A methodology to study intracellular distribution of nanoparticles in brain endothelial cells, *Int. J. Pharm.*, **298**, 310–314.

58. Garcia-Garcia E., Gil S., Andrieux K., Desmaële D., Nicolas V., Taran F., Georgin D., Andreux J. P., Roux F., and Couvreur P. (2005b). A relevant *in vitro* rat model for the evaluation of blood–brain barrier translocation of nanoparticles, *Cell Mol. Life Sci.*, **62**, 1400–1408.

59. Gelperina S. E., Khalansky A. S., Skidan I. N., Smirnova Z. S., Bobruskin A. I., Severin S. E., Turowski B., Zanella F. E., and Kreuter J. (2002). Toxicological studies of doxorubicin bound to polysorbate 80-coated poly(butyl cyanoacrylate) nanoparticles in healthy rats and rats with intracranial glioblastoma, *Toxicol. Lett.*, **126**, pp. 131–141.

60. Gessner A., Olbrich C., Schröder W., Kayser O., and Müller R. H. (2001). The role of plasma proteins in brain targeting: species dependent protein adsorption patterns on brain-specific lipid drug conjugate (LDC) nanoparticles, *Int. J. Pharm.*, **214**, pp. 87–91.

61. Gomes I. and Sharma S. K. (2004). Uptake of liposomally entrapped adenosine 3′-5′-cyclic monophosphate in muose brain, *Neurochem. Res.*, **29**, pp. 441–446.

62. Goppert T. M. and Müller R. H. (2005). Polysorbate-stabilized solid lipid nanoparticles as colloidal carriers for intravenous targeting of drugs to the brain: comparison of plasma protein adsorption patterns, *J. Drug Targeting*, **13**, pp. 179–187.

63. Gref R., Domb A., Quellec P., Blunk T., Müller R. H., Verbavatz J. M., and Langer R. (1995). The controlled intravenous delivery of drugs using PEG-coated sterically stabilized nanospheres, *Adv. Drug Del. Rev.*, **16**, pp. 215–233.

64. Gref R., Lück M., Quellec P., Marchand M., Dellacherie E., Harnisch S., Blunk T., and Müller R. H. (2000). Stealth corona-core nanoparticles surface modified by polyethylene glycol (PEG): influence of the corona (PEG chain length and surface density) and of the core composition on phagocytic uptake and plasma protein adsorption, *Coll. Surf. B: Biointerf.*, **18**, pp. 301–313.

65. Grislain L., Couvreur P., Lenaerts V., Roland M., Deprez-Decampeneere D., and Speiser P. (1983). Pharmacokinetics and distribution of a biodegradable drug-carrier, *Int. J. Pharm.*, **15**, pp. 335–345.

66. Hans M. L. and Lowman A. M. (2002). Biodegradable nanoparticles for drug delivery and targeting. *Curr. Opin. Solid State Mat. Sci.*, **6**, pp. 319–327.

67. Harris J. M. and Chess R. B. (2003). Effect of pegylation on pharmaceuticals, *Nat. Rev. Drug Discovery*, **2**, pp. 214–221.

68. Hassan E. E. and Gallo J. M. (1993). Targeting anticancer drugs to the brain. I: enhanced brain delivery of oxantrazole following administration in magnetic cationic microspheres, *J. Drug Targeting*, **1**, pp. 7–14.

69. Havrankova J., Brownstein M., and Roth J. (1981). Insulin and insulin receptors in rodent brain, *Diabetologia*, **20**, pp. 268–273.

70. Hu K., Li J., Shen Y., Lu W., Gao X., Zhang Q., and Jiang X. (2009). Lactoferrin-conjugated PEG–PLA nanoparticles with improved brain delivery: *in vitro* and *in vivo* evaluations, *J. Control. Re*lease, **134**, pp. 55–61.

71. Husain S. R. and Puri R. K. (2003). Interleukin 13 receptor directed cytotoxin for malignant glioma therapy: from bench to bedside, *J. Neurooncol.*, **65**, pp. 37–48.

72. Huwyler J., Wu D., and Pardridge W. M. (1996). Brain drug delivery of small molecules using immunoliposomes, *Proc. Natl. Acad. Sci.*, **93**, pp. 14164–14169.

73. Huwyler J., Yan J., and Pardridge W. M. (1997). Receptor mediated delivery of daunomycin using immunoliposomes: pharmacokinetics and tissue distribution in the rat, *J. Pharm. Exp. Ther.*, **282**, pp. 1541–1546.

74. Ishida T., Maeda R., Ichihara M., Mukai Y., Motoki Y., Manabe Y., Irimura K., and Kiwada H. (2002). The accelerated clearance on repeated injection of pegylated liposomes in rats: laboratory and histopathological study, *Cell Mol. Biol. Lett.*, **7**, pp. 286–295.

75. Ishida T., Maeda R., Ichihara M., Irimara K., and Kiwada H. (2003a). Accelerated clearance of PEGylated liposomes in rats after repeated injections, *J. Control. Re*lease, **88**, pp. 35–42.

76. Ishida T., Masuda K., Ichikawa T., Ichihara M., Irimara K., and Kiwada H. (2003b). Accelerated clearance of a second injection of PEGylated liposomes in mice, *Int. J. Pharm.*, **255**, pp. 167–174.

77. Ishida T., Ichikawa T., Ichihara M., Sadzuka Y., and Kiwada H. (2004). Effect of the physicochemical properties of initially injected liposomes on the clearance of subsequently injected PEGylated liposomes in mice, *J. Control. Re*lease, **95**, pp. 403–412.

78. Ishida T., Harada M., Wang X. Y., Ichihara M., Irimara K., and Kiwada H. (2005). Accelerated blood clearance of PEGylated liposomes following preceding liposome injection: effects of lipid dose and PEG surface-density and chain length of the first-dose liposomes, *J. Control. Re*lease, **105**, pp. 305–317.

79. Ishida T., Ichihara M., Wang X., Yamamoto K., Kimura J., Majima E., and Kiwada H. (2006a). Injection of PEGylated liposomes in rats elicits PEG-specific IgM, which is responsible for rapid elimination of a second dose of PEGylated liposomes, *J. Control. Re*lease, **112**, pp. 15–25.

80. Ishida T., Ichihara M., Wang X., and Kiwada H. (2006b). Spleen plays an important role in the induction of accelerated blood clearance of PEGylated liposomes, *J. Control. Re*lease, **115**, pp. 243–250.

81. Ito A., Shinkai M., Honda H., and Kobayashi T. (2005). Medical application of functionalized magnetic nanoparticles, *J. Biosci. Bioeng.*, **100**, pp. 1–11.

82. Jain S., Mishra V., Singh P., Dubey P. K., Saraf D. K., and Vyas S. P. (2003). RGD-anchored magnetic liposomes for monocytes/neutrophils-mediated brain targeting, *Int. J. Pharm.*, **261**, pp. 43–55.

83. Jefferies W. A., Brandon M. R., Hunt S. V., Williams A. F., Gatter K. C., and Mason D. Y. (1984). Transferrin receptor on endothelium of brain capillaries, *Nature*, **312**, pp. 162–163.

84. Kabanov A. V., Batrakova E. V., Melik-Nubarov N. S., Fedoseev N. A., Dorodnich T. Y., Alakhov V. Y., Chekhonin V. P., Nazarova I. R., and Kabanov V. A. (1992). A new class of drug carriers: micelles of poly (oxyethylene)-poly (oxypropylene) block copolymers as micro-containers for drug targeting from blood in brain, *J. Control. Re*lease, **22**, pp. 141–158.

85. Kakinuma K., Tanaka R., Takahashi H., Watanabe M., Nakagawa T., and Kuroki M. (1996). Targeting chemotherapy for malignant brain tumor using thermosensitive liposome and localized hyperthermia, *J. Neurosurg.*, **84**, pp. 180–184.

86. Kante B., Couvreur P., Dubois-Krack G., de Meester C., Guiot P., Roland M., Mercier M., and Speiser P. (1982). Toxicity of polyalkylcyanoacrylate nanoparticles I: free nanoparticles, *J. Pharm. Sci.*, **71**, pp. 786–790.

87. Kattan J., Droz J. P., Couvreur P., Marino J. P., Boutan-Laroze1 A., Rougier P., Brault P., Vranckx H., Grognet J. M., Morge X., and Sancho-Garnier H. (1992). Phase I clinical trial and pharmacokinetic evaluation of doxorubicin carried by polyisohexylcyanoacrylate nanoparticles, *Invest. New Drugs*, **10**, pp. 191–199.

88. Kihlberg J., Ahman J., Walse B., Drakenberg T., Nilsson A., Soederberg-Ahlm C., Bengtsson B., and Olsson H. (1995). Glycosilated peptide hormones: pharmacological properties and conformational studies of analogues of [1-desamino, 8-D-arginine] vasopressin, *J. Med. Chem.*, **38**, pp. 161–169.

89. Kim H. R., Andrieux K., Gil S., Taverna M., Chacun H., Desmaële D., Taran F., Georgin D., and Couvreur P. (2007a). Translocation of poly(ethylene glycol-co-hexadecyl)cyanoacrylate nanoparticles into rat brain endothelial cells: role of apolipoproteins in receptor-mediated endocytosis, *Biomacromol.*, **8**, pp. 793–799.

90. Kim H. R., Gil S., Andrieux K., Nicolas V., Appel M., Chacun H., Desmaële D., Taran F., Georgin D., and Couvreur P. (2007b). Low-density lipoprotein receptor-mediated endocytosis of PEGylated nanoparticles in rat brain endothelial cells, *Cell Molec. Life Sci.*, **64**, pp. 356–364.

91. Kim H. R., Andrieux K., Delomenie C., Chacun H., Appel M., Desmaële D., Taran F., Georgin D., Couvreur P., and Taverna M. (2007c). Analysis of plasma protein adsorption onto PEGylated nanoparticles by complementary methods: 2-DE, CE and Protein Lab-on-chip system, *Electrophoresis*, **28**, pp. 2252–2261.

92. Ko Y. T., Bhattacharya R., and Bickel U. (2009). Liposome encapsulated polyethylenimine/ODN polyplexes for brain targeting. *J. Control. Re*lease, **133**, pp. 230–237.

93. Kobayashi K., Han M., Watarai S., and Yasuda T. (1996). Availability of liposomes as drug carriers to the brain, *Acta Med. Okayama*, **50**, pp. 67–72.

94. Kopelman R., Lee Koo Y.-E., Philbert M., Moffat B. A., Ramachandra Reddy G., McConville P., Hall D. E., Chenevert T. L., Swaroop Bhojani M., Buck S. M., Rehemtulla A., and Ross B. D. (2005). Multifunctional nanoparticle platforms for *in vivo* MRI enhancement and photodynamic therapy of a rat brain cancer, *J. Magn. Magn. Mat.*, **293**, pp. 404–410.

95. Koziara J. M., Lockman P. R., Allen D. D., and Mumper R. J. (2003). *In situ* blood-brain barrier transport of nanoparticles, *Pharm. Res.*, **20**, pp. 1772–1778.

96. Koziara J. M., Lockman P. R., Allen D. D., and Mumper R. J. (2004). Paclitaxel nanoparticles for the potential treatment of brain tumors, *J. Control. Re*lease, **30**, pp. 259–269.

97. Kreuter J., Alyautdin R. N., Kharkevich D. A., and Ivanov A. A. (1995). Passage of peptides through the blood-brain barrier with colloidal polymer particles (nanoparticles), *Brain Res.*, **674**, pp. 171–174.

98. Kreuter J., Petrov V. E., Kharkevich D. A., and Alyautdin R. N. (1997). Influence of the type of surfactant on the analgesic effects induced by the peptide dalargin after its delivery across the blood-brain barrier using surfactant-coated nanoparticles, *J. Control. Re*lease, **49**, pp. 81–87.

99. Kreuter J. (2001). Nanoparticulate systems for brain delivery of drugs, *Adv. Drug Del. Rev.*, **47**, pp. 65–81.

100. Kreuter J. (2002a). Transport of drugs across the blood–brain barrier by nanoparticles, *Curr. Med. Chem.*, **2**, pp. 241–249.

101. Kreuter J., Shamenkov D., Petrov V., Ramge P., Cychutek K., Koch-Brandt C., and Alyautdin R. (2002b). Apolipoprotein-mediated transport of nanoparticle-bound drugs across the blood-brain barrier, *J. Drug Targeting*, **10**, pp. 317–325.

102. Kreuter J., Ramge P., Petrov V., Hamm S., Gelperina S. E., Engelhardt B., Alyautdin R., von Briesen H., and Begley D. J. (2003). Direct evidence that polysorbate-80–coated poly(butylcyanoacrylate) nanoparticles deliver drugs to the CNS via specific mechanisms requiring prior binding of drug to the nanoparticles, *Pharm. Res.*, **20**, pp. 409–416.

103. Kreuter J., Hekmatara T., Dreis S., Vogel T., Gelperina S., and Langer K. (2007). Covalent attachment of apolipoprotein A-I and B-100 to albumin nanoparticles enables drug transport into the brain, *J. Control. Re*lease, **118**, pp. 54–58.

104. Kroll R. A., Pagel M. A., Muldoon L. L., Roman-Goldstein S., and Neuwelt E. A. (1996). Increasing volume distribution to the brain with interstitial infusion: dose, rather than convection, might be the most important factor, *Neurosurgery*, **38**, pp. 752–754.

105. Kurihara A. (1999). Epidermal growth factor radiopharmaceuticals: ^{111}In chelation conjugation to a blood brain barrier delivery vector via a biotin-polyethylene linker, pharmacokinetics and *in vivo* imaging of experimental brain tumors, *Bioconj. Chem.*, **10**, pp. 502–511.

106. Laverman P., Carstens M. G., Boerman O. C., Dams E. M., Oyen W. J. G., van Rooijen N., Corstens F. H. M., and Storm G. (2001a). Factors affecting the accelerated blood clearance of polyethylene glycol-liposomes upon repeated injection, *J. Pharmacol. Exp. Ther.*, **298**, pp. 607–612.

107. Laverman P., Boerman O. C., Oyen W. J. G., Corstens F. H. M., and Storm G. (2001b). *In vivo* applications of PEG liposomes: unexpected observations, *Crit. Rev. Ther. Drug Carr. Syst.*, **18**, pp. 551–566.

108. Le Ray A. M., Vert M., Gautier J. C., and Benoît J. P. (1994). Fate of [14C]poly(-lactide-co-glycolide) nanoparticles after intravenous and oral administration to mice, *Int. J. Pharm.*, **106**, pp. 201–211.

109. Lee H. J., Engelhardt B., Lesley J., Bickel U., and Pardridge W. M. (2000). Targeting rat anti-mouse transferrin receptor monoclonal antibodies through blood–brain barrier in mouse, *J. Pharmacol. Exp. Ther.*, **292**, pp. 1048–1052.

110. Lee R. J. and Low P. S. (1995). Folate-mediated tumor cell targeting of liposome-entrapped doxorubicin *in vitro*, *Biochim. Biophys. Acta*, **1233**, pp. 134–144.

111. Lherm C., Müller R. H., Puisieux F., and Couvreur P. (1992). Alkylcyanoacrylate drug carriers: II. Cytotoxicity of cyanoacrylate nanoparticles with different alkyl chain length, *Int. J. Pharm.*, **84**, pp. 13–22.

112. Li S. (1999). Hydrolytic degradation characteristics of aliphatic polyesters derived from lactic and glycolic acids, *J. Biomed. Mater. Res.*, **48**, pp. 342–353.

113. Li Y. P., Pei Y. Y., Zhang X. Y., Gu Z. H., Zhou Z. H., Yuan W. F., Zhou J. J., Zhu J. H., and Gao X. J. (2001). PEGylated PLGA nanoparticles as protein carriers: synthesis, preparation and biodistribution in rats, *J. Control. Re*lease, **71**, pp. 203–211.

114. Linker R. A., Weller C., Luhder F., Mohr A., Schmidt J., Knauth M., Metselaar J. M., and Gold R. (2008). Liposomal glucocorticosteroids in treatment of chronic autoimmune demyelination: long-term protective effects and enhanced efficacy of methylprednisolone formulations, *Exp. neurology*, **211**, pp. 397–405.

115. Lobenberg R., Araujo L., von Briesen H., Rodgers E., and Kreuter J. (1998). Body distribution of azidothymidine bound to hexyl-cyanoacrylate nanoparticles after I.V. injection to rats, *J. Control. Re*lease, **50**, pp. 21–30.

116. Lockman P. R., Oyewumi M. O., Koziara J. M., Roder K. E., Mumper R. J., and Allen D. D. (2003a). Brain uptake of thiamine-coated nanoparticles, *J. Control. Re*lease, **93**, pp. 271–282.

117. Lockman P. R., Koziara J., Roder K. E., Paulson J., Abbruscato T. J., Mumper R. J., and Allen D. D. (2003b). *In vivo* and *in vitro* assessment of baseline blood-brain barrier parameters in the presence of novel nanoparticles, *Pharm. Res.*, **20**, pp. 705–713.

118. Lu W., Zhang Y., Tan Y. Z., Hu K. L., Jiang X. G., and Fu S. K. (2005). Cationic albumin-conjugated pegylated nanoparticles as novel drug carrier for brain delivery, *J. Control. Re*lease, **107**, pp. 428–448.

119. Lübbe A. S., Bergermann C. H., Riess H., Schriever F., Reichardt P., Possinger K., Matthias M., Dörken B., Herrmann F., Gürtler R.,

Hohenberger P., Haas N., Sohr R., Sander B., Lemke A. J., Ohlendorf D., Huhnt W., and Huhn D. (1996). Clinical experiences with magnetic drug targeting: a phase I study with 4′-epidoxorubicin in 14 patients with advanced solid tumors, *Cancer Res.*, **56**, pp. 4686–4693.

120. Lukowski G., Müller R. H., Müller B. W., and Dittgen M. (1992). Acrylic acid copolymer nanoparticles for drug delivery: I. Characterization of the surface properties relevant for *in vivo* organ distribution, *Int. J. Pharm.*, **84**, pp. 23–31.

121. Lukyanov A. N., Elbayoumi T. A., Chakilam A. R., and Torchilin V. P. (2004). Tumor-targeted liposomes: doxorubicin-loaded long-circulating liposomes modified with anti-cancer antibody, *J. Control. Re*lease, **100**, pp. 135–144.

122. Madhankumar A. B., Slagle-Webb B., Wang X., Yang Q. X., Antonetti D. A., Miller P. A., Sheehan J. M., and Connor J. R. (2009). Efficacy of interleukin-13 receptor–targeted liposomal doxorubicin in the intracranial brain tumor model, *Mol. Cancer Ther.*, **8**, pp. 648–654.

123. Maruyama K., Takahashi N., Tagawa T., Nagaike K., and Iwatsuru M. (1997). Immunoliposomes bearing polyethyleneglycol-coupled Fab′ fragment show prolonged circulation time and high extravasation into targeted solid tumors *in vivo*, *FEBS Lett.*, **413**, 177–180.

124. Michaelis K., Hoffmann. M. M., Dreis. S., Herbert. E., Alyautdin. R. N., Michaelis M., Kreuter J., and Langer K. (2006). Covalent linkage of apolipoprotein E to albumin nanoparticles strongly enhances drug transport into the brain, *J. Pharm. Exp. Ther.*, **317**, pp. 1246–1253.

125. Miller D., Keller B., and Borchardt R. (1994). Identification and distribution of insulin-receptors on cultured bovine brain microvessels endothelial cells: possible function in insulin processing in the blood-brain barrier, *J. Cell Physiol.*, **161**, pp. 333–341.

126. Mishra V., Mahor S., Rawat A., Gupta P. N., Dubey P., Khatri K., and Vyas S. P. (2006). Targeted brain delivery of AZT via transferrin anchored pegylated albumin nanoparticles, *J. Drug Targeting*, **14**, pp. 45–53.

127. Moghimi S. M., Hunter A. C., and Murray J. C. (2001). Long-circulating and target-specific nanoparticles: theory to practice, *Pharmacol. Rev.*, **53**, pp. 283–318.

128. Moghimi S. M., and Szebeni J. (2003). Stealth liposomes and long circulating nanoparticles: critical issue in pharmacokinetics, opsonization and protein-binding properties, *Prog. Lipid Res.*, **42**, pp. 463–478.

129. Mora M., Sagristà M. L., Trombetta D., Bonina F. P., De Pasquale A., and Saija A. (2002). Design and characterization of liposomes containing

long-chain N-AcylPEs for brain delivery: penetration of liposomes incorporating GM1 into the rat brain, *Pharm. Res.*, **19**, pp. 1430–1438.

130. Mornet S., Vasseur S., Grasset F., and Duguet E. (2006). Magnetic nanoparticle design for medical applications, *Progr. Solid State Chem.*, **34**, pp. 237–247

131. Morris C. M., Keith A. B., Edwardson J. A., and Pullen R. G. (1992). Uptake and distribution of iron and transferrin in the adult rat brain, *J. Neurochem.*, **59**, pp. 300–306.

132. Müller R. H., Lherm C., Herbert J., and Couvreur P. (1990). *In vitro* model for the degradation of alkylcyanoacrylate nanoparticles, *Biomaterials*, **11**, pp. 590–595.

133. Müller R. H., Lherm C., Herbort J., Blunk T., and Couvreur P. (1992). Alkylcyanoacrylate drug carriers: I. Physicochemical characterization of nanoparticles with different alkyl chain length, *Int. J. Pharm.*, **84**, pp. 1–11.

134. Muthu M. S. and Singh S. (2009). Targeted nanomedicines: effective treatment modalities for cancer, AIDS and brain disorders, *Nanomedicine*, **4**, pp. 105–118.

135. Naoi M. and Yagi K. (1980). Incorporation of enzyme through blood brain barrier into the brain by means of liposomes, *Biochem. Int.*, **1**, 591–596.

136. Negri L., Lattanti R., Tabacco F., Scolaro B., and Rocchi R. (1998). Glycodermorphins: opioid peptides with potent and prolonged analgesic activity and enhanced blood-brain barrier penetration, *Brit. J. Pharmacol.*, **124**, pp. 1516–1522.

137. Nerurkar M. M., Ho N. F. H., Burton P. S., Vidmar T. J., and Borchardt R. T. (1997). Mechanistic roles of neutral surfactants on concurrent polarized and passive membrane transport of a model peptide in Caco-2 cells, *J. Pharm. Sci.*, **86**, pp. 813–821.

138. Newton H. B. (2006). Advances in strategies to improve drug delivery to brain tumors, *Exp. Rev. Neurother.*, **6**, pp. 1495–1509.

139. Olivier J. C., Fenart L., Chauvet R., Pariat C., Cecchelli R., and Couet W. (1999). Indirect evidence that drug brain targeting using polysorbate 80-coated polybutylcyanoacrylate nanoparticles is related to toxicity, *Pharm. Res.*, **16**, pp. 1836–1842.

140. Olivier J. C., Huertas R., Jeong Lee H., Calon F., and Pardridge W. M. (2002). Synthesis of pegylated immunonanoparticles, *Pharm. Res.*, **19**, pp. 1137–1143.

141. Pang Z., Lu W., Gao H., Hu K., Chen J., Zhang C., Gao X., Jiang X., and Zhu C. (2008). Preparation and brain delivery property of biodegradable polymersomes conjugated with OX26, *J. Control. Release,* **128**, pp. 120–127.

142. Pankhurst Q. A., Connolly J., Jones S. K., and Dobson J. (2003). Applications of magnetic nanoparticles in biomedicine, *J. Phys. D: Appl. Phys.*, **36**, R167–R181.

143. Pardridge W. M., Eisenberg J., and Yang J. (1987). Human blood-brain barrier transferrin receptor, *Metabolism*, **36**, pp. 892–895.

144. Pardridge W. M., Buciak J. L., and Friden P. M. (1991). Selective transport of an anti-transferrin receptor antibody through the blood–brain barrier *in vivo*, *J. Pharmacol. Exp. Ther.*, **259**, pp. 66–70.

145. Pardridge W. M. (1995a). Vector-mediated peptide drug delivery to the brain, *Adv. Drug Del. Rev.*, **15**, pp. 109–146.

146. Pardridge W. M., Kang Y. S., Buciak J. L., and Yang J. (1995b). Human insulin receptor monoclonal antibody undergoes high affinity binding to human brain capillaries *in vitro* and rapid transctosis through the blood-brain barrier, *Pharm. Res.*, **12**, 807–816.

147. Pardridge W. M. (2001). *Brain Drug Targeting: The Future of Brain Drug Development.* Cambridge University Press: Cambridge, pp. 1–370.

148. Pardridge W. M. (2002). Drug and gene targeting to the brain with molecular Trojan horses, *Nat. Rev. Drug Discov.*, **1**, pp. 131–139.

149. Pardridge W. M. (2005). The blood-brain barrier: bottleneck in brain drug development, *NeuroRX*, **2**, pp. 3–14.

150. Pardridge W. M. and Olivier J. C. (2005). Immunonanoparticles, US Patent 20050042298.

151. Peira E., Marzola P., Podio V., Aime S., Sbarbati A., and Gasco M. R. (2003). *In vitro* and *in vivo* study of solid lipid nanoparticles loaded with superparamagnetic iron oxide, *J. Drug Targeting*, **11**, pp. 19–24.

152. Pereverzeva E., Treschalin I., Bodyagin D., Maksimenko O., Langer K., Dreis S., Asmussen B., Kreuter J., and Gelperina S. (2007). Influence of the formulation on the tolerance profile of nanoparticle-bound doxorubicin in healthy rats: focus on cardio- and testicular toxicity, *Int. J. Pharm.*, **337**, pp. 346–356.

153. Pereverzeva E., Treschalin I., Bodyagin D., Maksimenko O., Kreuter J., and Gelperina S. (2008). Intravenous tolerance of a nanoparticle-based formulation of doxorubicin in healthy rats, *Toxicol. Lett.*, **178**, pp. 9–19.

154. Petri B., Bootz A., Khalansky A., Hekmatara T., Müller R., Uhl R., Kreuter J., and Gelperina S. (2007). Chemotherapy of brain tumour using

doxorubicin bound to surfactant-coated poly(butyl cyanoacrylate) nanoparticles: revisiting the role of surfactants, *J. Control. Re*lease, **117**, pp. 51–58.

155. Plate K. H., Breier G., Weich H. A., and Risau W. (1992). Vascular endothelial growth factor is a potential tumor angiogenesis factor in human gliomas *in vivo*, *Nature*, **359**, pp. 845–848.

156. Polt R., Porreca F., Szabò L. Z., Bilsky E. J., Davis P., Abbruscato T. J., Davis T. P., Harvath R., Yamamura H. I., and Hruby V. J. (1994). Glycopeptide enkephalin analogues produce analgesia in mice: evidence for penetration of the blood-brain barrier, *Proc. Natl. Acad. Sci.*, **91**, pp. 7114–7118.

157. Polt R. and Palian M. M. (2001). Glycopeptide analgesics, *Drugs Future*, **26**, pp. 561–576.

158. Polt R., Dhanasekaran M., and Keyari C. M. (2005). Glycosylated neuropeptides: a new vista for neuropsychopharmacology? *Med. Res. Rev.*, **25**, pp. 557–585.

159. Prigent S. A., Stanley K. K., and Siddle K. (1990). Identification of epitopes on the human insulin receptor reacting with rabbit polyclonal antisera and mouse monoclonal antibodies, *J. Biol. Chem.*, **265**, pp. 9970–9977.

160. Pulfer S. K. and Gallo J. M. (1998). Enhanced brain tumor selectivity of cationic magnetic polysaccharide microspheres, *J. Drug Targeting*, **6**, pp. 215–227.

161. Pulfer S. K., Ciccotto S. L., and Gallo J. M. (1999). Distribution of small magnetic particles in brain tumor-bearing rats, *J. Neurooncol.*, **41**, pp. 99–105.

162. Qian Z. M., Li H., Sun H., and Ho K. (2002). Targeted drug delivery via the transferrin receptor mediated endocytosis pathway, *Pharmacol. Rev.*, **54**, pp. 561–587.

163. Ramge P., Unger R. E., Oltrogge J. B., Zenker D., Begley D., Kreuter J., and Von Briesen H. (2000). Polysorbate-80 coating enhances uptake of polybutylcyanoacrylate (PBCA)-nanoparticles by human and bovine primary brain capillary endothelial cells, *Eur. J. Neurosci.*, **12**, pp. 1931–1940.

164. Raub T. J., Kuentzel S. L., and Sawada G. A. (1992). Permeability of bovine brain microvessel endothelial cells *in vitro*: barrier tightening by a factor released from astroglioma cells, *Exp. Cell Res.*, **199**, pp. 330–340.

165. Reddy L., Sharma R., Chuttani K., Mishra A., and Murthy R. (2004). Etoposide-incorporated tripalmitin nanoparticles with different

surface charge: formulation, characterization, radiolabeling, and biodistribution studies, *AAPS J.*, **6**, Article 23 (http://www.aapsj.org).

166. Ricci M., Blasi P., Giovagnoli S., and Rossi C. (2006). Delivering drugs to the central nervous system: a medicinal chemistry or a pharmaceutical technology issue? *Curr. Med. Chem.*, **13**, pp. 1707–1725.

167. Sachdeva M. S. (1998). Drug targeting systems for cancer chemotherapy, *Exp. Opin. Invest. Drugs*, **7**, pp. 1849–1864.

168. Sakane T., Tanaka C., Yamamoto A., Hashida M., Sezaki H., Ueda H., and Takagi H. (1989). The effect of polysorbate 80 on brain uptake and analgesic effect of D-kyotorphin, *Int. J. Pharm.*, **57**, pp. 77–83.

169. Sauer I., Dunay I. R., Weisgraber K., Bienert M., and Dathe M. (2005). An apolipoprotein E-derived peptide mediates uptake of sterically stabilized liposomes into brain capillary endothelial cells, *Biochemistry*, **44**, pp. 2021–2029.

170. Sauer I., Nikolenko H., Keller S., Ajaj K. A., Bienert M., and Dathe M. (2006). Dipalmitoylation of a cellular uptake-mediating apolipoprotein E-derived peptide as a promising modification for stable anchorage in liposomal drug carriers, *Biochim. Biophys. Acta*, **1758**, pp. 552–561.

171. Saul J. M., Annapragada A., Natarajan J. V., and Bellamkonda R. V. (2003). Controlled targeting of liposomal doxorubicin via the folate receptor *in vitro*, *J. Control. Re*lease, **92**, pp. 49–67.

172. Schmidt J., Metselaar J. M., Wauben M. H. M., Toyka K. V., Storm G., and Gold R. (2003). Drug targeting by long-circulating liposomal glucocorticosteroids increases therapeutic efficacy in a model of multiple sclerosis, *Brain*, **126**, pp. 1895–1904.

173. Schneider S. W., Ludwig T., Tatenhorst L., Braune S., Oberleithner H., Senner V., and Paulus W. (2004). Glioblastoma cells release factors that disrupt blood-brain barrier features, *Acta Neuropathol.*, **107**, pp. 272–276.

174. Schnyder A., Krahenbuhl S., Drewe J., and Huwyler J. (2005).Targeting of daunomycin using biotinylated immunoliposomes: pharmacokinetics, tissue distribution and *in vitro* pharmacological effects, *J. Drug Targeting*, **13**, pp. 325–335.

175. Segovia J., Vergara P., and Brenner M. (1998). Differentiation-dependent expression of transgenes in engineered astrocyte cell lines, *Neurosci. Lett.*, **242**, pp. 172–176.

176. Shen F., Ross J. F., Wang X., and Ratnam M. (1994). Identification of a novel folate receptor, a truncated receptor, and receptor type beta in hematopoietic cells: cDNA cloning, expression, immunoreactivity, and tissue specificity, *Biochemistry*, **33**, 1209–1215.

177. Shi N. and Pardridge W. M. (2000). Noninvasive gene targeting to the brain, *Prot. Natl. Acad. Sci.*, **97**, pp. 7567–7572.

178. Shi N., Boado R. J., and Pardridge W. M. (2001a). Receptor-mediated gene targeting to tissues *in vivo* following intravenous administration of pegylated immunoliposomes, *Pharm. Res.*, **18**, pp. 1091–1095.

179. Shi N., Zhang Y., Zhu C., Boado R. J., and Pardridge W. M. (2001b). Brain specific expression of an exogenous gene after I.V. administration, *Prot. Natl. Acad. Sci.*, **98**, pp. 12754–12759.

180. Shin S. U., Friden P., Moran M., Olson T., Kang Y. S., Pardridge W. M., and Morrison S. L. (1995). Transferrin-antibody fusion proteins are effective in brain targeting, *Proc. Natl. Acad. Sci.*, **92**, pp. 2820–2824.

181. Siegal T., Rubinstein R., Bokstein F., Schwartz A., Lossos A., Shalom E., Chisin R., and Gomori J. M. (2000). *In vivo* assessment of the window of barrier opening after osmotic blood-brain barrier disruption in humans, *J. Neurosur.*, **92**, pp. 599–605.

182. Simeonova M., Ivanova T., Raikova E., Georgieva M., and Raikov Z. (1988). Tissue distribution of polybutylcyanoacrylate nanoparticles carrying spin-labelled nitrosourea, *Int. J. Pharm.*, **43**, pp. 267–271.

183. Smith M. W. and Gumbleton M. (2006). Endocytosis at the blood-brain barrier: from basic understanding to drug delivery strategies, *J. Drug Targeting*, **14**, pp. 191–214.

184. Soma C. E., Dubernet C., Bentolila D., Benita S., and Couvreur P. (2000). Reversion of multidrug resistance by co-encapsulation of doxorubicin and cyclosporin A in polyalkylcyanoacrylate nanoparticles, *Biomaterials*, **21**, pp. 1–7.

185. Soni V., Kohli D. V., and Jain S. K. (2005). Transferrin coupled liposomes as drug delivery carriers for brain targeting of 5-fluorouracil, *J. Drug Targeting*, **13**, pp. 245–250.

186. Soni V., Kohli D. V., and Jain S. K. (2008). Transferrin-conjugated liposomal system for improved delivery of 5-fluorouracil to brain, *J. Drug Targeting*, **16**, pp. 73–78.

187. Soppimath K. S., Aminabhavi T. M., Kulkarni A. R., and Rudzinski W. E. (2001). Biodegradable polymeric nanoparticles as drug delivery devices, *J. Control. Re*lease, **70**, pp. 1–20.

188. Steiniger S. C. J., Kreuter J., Khalansky A. S., Skidan I. N., Bobruskin A. I., Smirnova Z. S., Severin S. E., Uhl R., Kock M., Geiger K. D., and Gelperina S. E. (2004). Chemotherapy of glioblastoma in rats using doxorubicin-loaded nanoparticles, *Int. J. Cancer*, **109**, pp. 759–767.

189. Stolnik S., Dunn S. E., Garnett M. C., Davies M. C., Coombes A. G., Taylor D. C., Irving M. P., Purkiss S. C., Tadros T. F., and Davis S. S. (1994).

Surface modification of poly(lactide-co-glycolide) nanospheres by biodegradable poly(lactide)-poly(ethylene glycol) copolymers, *Pharm. Res.*, **11**, pp. 1800–1808.

190. Stolink S., Heald C. R., Neal J., Garnett M. C., Davis S. S., Illum L., Purkis S. C., Barlow R. J., and Gellert P. R. (2001). Polylactide-poly(ethylene glycol) micellar-like particles as potential drug carriers: production, colloidal properties and biological performance, *J. Drug Targeting*, **9**, pp. 361–378.

191. Sun W., Xie C., Wang H., and Hu Y. (2004). Specific role of polysorbate 80 coating on the targeting of nanoparticles to the brain, *Biomaterials*, **25**, pp. 3065–3071.

192. Swindler D. R. and Erwin J. (eds) (1986). *Comparative Primate Biology*, New York: Alan R. Liss.

193. Taylor E. M., Crowe A., and Morgan E. H. (1991). Transferrin and iron uptake by the brain: effects of altered iron status, *J. Neurochem.*, **57**, pp. 1584–1592.

194. Torchilin V. P. (1998). Polymer-coated long-circulating microparticulate pharmaceuticals, *J. Microencapsul.*, **15**, pp. 1–19.

195. Torchilin V. P. (2006). Multifunctional nanocarriers, *Adv. Drug Del. Rev.*, **58**, pp. 1532–1555.

196. Tosi G., Costantino L., Rivasi F., Ruozi B., Leo E., Vergoni A. V., Tacchi R., Bertolini A., Vandelli M. A., and Forni F. (2007). Targeting the central nervous system: *in vivo* experiments with peptide-derivatized nanoparticles loaded with loperamide and rhodamine-123, *J. Control. Re*lease, **122**, pp. 1–9.

197. Tosi G., Costantino L., Ruozi B., Forni F., and Vandelli M. A. (2008). Polymeric nanoparticles for the drug delivery to the central nervous system, *Exp. Opin. Drug Del.*, **5**, pp. 155–174.

198. Trinder D., Morgan E. H., and Baker E. (1988). The effects of an antibody to the rat transferrin receptor and of rat serum albumin on the uptake of diferric transferrin by rat hepatocytes, *Biochim. Biophys. Acta*, **943**, pp. 440–446.

199. Tröester S. D. and Kreuter J. (1992). Influence of the surface properties of low contact angle surfactants on the body distribution of 14C-poly(methyl methacrylate) nanoparticles, *J. Microencaps.*, **9**, pp. 19–28.

200. Tusij A. (2000). *The Blood-Brain Barrier and Drug Delivery to the CNS*, New York: Marcel Dekker.

201. Ueda F., Raja K. B., Simpson R. J., Trowbridge I. S., and Bradbury M. W. (1993). Rate of 59Fe uptake into brain and cerebrospinal fluid and

the influence thereon of antibodies against the transferrin receptor, *J. Neurochem.*, **60**, pp. 106–113.

202. Ulbrich K., Hekmatara T., Herbert E., and Kreuter J. (2009). Transferrin- and transferrin-receptor-antibody-modified nanoparticles enable drug delivery across the blood–brain barrier (BBB), *Eur. J. Pharm. Biopharm.*, **71**, pp. 251–256.

203. Ullrich A., Bell J. R., Chen E. Y., Herrera R., Petruzzelli L. M., Dull T. J., Gray A., Coussens L., Liao Y. C., Tsubokawa M., Mason A., Seeburg P. H., Grunfeld C., Rosen O. M., and Ramachandran J. (1985). Human insulin receptor and its relationship to the tyrosine kinase family of oncogenes, *Nature*, **313**, pp. 756–761.

204. Umezawa F. and Eto Y. (1988). Liposome targeting to mouse brain: mannose as a recognition marker, *Biochim. Biophys. Res. Commun.*, **153**, pp. 1038–1044.

205. Vauthier C., Dubernet C., Chauvierre C., Brigger I., and Couvreur P. (2003). Drug delivery to resistant tumors: the potential of poly(alkyl cyanoacrylate) nanoparticles, *J. Control. Re*lease, **93**, pp. 151–160.

206. Vauthier C., Labarre D., and Poncheli G. (2007). Design aspects of poly(alkylcyanoacrylate) nanoparticles for drug delivery, *J. Drug Targeting*, **15**, pp. 641–663.

207. Verdun C., Brasseur F., Vranckx H., Couvreur P., and Roland M. (1990). Tissue distribution of doxorubicin associated with polyisohexylcyanoacrylate nanoparticles, *Cancer Chemother. Pharmacol.*, **26**, pp. 13–18.

208. Vergoni A. V., Tosi G., Tacchi R., Vandelli M. A., Bertolini A., and Costantino L. (2009). Nanoparticles as drug delivery agents specific for CNS: *in vivo* biodistribution, *Nanomed. Nanotech. Biol. Med.*, doi:10.1016/j.nano.2009.02.005.

209. Verrecchia T., Spenlehauer G., Bazile D. V., Murry-Brelier A., Archimbaud Y., and Veillard M. (1995). Non-stealth (poly(lactic acid/albumin)) and stealth (poly(lactic acid-polyethylene glycol)) nanoparticles as injectable drug carriers, *J. Control. Re*lease, **36**, pp. 49–61.

210. Vinogradov S. V., Batrakova E. V., and Kabanov A. V. (2004). Nanogels for oligonucleotide delivery to the brain, *Bioconjugate Chem.*, **15**, pp. 50–60.

211. Visser C. C., Stefanovic S., Voorwinden L. H., van Bloois L., Gaillard P. J., Danhof M., Crommelin D. J. A., and De Boer A. G. (2005). Targeting liposomes with protein drugs to the blood–brain barrier *in vitro*, *Eur. J. Pharm. Sci.*, **25**, pp. 299–305.

212. Von Burkersroda F., Gref R., and Gopferich A. (1997). Erosion of biodegradable block copolymers made of poly(D,L-lactid acid) and poly(ethylene glycol), *Biomaterials*, **18**, pp. 1599–1607.

213. Vyas S. P., Singh A., and Sihorkar V. (2001). Ligand-receptor mediated drug delivery: an emerging paradigm in cellular drug targeting. *Crit. Rev. Ther. Drug Carr. Syst.*, **189**, pp. 1–76.

214. Wang A. Z., Gu F., Zhang L., Chan J. M., Radovic-Moreno A., Shaikh M. R., and Farokhzad O. C. (2008). Biofunctionalized targeted nanoparticles for therapeutic applications, *Exp. Opin. Biol. Ther.*, **8**, pp. 1063–1070.

215. Wang S., Lee R. J., Cauchon G., Gorenstein D. G., and Low P. S. (1995). Delivery of antisense oligodeoxyribonucleotides against the human epidermal growth factor receptor into cultured KB cells with liposomes conjugated to folate via polyethylene glycol, *Prot. Natl. Acad. Sci.*, **92**, pp. 3318–3322.

216. Waser P. G., Müller U., Kreuter J., Berger S., Munz K., Kaiser E., and Pfluger B. (1987). Localization of colloidal particles (liposomes, hexylcyanoacrylate nanoparticles and albumin nanoparticles) by histology and autoradiography in mice, *Int. J. Pharm.*, **39**, pp. 213–227.

217. Weiss N., Miller F., Cazaubon S., and Couraud P. O. (2009). The blood-brain barrier in brain homeostasis and neurological diseases, *Biochim. Biophys. Acta*, **1788**, pp. 842–857.

218. Weitman S. D., Lark H., Coney L. R., Fort D. W., Frasca V., Zurawski V. R., and Kamen B. A. (1992). Distribution of the folate receptor GP38 in normal and malignant cell lines and tissues, *Cancer Res.*, **52**, pp. 3396–3401.

219. White M. F. (2003). Insulin signaling in health and disease, *Science*, **302**, pp. 1710–1711.

220. Woodcock D. M. (1992). Reversal of multidrug resistance by surfactants, *Br. J. Cancer*, **66**, pp. 62–68.

221. Wu D. and Pardridge W. M. (1996). CNS pharmacologic effect in conscious rats after intravenous injection of a biotinylated vasoactive intestinal peptide analogue coupled to a blood–brain barrier drug delivery system, *J. Pharmacol. Exp. Ther.*, **279**, pp. 77–83.

222. Wu D., Yang J., and Pardridge W. M. (1997). Drug targeting of a peptide radiopharmaceutical through the primate blood–brain barrier *in vivo* with a monoclonal antibody to the human insulin receptor, *J. Clin. Invest.*, **100**, pp. 1804–1812.

223. Wu D. and Pardridge W. M. (1998). Pharmacokinetics and blood–brain barrier transport of an anti-transferrin receptor monoclonal antibody (OX26) in rats after chronic treatment with the antibody, *Drug Metab. Dispos.*, **26**, pp. 937–939.

224. Wu D. and Pardridge W. M. (1999). Neuroprotection with non-invasive neurotrophin delivery to brain, *Proc. Natl. Acad. Sci.*, **96**, pp. 254–259.

225. Xie Y., Ye L., Zhang X., Cui W., Lou J., Nagai T., and Hou X. (2005). Transport of nerve growth factor encapsulated into liposomes across the blood-brain barrier: *in vitro* and *in vivo* studies, *J. Control. Re*lease, **105**, pp. 106–119.

226. Yagi K., Naoi M., and Arichi S. (1982). Incorporation of enzyme into the brain by means of liposomes of novel composition, *J. Appl. Biochem.*, **4**, pp. 121–125.

227. Yamauchi K., Tozuka M., Hidaka H., Hidaka E., Kondo Y., and Katsuyama T. (1999). Characterization of apolipoprotein E-containing lipoproteins in cerebrospinal fluid: effect of phenotype on the distribution of apolipoprotein E, *Clin. Chem.*, **45**, 1431–1438.

228. Yamazaki T., Sato Y., Hanai M., Mochimaru J., Tsujino I., Sawada U., and Horie T. (2000). Non-ionic detergent tween 80 modulates VP-16 resistance in classical multidrug resistant K562 cells viaenhancement of VP-16 influx, *Cancer Lett.*, **149**, pp. 153–161.

229. Yang S. C., Zhu J. B., Lu Y., Liang B. W., and Yang C. Z. (1999a). Body distribution of camptothecin solid lipid nanoparticles after oral administration, *Pharm. Res.*, **16**, pp. 751–757.

230. Yang S. C., Lu L. F., Cai Y., Zhu J. B., Liang B. W., and Yang C. Z. (1999b). Body distribution in mice of intravenously injected camptothecin solid lipid nanoparticles and targeting effect on brain, *J. Control. Re*lease, **59**, pp. 299–307.

231. Yellen B. B., Forbes Z. G., Halverson D. S., Fridman G., Barbee K. A., Chorny M., Levy R., and Friedman G. (2005). Targeted drug delivery to magnetic implants for therapeutic applications, *J. Magn. Magn. Mater.*, **293**, pp. 647–654.

232. Zara G. P., Cavalli R., Bargoni A., Fundaro A., Vighetto D., and Gasco M. R. (2002). Intravenous administration to rabbits of non-stealth and stealth doxorubicin loaded solid lipid nanoparticles at increasing concentrations of stealth agent: pharmacokinetics and distribution of doxorubicin in brain and other tissues, *J. Drug Targeting*, **10**, pp. 327–335.

233. Zhang X., Xie J., Li S., Wang X., and Hou X. (2003). The study on brain targeting of the anphotericin B liposomes, *J. Drug Targeting*, **11**, pp. 117–122.

234. Zhang Y., Lee H. J., Boado R. J., and Pardridge W. M. (2002a). Receptor-mediated delivery of an antisense gene to human brain cancer cells, *J. Gene Med.*, **4**, pp. 183–194.

235. Zhang Y., Zhu C., and Pardridge W. M. (2002b). Antisense gene therapy of brain cancer with an artificial virus gene delivery system, *Mol. Ther.*, **6**, pp. 67–72.

236. Zhang Y., Schlachetzki F., and Pardridge W. M. (2003a). Global non viral gene transfer to the primate brain following intravenous administration, *Mol. Ther.*, **7**, pp. 11–18.

237. Zhang Y., Calon F., Zhu C., Boado R., and Pardridge W. M. (2003b). Intravenous non viral gene therapy causes normalization of striatal tyrosine hydroxylase and reversal of motor impairment in experimental Parkinsonism, *Hum. Gene Ther.*, **14**, pp. 1–12.

238. Zhang Y., Schlachetzki F., Zhang Y. F., Boado R. J., and Pardridge W. M. (2004). Normalization of striatal tyrosine hydroxylase and reversal of motor impairment in experimental parkinsonism with intravenous non viral gene therapy and a brain specific promoter, *Human Gene Ther.*, **15**, pp. 339–350.

239. Zhang Y. and Pardrdge W. M. (2008). Near complete rescue of experimental parkinson's desease with intravenous, non-viral GDNF gene terapy, *Pharm. Res.*, **26**, pp. 1059–1063.

Chapter 4

Pegylated Zinc Protoporphyrin: A Micelle-Forming Polymeric Drug for Cancer Therapy

Jun Fang,[a] Hideaki Nakamura,[a] Takahiro Seki,[a] Haibo Qin,[a,b] G. Y. Bharate,[a,c] and Hiroshi Maeda[a,c,d,*]

[a]*Laboratory of Microbiology & Oncology, Faculty of Pharmaceutical Sciences, Sojo University, Ikeda 4-22-1, Kumamoto 860-0082, Japan*
Departments of [b]Applied Microbiology and [c]Applied Chemistry, School of Engineering, Sojo University, Ikeda 4-22-1, Kumamoto 860-0082, Japan
[d]*Bio-Dynamics Research Laboratory, Kumamoto University Cooperative Research Center 2081-7 Tabaru, Mashiki-machi, Kumamoto 861-2202, Japan*
*hirmaeda@ph.sojo-u.ac.jp

4.1 Introduction

Cancer has been the first or second main cause of death of humans in developed countries in the past few decades. Great many efforts have been undertaken for the control of cancer; toward this goal, chemotherapy plays an important role. However, the decisive effect against cancer was limited, although so many anticancer drugs have been developed. One of the major problems that limit successful cancer chemotherapy is the lack of selectivity to tumors; instead, these agents also cause damage to normal tissues and organs, which induces adverse effects to certain organs, leading to dose-limiting toxicity. To overcome these obstacles, since the 1970s, many strategies have been challenged to make anticancer drugs more selective to tumors. One method to achieve this goal is to utilize antibodies directed to specific tumor epitopes of certain proteins or

Nanotechnology in Health Care
Edited by Sanjeeb K. Sahoo

ISBN 978-981-4267-21-2 (Hardcover), 978-981-4267-35-9 (eBook)
www.panstanford.com

enzymes, such as trastuzumab, rituximab, radiolabeled antibodies ibritumomab, tiuxetan (Zevalin), tositumomab (Bexxar), and bevacizumab (Avastin) [1]. These drugs exhibit promising anticancer effects with lesser toxicity in mice tumor models compared to conventional anticancer drugs. However, it is now realized that the success rate or response rate of these molecular target drugs is no better than 10% in clinical settings. Although some success is seen in imatinib (Gleevec), most of the advanced molecular target drugs are disappointing. Factors causing therapeutic failure are mostly related to the heterogeneity of tumor antigens and, secondly, the emergence of resistant subclones. Recent progress in cancer genomics showed that excessively high incidence of mutation occurred in cancer genomes [2–5]. In addition, there may be the likelihood that the tumor-associated antigens are shed into the blood circulation. As a result, the antibody might encounter the tumor antigens before it reaches the target tumor, and hence the therapeutic efficacy will be reduced, if not abolished.

In the 1980s, Matsumura and Maeda marked a major break through in the development of anticancer drugs. They discovered another approach to selective targeting of anticancer drugs to tumors, based on the unique pathophysiological characteristics of tumor vasculature. They found that compared with normal tissues, tumor has highly leaky blood vessels as well as poor lymphatic recovery. Accordingly, macromolecules with molecular weight larger than 40 kDa will be delivered to the tumor interstitium selectively as a result of extravasation (or leakiness), and they will remain there for long time. They called the phenomenon the enhanced permeability and retention (EPR) effect of macromolecules and lipids in solid tumor tissues [6–14].

Poly(styrene-co-maleic acid-half-*n*-butylate) [SMA]-conjugated neocarzinostatin (NCS), or SMANCS, developed by Maeda *et al.*, is the first clinically approved polymeric drug that takes advantage of the EPR effect. They showed that SMANCS has a long plasma half-life and pronounced tumor-targeting efficiency, showing dramatic therapeutic effect against primary hepatoma, with much better survival scores, and, especially a notable improved quality of life with very few side effects compared with conventional anticancer drugs [6–9]. Afterward, many polymeric drugs with EPR effects were developed, some of which are now in clinical use or in clinical trials, such as Doxil (stealth liposomes containing doxorubicin) and poly-L-glutamic acid conjugates and micellar nanoparticles of paclitaxel, camptothecin, and cisplatin [15]. The EPR effect is thus becoming a gold standard for the design and development of new anticancer drugs [8, 12, 13].

In this chapter, we will describe a promising polymeric drug candidate pegylated zinc protoporphyrin (PZP), which we developed more recently and which can take advantage of the EPR effect. We describe herein the synthesis, parmakoninetics, and *in vitro* and *in vivo* anticancer effect. The versatile modes of actions of PZP such as the depletion of the antioxidative system in tumor cells (oxidation therapy), photodynamic therapy (PDT), and oncogene-related anticancer mechanisms will also be discussed.

4.2 Tumor-Targeted Oxidation Therapy Based on the EPR Effect

In our laboratory, we have investigated a unique antitumor strategy by utilizing cytotoxic reactive oxygen species (ROS) to kill cancer cells, which are termed "oxidation therapy" [16–20]. For the induction of ROS in a tumor, one method is to use ROS-generating enzymes, for example D-amino acid oxidase (DAO) or xanthine oxidase (XO); another method is the inhibition of the antioxidant system in the tumor. For this sample, we developed PZP to inhibit an important antioxidant enzyme heme oxygenase-1 (HO-1, also called HSP32 and survival factor) in the tumor. In both systems, the therapeutic principles are macromolecules through polymer conjugation, which take advantage of the EPR effect.

ROS are oxygen-derived species with unpaired valence electrons, including superoxide anion (O_2•–), hydroxyl radicals (•OH), hydrogen peroxide (H_2O_2), singlet oxygen, alkylperoxides, and hypochloride (HCLO). They are generally highly reactive molecules and potentially hazardous endogenous products. ROS involves various cellular functions and is indispensable for cell growth and development as well as drug metabolism [21, 22]. On the other hand, because of its highly reactive nature, ROS can react quickly and modify or damage various molecules in cells, including proteins [23], nucleic acids [24], and lipids [25]. The results induce cell death in one way or the other. There are a variety of antioxidative defense systems in cells to counteract the insults of ROS to cells under physiological conditions and thus diminish the toxicity of ROS. Some of these antioxidative systems are superoxide dismutase (SOD), catalase, glutathione peroxidase, and thioredoxin. There are also other enzymes or compounds that scavenge the free radicals directly or indirectly (e.g., HO-1, ascorbate, tocopherol, and glutathione), by which the cellular ROS insults are reduced to nontoxic level [26]. It is very intriguing on the contrary that cancer cells are more frequently deficient in many crucial antioxidative enzymes, such as catalase, glutathione peroxidase, and SOD [27–31], whereas HO-1, on the contrary, is upregulated, probably serving as a major antioxidative defense enzyme in tumors, where potent antioxidant bilirubin is generated from biliverdin, a product of heme metabolism by HO-1. This means tumor cells may be highly vulnerable to ROS in theory if HO-1 is suppressed. We showed this hypothesis is valid by *in vitro* experiments using various normal and tumor cells [31]. In concordant to this notion, many conventional anticancer drugs, including neocarzinostatin, vinblastine, doxorubicin, camptothecin, cisplatin, and inostamycin, exhibit antitumor activity via ROS generation if not totally [32].

Under these circumstances, the above-mentioned oxidation therapy was developed. In that system, we further improved this antitumor strategy by utilizing macromolecular agents that will target tumor more selectively, that is, pegylated DAO (PEG-DAO), pegylated XO (PEG-XO), and PZP [16–20, 33, 34]. These agents are either ROS-generating systems or inhibitors of antioxidant enzyme HO-1, all of which will eventually damage tumor cells. In this chapter, we will focus on PZP, which inhibits HO-1 (HSP32) activity in tumors.

4.3 PEG-Zinc Protoporphyrin (PZP): A Micellar Form of HO-1 Inhibitor with Potential Anticancer Activity

4.3.1 HO-1 (HSP32) as an Anticancer Target and Use of Zinc Protoporphyrin

HO is a key enzyme of heme degradation, generating biliverdin, carbon monoxide (CO), and free iron [35, 36]. Biliverdin is subsequently reduced to bilirubin by biliverdin reductase (Fig. 4.1). Three isoforms of HO have been identified in mammalian cells: HO-1, HO-2, and HO-3 [35], among which HO-1 is the inducible form enzyme, which is however highly expressed in the liver and spleen. More important, it is known that HO-1 plays important roles in cell growth and cell death, by protecting cells against harmful oxidative stress and apoptosis [35]. HO-1 induction is triggered by a variety of stress or stimuli, including hypoxia, heavy metals, heme compound,

UV irradiation, ROS such as H_2O_2, and nitric oxide (NO) [35, 37, 38]. The mechanism of the antioxidative and antiapoptotic effects of HO-1 is proposed to be multiple: (i) decreasing the prooxidant level (heme) through heme degradation; (ii) increasing the antioxidant level (bilirubin); (iii) producing the antioxidative, antiapoptotic molecule CO; and (iv) inducing ferritin, which removes and detoxifies free ferric ion, a potent catalyzer of hydroxyl radical generation [35, 39] (Fig. 4.1).

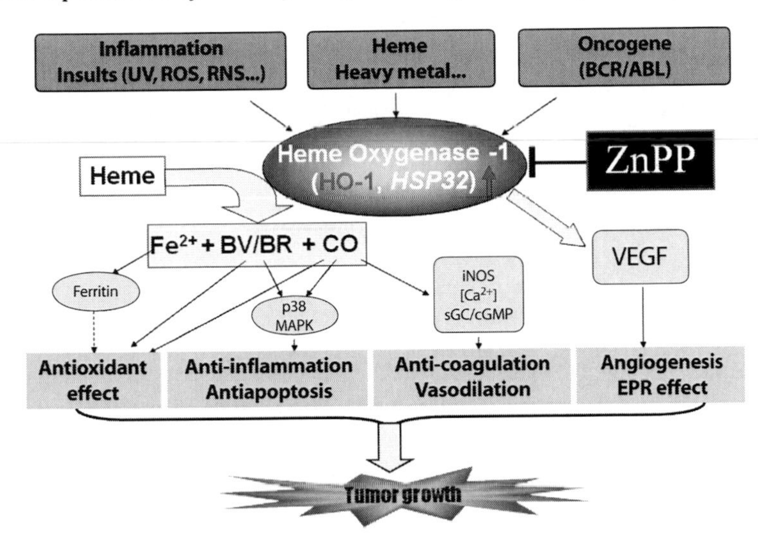

Figure 4.1 A schematic representation of the cytoprotective role of HO-1 and mechanisms of the antitumor effect of ZnPP. Heme oxygenase-1 (HO-1, HSP32) is induced by various stimuli, including ROS, heme, and heavy metal; its expression is also involved in the oncogene BCR/ABL pathway. Upregulated HO-1 subsequently results in increased production of bilirubin, carbon monoxide (CO), and free iron through the degradation of heme. Bilirubin and CO exhibit potent antioxidative activity and also show antiapoptotic and anticoagulation activity via different signaling cascades. Free iron also shows antioxidative effect by inducing ferritin expression. HO-1 itself is also involved in VEGF-induced angiogenesis. Taken together, tumor growth is greatly enhanced through HO-1 expression. Thus, the inhibition of HO-1 activity by use of the inhibitor ZnPP becomes a promising anticancer therapy. (Abbreviations used: BV, biliverdin; BR, bilirubin; CO, carbon monoxide; VEGF, vascular endothelial growth factor; ZnPP, zinc protoporphyrin. (Modified from Ref. 35 with permission.) See also Color Insert.

Therefore, under physiological condition, HO-1 serves as a key enzyme to defend against oxidative stress [35, 36], which is beneficial for cell growth and survival. However, on the contrary, it is also known to play crucial roles in many tumors of both humans and experimental animals, to support tumor growth by virtue of its antiapoptotic and antioxidative effects [35, 37, 38, 40, 41]. In this context, HO-1 is thus considered to be a survival factor of tumor cells and can be a target for cancer treatment. In other words, the impairment or inhibition of this crucial defensive enzyme in tumor cells would be a potential therapeutic target, which is the second approach in oxidation therapy. This antitumor strategy was confirmed to be effective in many experimental solid tumors with use of HO inhibitor zinc protoporphyrin (ZnPP), especially its pegylated derivative [37, 38, 41, 42, and unpublished data] as a novel anticancer drug.

4.3.2 Synthesis and Physiochemical Characteristics of PZP

One problem with free ZnPP is its poor water solubility *per se* for injection. To overcome this drawback, a pegylated ZnPP (PZP) was synthesized, which not only exhibits good water solubility, but also forms micelle of macromolecular nature in aqueous solution, thus achieving tumor-seeking capability by the EPR effect [40, 41].

4.3.2.1 Synthesis and micelle formation of PZP

A scheme of synthesis of PZP is shown in Fig. 4.2. Two carboxyl groups on the protoporphyrin IX ring are relatively inactive for conjugation, so we introduced a spacer using ethylene diamine in protoporphyrin IX, and the two amino groups introduced become the target of pegylation by succinimidyl polyethylene glycol (PEG). Subsequently, zinc was inserted into the protoporphyrin ring in a chloroform solution using zinc acetate, resulting in PZP.

The molecular weight of PZP depends on the size of the PEG used, that is, ~11 kDa when a PEG chain of Mw 5 kDa was used. However, its apparent molecular size in a physiological aqueous solution was found to be larger than 70 kDa based on gel chromatography on Sephadex G-75 column [40]. This suggests that PZP formed micelles in the aqueous solution and it is a multimolecular complex, where a core of hydrophobic ZnPP may be clustered together with a hydrophilic PEG chain stretching outward (Fig. 4.2). Moreover, in a recent study, PZP made of PEG of 2 kDa showed an apparent molecular weight of 115 kDa in an aqueous solution, by Sephacryl HR 200 chromatography (Fig. 4.3A and B), whereas the dynamic light scattering of this PZP showed a hydrodynamic diameter of about 180 nm (Fig. 4.3C). These findings strongly indicate the multimolecular formation of PZP micelles.

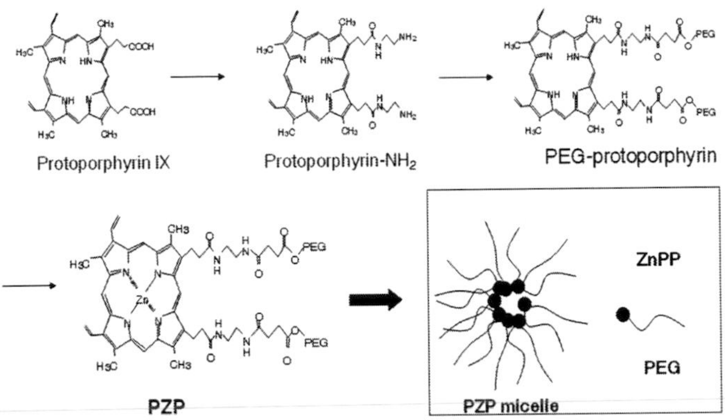

Protoporphyrin IX → Protoporphyrin-NH_2 → PEG-protoporphyrin

→ PZP ➡ PZP micelle (ZnPP, PEG)

Figure 4.2 A scheme of PEG-ZnPP synthesis and micelle formation of PZP. •, ZnPP; ~, PEG chain. Head group of ZnPP (•) clustered together to from micelle. (Reproduced from Ref. 40 with permission.)

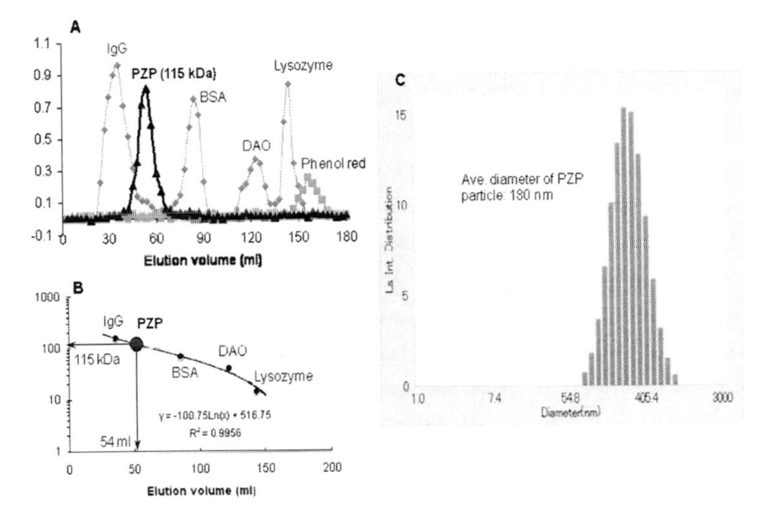

Figure 4.3 Sephadex chromatography (A), plotting of elution volume vs. Mw (B), and dynamic light scattering (C) of PZP. In (A), Sephadex G-100 gel chromatography of PZP was performed using known molecular size protein markers as reference standards (IgG, human immunoglobulin, 155 kDa; BSA, bovine serum albumin, 68 kDa; DAO, D-amino acid oxidase, 39 kDa; lysozyme, 14 kDa). Molecular weight vs. elution volume curve was drawn in (B), and the molecular weight of PZP was calculated. The eluent solution used is bicarbonate buffer (50 mM, pH 8.2) with a flow rate of 55 ml/h. Absorbance at 280 nm was utilized for IgG, BSA, DAO, and lysozyme; 420 nm is for PZP; and 560 nm is for phenol red. (C) Dynamic light scattering of PZP in PBS at 25°C. The concentration of PZP was 2 mg/ml.

4.3.2.2 Spectroscopy of PZP

The UV spectrum of PZP is shown in Fig. 4.4A. Before zinc chelation, the PEG-protoporphyrin conjugate shows a peak absorption at 406 nm accompanying minor four bands of 505, 540, 575, and 627 nm in the visible region, which correspond to the Soret band and bands numbered I (627 nm), II (575 nm), III (540 nm), and IV (505 nm), respectively, for the protoporphyrin ring as reported previously [43]. After zinc insertion, a red shift (422 nm) of the Soret band was observed in PZP, compared to PEG-protoporphyrin (Fig. 4.4A). In addition, a marked difference was also found in the visible region. In other words, four minor bands (I~IV) in protoporphyrin in PZP become two bands at 548 and 584 nm (Fig. 4.4A). These findings are consistent with a previous report that divalent metal insertion into a porphyrin ring induces a red shift of the Soret band and the formation of two minor peaks, alpha (584 nm) and beta (548 nm) [43]. Furthermore, the spectrum of PZP showed good agreement with free ZnPP (Fig. 4.4A). These results suggested zinc was chelated into the protoporphyrin ring.

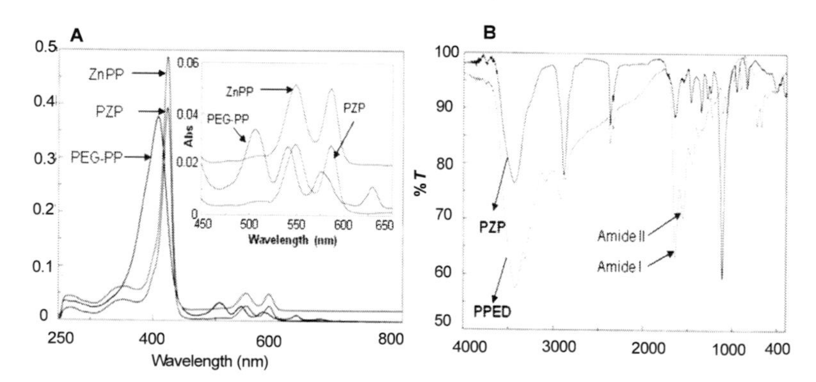

Figure 4.4 UV spectra (A) and IR spectra (B) of PZP. Samples are dissolved in dimethyl sulfoxide for UV detection at 2 μM (ZnPP or protoporphyrin equivalent). Inset of (A) shows the amplified absorption UV spectra from 450 nm to 650 nm. PEG-PP represents PEG conjugated protoporphyrin. In (B), after the reaction of protoporphyrin with ethylene diamine, clear appearance of amide I (1641 cm^{-1}) and amide II (1552 cm^{-1}) was observed in bis(ethylenediamine) protoporphyrin (PPED). In PZP, excess amount of PEG over amide bond overshadowed the absorption of amide I and II. See also Color Insert.

The formation of an amide bond in protoporphyrin was demonstrated by infrared spectroscopy. After introducing amide groups via ethylene diamine onto the two carboxyl groups of protoporphyrin, clear peaks corresponding to amide I (1641 cm^{-1}) and amide II (1552 cm^{-1}) were observed [40] (Fig. 4.4B).

4.3.2.3 Stability of PZP micelles

As mentioned above, PZP forms micelles in aqueous solutions, as evidenced by gel permeation chromatography showing an apparent solution behavior size of 115 kDa and dynamic light scattering showing a mean particle size of 180 nm. This was further supported by a study using fluorescence spectroscopy. Free ZnPP in DMSO showed a strong fluorescence at 580–620 nm upon excitation at 420 nm; similarly, intense fluorescence was observed for PZP when dissolved in DMSO where no micelles would be formed. However, when dissolved in aqueous solutions, the fluorescence of PZP was almost quenched (Fig. 4.5A). This suggests that PZP behaves as a micellar structure in an aqueous solution and its π–π interaction quenches fluorescence due to energy transfer. Similar phenomena have been reported for the micellar drugs using styrene maleic acid copolymer (SMA) containing doxorubicin, pirarubicin, and ZnPP, in our previous work [42, 44–46]. The micelle formation of PZP in aqueous solutions is considered the consequence of self-assembly of porphyrins, as reported before, in which noncovalent interaction, including hydrogen bonding, electrostatic interactions, and van der Waals interaction, plays major roles in complex formation and contributes to the stability of the micelle [47]. The formation of supramolecular assemblies through the self-association of a PEG conjugate in an aqueous medium was also found in several other block copolymers containing PEG and other polymers, such as polyaspartic acid or propylene oxide [48–51].

Using fluorescence spectroscopy, we investigated the stability of PZP micelles in various buffers with different pHs (phosphate buffer between pH 6.0 to 11.0). As shown in Fig. 4.5B, the quenched states of fluorescence intensity of PZP were observed over the range from pH 6.0 to pH 10.5, indicating the compact micellar structures that are stable over this pH range. Above this pH range, a significant increase in fluorescence intensity was found, suggesting the disruption of micelles and thus the rapid release of ZnPP as free form (Fig. 4.5B). Accordingly, the inflection point for PZP was calculated as pH 11.0 ± 0.3.

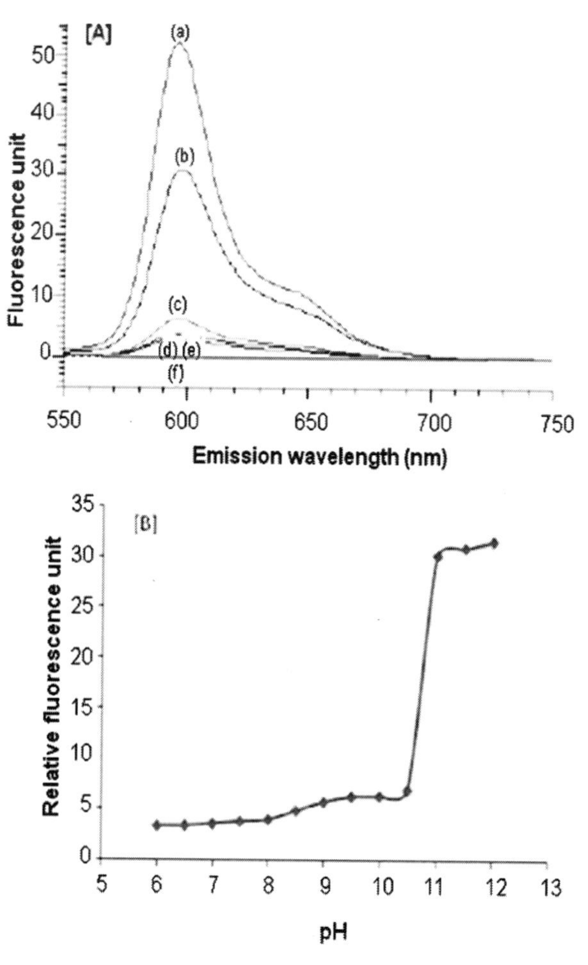

Figure 4.5 Fluorescence emission spectra of PZP in different solutions (A) and the stability of PZP micelle as seen by the increase of fluorescence spectra (B). Fluorescence spectra were recorded with excitation at 420 nm (corresponding to ZnPP) and emission from 550 nm to 750 nm. The concentration for each measurement of PZP or ZnPP was 1 μM. (A) shows the fluorescence spectra of ZnPP and PZP in 0.1 M sodium phosphate buffer with different pHs: (a) ZnPP at pH 7.5; (b) PZP at pH 11.0; (c) PZP at pH 9.5; (d) PZP at pH 7.5; (e) PZP at pH 6.5; and (f) PZP in deionized water. In (B), the degradation of PZP micelles is seen by the generation of fluorescence intensity (at 596 nm) at different pHs, indicating the micelles are disrupted above pH 10.5.

4.3.2.4 Inhibitory activity of PZP against HO-1

It is also important for PZP to have potent HO-1 inhibitory activity. As expected, PZP exhibited comparable HO inhibition activity with K_i of 0.12 μM, comparable to free ZnPP (K_i of 0.11 μM) [40]. However, a preincubation time of about 30 min or longer was needed to achieve complete inhibitory activity for PZP, which suggested that ZnPP must be liberated from PZP. That would compete with the substrate binding site in HO-1. For a higher HO-1 inhibitory activity of PZP, enzymatic cleavage of the amide bond between ZnPP and PEG is considered necessary. Because there are many protease (e.g., catepsin) in tumor tissues [52], which can cleave the amide bond, PZP will undergo cleavage after being internalized in tumors, to exhibit HO-1 inhibitory activity more quickly and tightly after releasing free ZnPP.

4.3.3 Biological Characteristics of PZP

4.3.3.1 Tumor cell selective cytotoxicity

The most desirable anticancer drugs are those that can kill cancer cells selectively without cytotoxicity to normal cells. One way to achieve this is to find out the target molecules that exist selectively in tumor cells, which is the subject of molecular targeted therapy. In this context, HO-1 is a good candidate because it is highly expressed in tumor cells *in vivo* and is a very important molecule for tumor survival [35, 37, 38]. In contrast, normal cells usually do not express HO-1 to that level. Our *in vitro* cytotoxicity assay supported this hypothesis — when compared with normal cells, tumor cells were found about three- to tenfold more susceptible to PZP treatment (Table 4.1).

Compared with the commonly used anticancer drugs, PZP behaves as macromolecules in aqueous milieu, as mentioned above (Fig. 4.3), and as a nanosized micelle, PZP thus exhibited superior *in vivo* pharmacokinetics (longer plasma residence time) and tumor accumulation (EPR effect), as discussed below in detail. These features of PZP will further increase tumor selectivity, greatly enhancing its antitumor efficacy and safety.

Table 4.1 Cytotoxic IC_{50} of PZP against normal and tumor cells[a]

Tumor cells	IC_{50} (μM)[b]	Normal cells	IC_{50} (μM)
DLD-1	14	CV-1	≥50
Sk-Hep	16	HBE140	>50
HT-29	5.8	RLF	>200
A431	15	Human hepatocyte	>50
HeLa	11	MDCK	>30
CNE	26.5	HRPE	>50
ES2	13.8		
KYSE-510	13		
ASPC1	12		
Lxc	10.8		
MCF-7	8		
Mean	13.6 ± 1.6	Mean	>50

[a]The cells used are: DLD-1, HT-29, SW480, human colon cancer cells; Sk-Hep, human liver cancer cells; A431, human epidermoid carcinoma cells; HeLa, human cervix cancer cells; CNE, Lxc, human laryngeal cancer cells; ES2, human ovarian cancer cells; KYSE-510, human esophageal cancer cells; MCF-7, human breast cancer cells; ASPC1, human pancreatic cancer cells; CV-1, monkey kidney fibroblast; HBE140, human bronchial epithelial cells; RLF, rat liver fibroblast; HRPE, human retinal pigment epithelial cell; MDCK, Madin-Darby canine kidney epithelial cells.

[b]IC_{50}, 50% inhibitory concentration.

4.3.3.2 *In vivo* pharmacokinetics, tumor uptake, and tissue delivery of PZP

As mentioned above, PZP is a macromolecule whose molecular weight (i.e., 144 kDa) is large enough to exert the EPR effect. As expected, when PZP was administered intravenously, it showed a much longer plasma circulation time of $t_{1/2}$, 40 times longer than nonconjugated free ZnPP [41]. In addition, PZP preferentially accumulated in the solid tumor in murine tumor models (about 5–10 times higher than normal organs at 48 h after an IV injection) due to the EPR effect [41]. More important, the high level of PZP accumulated in the tumor was sustained for a long time, that is, 72 h [41]. Superior *in vivo* pharmacokinetics and tumor-selective accumulation of PZP were also observed in our recently prepared PZP2000 (Fig. 4.6).

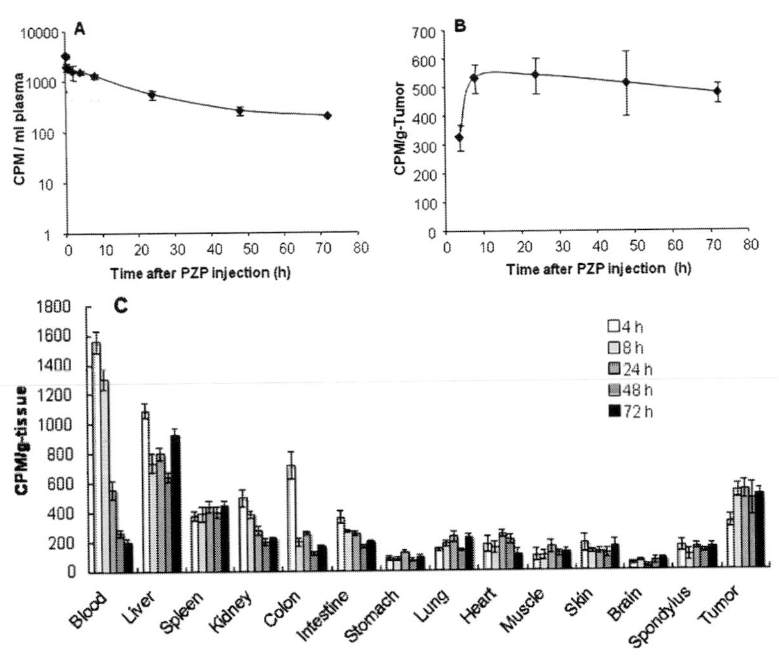

Figure 4.6 Pharmacokinetics of ^{65}Zn radiolabelled PZP with PEG of 2000 Da. (A) the plasma level of PZP after IV injection (about 12,000 cpm/mouse, 3 mg/kg of ZnPP equivalent); (B) intratumor accumulation of PZP after IV injection. (C) shows the body distribution of PZP at different times after IV injection. Results are expressed as means; error bars, ±SE ($n = 3 - 4$).

Many antitumor agents require intracellular uptake for their activities. Most conventional anticancer drugs of low molecular weight enter cells by free diffusion or by transporter of corresponding molecules. However, macromolecular drugs undergo endocytosis as the major mechanism of cellular uptake [53, 54]. Our studies using PZP showed that the uptake of PZP was slower than that of free ZnPP by a flow-cytometry based on the fluorescence of ZnPP that is taken up into the tumor cells (unpublished data). More important, the internalization of PZP gradually increased in a time-dependent manner when cultured at 37°C (Fig. 4.7) [55]. However, at 25°C, the uptake of PZP was significantly slower, and there is almost no uptake at 4°C (unpublished data). In addition, the internalization of PZP was also found localized in the lysosome as revealed by the use of LysoTracker® under a confocal laser microscope (unpublished data). This data clearly showed that the uptake of PZP is an endocytosis-dependent phenomenon.

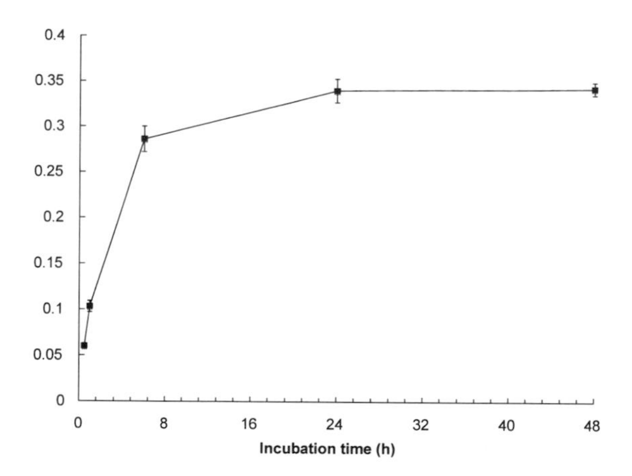

Figure 4.7 The cellular uptake of PZP as observed by fluorescence intensity. K562 CML cells were cultured in RPMI containing 10% fetal calf serum (pH 7.4) at 37°C and treated with PZP (5 μM) for various time periods as indicated. Thereafter, cellular uptake of PZP expressed as μM ZnPP incorporated in 10^6 cells were determined spectrophotometrically. (Modified from Ref. 55 with permission.)

For the development of PZP toward clinical application, ADME (absorption, distribution, metabolism, excretion) of PZP was investigated. As to tissue distribution, PZP was found in high levels in the liver and spleen in addition to the tumor (Fig. 4.6C). This is probably due to the high affinity of heme and its derivatives (i.e., PZP) to these organs (liver and spleen), because they are the major organs for heme catabolism. However, its concentrations in other normal tissues and organs were $1/5 \sim 1/10$ of that in tumors.

Regarding the degradation of PZP *in vivo*, a study of size exclusion chromatography using Bio-Beads S-X1 column with chloroform as eluant was carried out, to detect intact PZP and its degradation products in plasma, urine feces, and various organs, including the ZnPP structure remained intact because it still exhibited the same fluorescence emission spectrum as that of ZnPP. It thus suggests that part of the PEG side chain was cleaved off eventually, resulting in a smaller size of PZP, which was eluted at a later time in the smaller size, which however is still active against HO-1. A similar phenomenon was found both in the liver and tumor (Fig. 4.8A). The degradation of PZP was also detected in the urine during excretion, suggesting that it needs to be further degraded for excretion via the renal route from the body, when compared to the excreted size in feces (Fig. 4.8A).

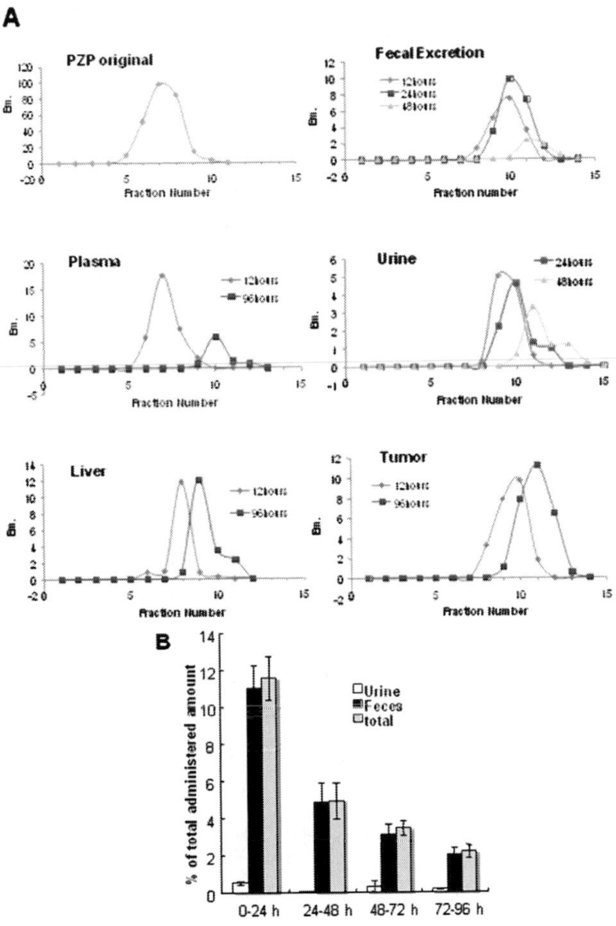

Figure 4.8 The *In vivo* fate of PZP. Degradation (A) and excretion (B) of PZP in tumor-bearing mice were determined by HPLC. For measuring the degradation of PZP in (A), sarcoma S180 bearing ddY mice received IV injection of PZP (20 mg/kg of ZnPP equivalent) followed by the collection of each specimen at 24 h, 48 h, or 96 h. The obtained tissues were then subjected to homogination, chloroform extraction of PZP, and gel chromatography (Bio-Beads® S-X1 column, inner diameter of 11 mm and height of 350 mm; mobile phase, chloroform; flow rate, 40 mL/h). The fluorescence intensity of each fraction (2 mL) was measured at excitation of 420 nm and emission from 550 nm to 700 nm. In (B), for excretion assay, mice received an IV injection of ^{65}Zn radiolabelled PZP (14,000 cpm/mouse,). After the scheduled time, the urine and feces were collected. Radioactivity in each sample was measured by using a gamma counter.

PZP is mainly excreted via the fecal route; about 10% of the PZP was excreted in the first 24 h; then it was excreted in gradually lesser amounts at the rate of about 3–5% per day (Fig. 4.8B).

4.3.3.3 Antitumor effect of PZP

Because of the prolonged circulation time and targeted tumor accumulation (the EPR effect), PZP exerted remarkable antitumor effect in the mouse solid tumor S-180 model [41]. A daily IV injection of PZP for six days resulted in significant growth delay of the S-180 tumor (Fig. 4.9A); two out of seven mice were found tumor free. Meanwhile, no or very little side effects were observed in the blood cell counts, liver biochemistry, kidney functions, and histological examination of various organs, including liver and spleen [41].

Furthermore, when combined with ROS or the ROS-generation system (i.e., PEG-DAO) with this inhibitor of oxystress protecting system (i.e., PZP), we found a synergistic or additive effect between them [56.]. PZP also showed a similar trend with conventional chemotherapeutic agents. That is, PZP-treated SW480 cells *in vitro* became much more vulnerable to the treatment of ROS or ROS-generating anticancer drugs such as doxorubicin and camptothecin [56]. IC_{50} (50% inhibitory concentration) values, when pretreated with PZP, were reduced to 25%, 39%, 83%, and 61% for H_2O_2, t-butyl hydroperoxide, camptothecin, and doxorubicin, respectively. In parallel, a marked *in vivo* antitumor effect was observed for PEG-DAO/D-proline (a substrate of DAO) plus PZP, with only one injection of PZP and three subsequent injections of PEG-DAO/D-proline, both of which were ineffective doses when administered alone (Fig. 4.9B) [56]. This data suggested that the therapeutic potential of combination therapy with conventional low molecular weight anticancer drugs and PZP appears promising. In support of the above hypothesis, we found decreased HO-1 activity by PZP treatment [41] that led to tumor cells more vulnerable to ROS.

4.3.4 Mechanisms Involved in the Antitumor Effect of PZP

4.3.4.1 Induction of apoptosis through inhibition of HO-1 activity

Because HO-1 is a major antioxidative enzyme with a potential antiapoptotic effect and is known as a survival factor [35, 36], the inhibition of HO-1 activity by PZP will result in increased levels of ROS in a tumor, which is mostly generated from infiltrated leukocytes and lead to the apoptosis of tumor cells. As expected, ZnPP- or PZP-treated tumor cells showed an increased amount of apoptosis by use of both TUNEL assay and flow-cytometric assay using Annexin-V, which was further confirmed by the increase of activated capase-3 [38, 41]. An *In vivo* experiment using PZP also showed that PZP significantly induced the apoptosis of tumor cells [41]. A similar finding was obtained with the use of siRNA of HO-1 [41]. The apoptosis-inducing effect of ZnPP/PZP was also reported by other different groups using different cell lines [57, 58].

Regarding the ZnPP- or PZP-induced apoptosis pathway, ROS appears the key molecule, as mentioned above, because when cells were treated with an antioxidant N-acetyl cysteine (NAC) or bilirubin, a potent antioxidant that is one of the major products of heme metabolism by HO, the cell death/apoptosis of tumor cells induced by the PZP was significantly reduced [38, 41.].

Furthermore, a ROS-mediated cellular response factor, apoptosis signal-regulating kinase 1 (ASK1), a member of the mitogen-activated protein kinase kinase kinase (MAPKKK) family, may play a crucial role in the following apoptosis cascade of PZP [59, 60]. That is, the excess of ASK1 that is activated by ROS such as H_2O_2 will activate both p38 and c-Jun N-terminal kinase (JNK) pathway, inducing a wide variety of cellular responses, including apoptosis [59–61].

However, it should be also noted that porphyrin derivatives, such as hemin and hematin as well as ZnPP and PZP, are also potential inducers of HO-1. We did find that HO-1 protein expression in the S-180 solid tumor was increased after PZP treatment [41]. However, the net HO-1 activity in tumor is significantly decreased [41]. This result suggests that the antitumor treatment of PZP will be effective as long as HO-1 activity is inhibited substantially. However, to achieve an optimal antitumor effect, the dose of PZP needs to be optimized to obtain the maximum HO-1 inhibition, preferably less induction of HO-1.

4.3.4.2 New insight into the antitumor mechanisms of PZP involving oncogene

Besides the antitumor mechanism based on the suppression of the antioxidative defense system by inhibiting HO-1 in tumor cells, PZP was found to down regulate the oncogene *BCR/ABL* in chronic

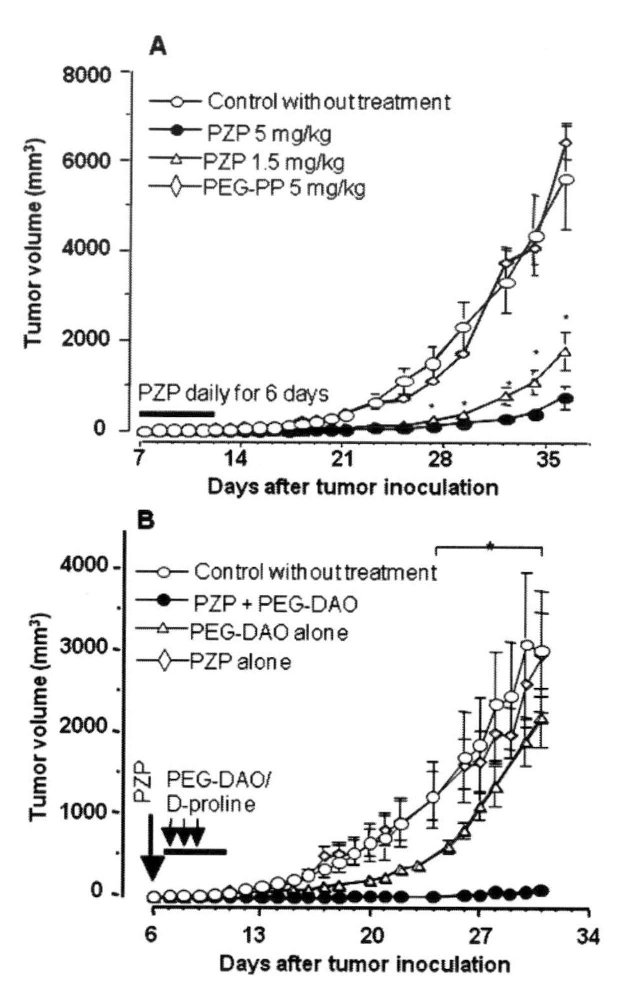

Figure 4.9 The antitumor effect of PZP (A) and PZP plus PEG-DAO (B) in the S180 tumor model. S180 cells (2×10^6 cells) were implanted s.c. in ddY mice. Six to ten days after inoculation, the mice were treated by each agent as indicated in the figure. The dose of PZP is expressed as ZnPP equivalent. The treatment protocol for the combination of PZP and PEG-DAO is that PZP (1.5 mg/kg ZnPP equivalent) was administered and 24 h later, PEG-DAO was injected intravenously for 3 days at a dose of 0.75 unit/mouse; D-proline was injected i.p. 4 h after PEG-DAO administration and, in addition, was injected daily for an extra 2 days after the cessation of PEG-DAO. The data are means ($n = 4 - 8$); bars, SE. *, $P < 0.001$. See references 41 and 56 for details.

myeloid leukemia (CML) cells, resulting in the apoptosis of the CML cells [62, 63]. Moreover, PZP was also found effective both on imatinib (Gleevec)-resistant human CML as well as acute lymphoblastic leukemia (ALL) cells [55, 64]. These findings may suggest the multiple functions of HO-1 (HSP32) and unique mechanisms in cancer chemotherapy.

In addition, there may be other mechanisms for PZP actions involving intracellular zinc signaling, as reported by Hirano *et al.* [65], in which porphyrin may serve as the carrier of zinc, though this needs to be demonstrated.

Accordingly, PZP not only induces ROS-related cytotoxicity via HO-1 inhibition but also leads to cancer cell death via other mechanisms without detrimental toxicity to the host *in vivo*.

4.3.5 PDT: An Enhanced and Unique Antitumor Strategy of PZP

More recently, we found that the antitumor effect of PZP could be greatly enhanced after exposure to visible light but not by a laser beam (i.e., 630 nm for Photofrin®) [42, 66]. In contrast to this laser-based PDT, our method uses a xenon light source or fluorescent bulb of blue light (see below). The mechanism is based on the fact that porphyrin derivatives are efficient photosensitizers generating singlet oxygen ($^1O_2$) upon excitation at about 415 nm [42]. The advantages of PZP over conventional photosensitizer (e.g., Photofrin®) are twofold. One is that ZnPP does not require a laser beam whereas Photofrin® requires a laser beam (at 630 nm). In contrast, with laser-based PDT, ZnPP/PZP generates $^1O_2$ under a conventional xenon light source that has a wider range of wavelength to be absorbed and excite protoporphyrin whereas a laser beam emits single chrometric narrow beam of 1 or 2 nm; thus, the total energy input may not be as high as obtaining sufficient effect (Fig. 4.10). In addition, the absorption maximum of the photosensitizer may not fit to the emission spectrum of the laser. An advantage believed in the laser-based PDT is that its long wavelength would penetrate deep into the tissue. However, we found that conventional endoscope can be a useful light source in our PDT system. The second point is that our photosensitizer PZP predominantly accumulates in tumor tissues so that the adverse side effect on normal skin is much less, while Photofrin®, being of small molecular weight and hydrophobic sensitizer, might accumulate in normal skin and become subject of damage. Thus, ambient room or outdoor light will generate adverse effects on the exposed skin in the case of conventional PDT whereas this adverse effect could be avoided in PZP-based PDT.

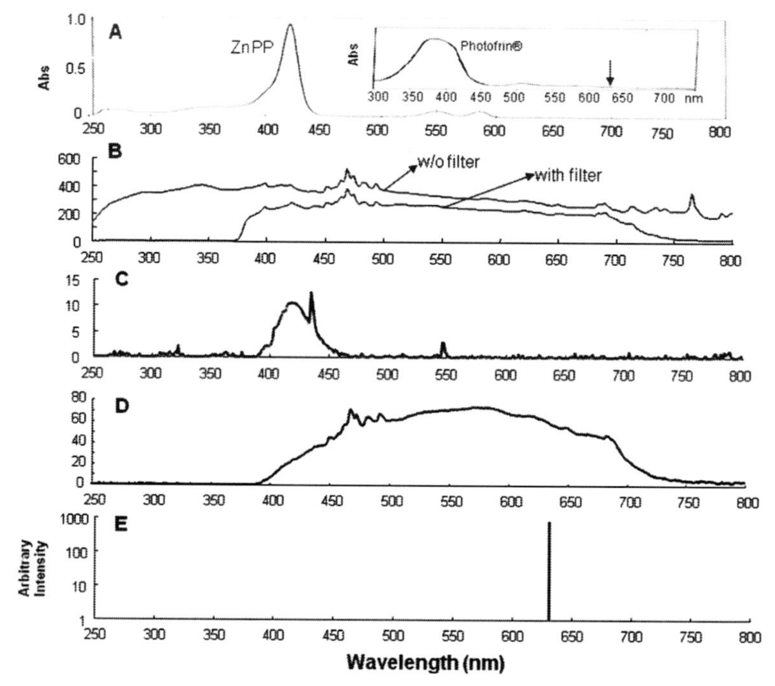

Figure 4.10 The relationship of the absorption and emission spectra of different photosensitizers and irradiating light sources used in PDT. (A) the UV absorption spectrum of ZnPP showing a peak absorbance at about 420 nm and that of photofrin® (inset). The arrow indicates the laser applied in photofrin® PDT. (B), (C), and (D) show the spectra of xenon light (Optical modulex II, Ushio Inc., Tokyo, Japan), a blue fluorescent blue light tube (Philips, TL-D 15W), and the light from endoscope, respectively. (E) is the typical emission spectrum of the laser used for Photofrin® PDT. Both xenon light (Ushio light source and endoscopic light source) and Philips fluorescent light show strong and wide band covering the entire absorption band to excite ZnPP (400–450 nm). The area is far greater than the laser for Photofrin® PDT that has an narrow band and does not fit to the maximum absorption area for the excitation of ZnPP and Photofrin®.

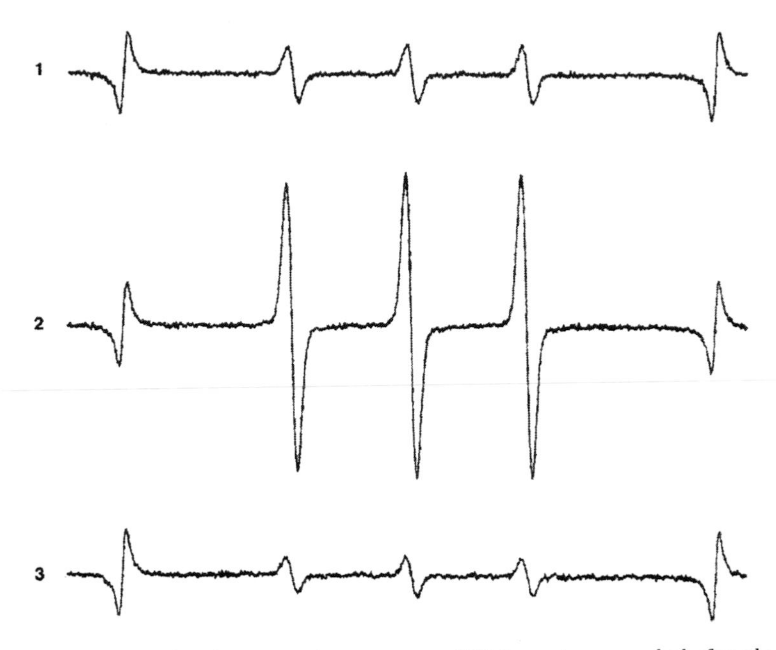

Figure 4.11 The electron spin resonance (ESR) spectra recorded after the irradiation of PZP in the presence of a spin-trapping agent for singlet oxygen hydro-TEMP (4-hydroxy-2,2,6,6-tetramethyl piperidine). (1) The ESR spectrum of an aqueous solution of 30 μM PZP and 50 mM hydroxy-TEMP was recorded before and (2) after irradiation with visible light (tungsten-xenon lamp) having luminous intensity of 50,000 LUX for 5 min. In (3), a solution with the same composition as above was irradiated with visible light in the presence of 5 mM sodium azide, a specific scavenger of singlet oxygen. No significant detection of signal in (3) indicates that the signal derived in (2) is singlet oxygen dependent. (Reproduced from Ref. 42 with permission.)

As expected, ZnPP or PZP efficiently generated highly reactive $^1O_2$ under illumination of visible light, laser, or xenon light (Fig. 4.11) [42, 66]. Under the irradiation of a tungsten xenon light such as the commonly used endoscopic light or the blue fluorescent light tube (Philips, TL-D 15W) having emission primarily above 400 nm, the PDT effect of PZP was investigated *in vivo*. In fact, the latter blue light is used for the treatment of neonatal icterus. PZP *per se* induced marked tumor regression, both in mouse tumor xenograft models and chemically induced rat breast cancers (unpublished data), and similar results were observed when SMA–encapsulated ZnPP micelles (SMA-ZnPP) were used in the same experimental setting [42]. In the same sets of experiments with light (xenon) exposure, results were further far improved [42 and unpublished data]. *In vitro* experiment using cells exposed to the light from a Philips light tube (~20 mW/cm^2/s) for 10 min showed that the IC_{50} of PZP was significantly reduced (i.e., 2.5 μM with light vs. 20 μM without light) (unpublished data). All these findings suggested the applicability of PZP as a new agent for PDT.

With regard to the cost of PDT, the laser apparatus for conventional PDT is very expensive (~500,000 US dollars/unit in Japan), whereas the xenon beam of endoscope is available in any hospital. Therefore, the application of PZP using endoscopic light appears more practical for superficial cancers of such as the esophagus, the breast, the bronchogenic origin (lung), the colon, the urinary bladder, and the cervix.

4.4 Cautions in PZP-Mediated Oxidation Therapy

Regarding oxidation therapy, that is, ROS-mediated antitumor therapy, it should be noted that the biological effects of ROS in cancer are dose-dependent phenomena within certain limits (namely, high levels of oxidative stress exhibit cytotoxicity as mentioned above) whereas low or intermediate levels of oxidative stress are more effective in inducing mutations and promoting proliferation of cells or affecting the signaling system, which ultimately leads to carcinogenesis or tumor progression [67, 68]. Various examples indicate that ROS is a class of endogenous signaling molecules but excess level is cytotoxic or detrimental or carcinogenic by triggering the mutation of the cells [69–71]. In other words, oxidative stress could modulate genetic expression of, for example, epidermal growth factor (EGF), tyrosine phosphorylation, protein kinase C (PKC) [72], and transcription factors, including NF-κB, activator protein 1 (AP-1), and NF-E2-related factor (Nrf2) [73–75], which results in the proliferation of tumor cells, that is, carcinogenesis and tumor metastasis [75, 76]. In addition, as described above, the ASK MAPKKK family also plays a crucial role in ROS-mediated cellular responses. It may also be probably involved in many ROS-mediated human diseases, including cancer [59, 60]. As for these signal transduction pathways, 8-nitroguanosine 3′,5′-cyclic monophosphate (8-nitro-cGMP), which is an NO-dependent nitrated derivative of cGMP, was recently found to play an important role in signal transduction via the S-guanylation of a redox-sensor signaling protein Kelch-like ECH-associated protein 1 (Keap1) [77]. The S-guanylation of Keap1 results in the inactivation of Keap1, which leads to the nuclear export of Nrf2 and the activation of transcriptional activity of Nrf2, to regulate the progression of inflammation and probably cancer.

Accordingly, it is critical to control the level of ROS carefully in oxidation therapy, because insufficient induction of ROS will inversely enhance tumor growth. Indeed, in contrast to our reports about oxidation therapy, Nishikawa *et al.* showed that tumor metastasis could be inhibited with the use of antioxidative enzymes catalase and SOD, by decreasing the ROS levels in tumors [78, 79]. To explain these observations, we anticipated that H_2O_2 modulates the vascular flow [80], the way NO does. It is also likely that the inhibition of reactive nitric species (or NO), which induces the EPR effect, could suppress tumor growth. We found that peroxynitrite (ONOO-) which is a reaction product of NO and O_2•–, could activate matrix metalloproteinase (MMP) [81, 82]. Because MMP is an important factor in tumor metastasis, the inhibition of either NO or O_2•– would suppress tumor metastasis. Taken together, these findings indicated the controversial aspects of ROS in cancer therapy: a high level of ROS (oxidation therapy) is beneficial for tumor treatment but a moderate level of ROS would trigger tumor growth.

4.5 Conclusion

The therapeutic concept based on the EPR effect has a great impact on cancer chemotherapy, that is, the greatly improved pharmacokinetics of polymeric or micellar drugs (e.g., prolonged $t_{1/2}$), and more important, enhanced tumor-targeting efficiency by the EPR effect, which will ensure better therapeutic outcomes with far fewer side effects. As a well-designed example of micellar drug, in this chapter, we focused on our promising antitumor agent PZP. By utilizing polymer conjugation of the active principle, ZnPP, which is an almost water-insoluble agent, it becomes moderately water soluble by forming micelles, making it possible to exert the EPR effect and have better clinical application. The application of PZP could also be extended to combination therapy with conventional anticancer drugs. Further, the advantages of new PDT using a conventional xenon beam light source such as endoscopic exposure were discussed. We thus anticipate the clinical development of PZP for various solid tumors in this direction.

In addition, it is important to note that the antitumor effect of PZP is presumably HO-1 dependent, namely, it kills tumor cells by inhibiting HO-1 activity, thus depriving the antioxidant system in tumor cells and inducing the apoptosis of tumor cells via oxystress. It has been reported that most tumor cells rely on HO-1 for their rapid growth and survival, suggesting it is an ideal target for cancer therapy.

References

1. Allen T. M. (2002). Ligand-targeted therapeutics in anticancer therapy. *Nat. Rev. Cancer*, **2**, pp. 750–763.
2. Sjöblom T., Jones S., Wood L. D., Parsons D. W., Lin J., Barber T. D., Mandelker D., Leary R. J., Ptak J., Silliman N., Szabo S., Buckhaults P., Farrell C., Meeh P., Markowitz S. D., Willis J., Dawson D., Willson J. K., Gazdar A. F., Hartigan J., Wu L., Liu C., Parmigiani G., Park B. H., Bachman K. E., Papadopoulos N., Vogelstein B., Kinzler K. W., and Velculescu V. E. (2006). The consensus coding sequences of human breast and colorectal cancers. *Science*, **314**, pp. 268–274.
3. Lin J., Gan C. M., Zhang X., Jones S., Sjöblom T., Wood L. D., Parsons D. W., Papadopoulos N., Kinzler K. W., Vogelstein B., Parmigiani G., and Velculescu V. E. (2007). A multidimensional analysis of genes mutated in breast and colorectal cancers. *Genome Res.*, **17**, pp. 1304–1318.
4. Wood L. D., Parsons D. W., Jones S., Lin J., Sjöblom T., Leary R. J., Shen D., Boca S. M., Barber T., Ptak J., Silliman N., Szabo S., Dezso Z., Ustyanksky V., Nikolskaya T., Nikolsky Y., Karchin R., Wilson P. A., Kaminker J. S., Zhang Z., Croshaw R., Willis J., Dawson D., Shipitsin M., Willson J. K., Sukumar S., Polyak K., Park B. H., Pethiyagoda C. L., Pant P. V., Ballinger D. G., Sparks A. B., Hartigan J., Smith D. R., Suh E., Papadopoulos N., Buckhaults P., Markowitz S. D., Parmigiani G., Kinzler K. W., Velculescu V. E., and Vogelstein B. (2007). The genomic landscapes of human breast and colorectal cancers. *Science*, **318**, pp. 1108–1113.
5. Leary R. J., Lin J. C., Cummins J., Boca S., Wood L. D., Parsons D. W., Jones S., Sjöblom T., Park B. H., Parsons R., Willis J., Dawson D., Willson J. K.,

Nikolskaya T., Nikolsky Y., Kopelovich L., Papadopoulos N., Pennacchio L. A., Wang T. L., Markowitz S. D., Parmigiani G., Kinzler K. W., Vogelstein B., and Velculescu V. E. (2008). Integrated analysis of homozygous deletions, focal amplifications, and sequence alterations in breast and colorectal cancers. *Proc. Natl. Acad. Sci. USA*, **105**, pp. 16224–16229.

6. Matsumura Y., and Maeda H. (1986). A new concept for macromolecular therapeutics in cancer chemotherapy: mechanism of tumoritropic accumulation of proteins and the antitumor agent SMANCS. *Cancer Res.*, **46**, pp. 6387–6392.
7. Maeda H. (2001). SMANCS and polymer-conjugated macromolecular drugs: advantages in cancer chemotherapy. *Adv. Drug Deliv. Rev.*, **46**, pp. 169–185.
8. Maeda H., Sawa T., and Konno T. (2001). Mechanism of tumor-targeted delivery of macromolecular drugs, including the EPR effect in solid tumor and clinical overview of the prototype polymeric drug SMANCS. *J. Control. Release*, **74**, pp. 47–61.
9. Fang J., Sawa T., and Maeda H. (2003). Factors and mechanism of "EPR" effect and the enhanced antitumor effects of macromolecular drugs including SMANCS. *Adv. Exp. Med. Biol.*, **519**, pp. 29–49.
10. Duncan R. (2003). The dawning era of polymer therapeutics. *Nat. Rev. Drug Discov.*, **2**, pp. 347–360.
11. Maeda H., Greish K., and Fang J. (2006). The EPR effect and polymeric drugs: a paradigm shift for cancer chemotherapy in the 21st century. *Adv. Polym. Sci.*, **193**, pp. 103–121.
12. Vicent M. J., and Duncan R. (2006). Polymer conjugates: nanosized medicines for treating cancer. *Trends Biotechnol.*, **24**, pp. 39–47.
13. Seki T., Fang J., and Maeda H. (2009). Tumor targeted macromolecular drug delivery based on the enhanced permeability and retention effect in solid tumor. In *Pharmaceutical Perspectives of Cancer Therapeutics*, AAPS-Springer Publishing (pp. 93–102).
14. H. Maeda, Bharate G.Y., and Daruwalla J. (2009). Polymeric drugs and nanomedicines for efficient tumor targeted drug delivery based on EPR-effect. *Eur. J. Phar. Biophar.*, **71**, pp. 409–419.
15. Matsumura Y., and Kataoka K. (2009). Preclinical and clinical studies of anticancer agent-incorporating polymer micelles. *Cancer Sci.*, **100**, pp. 572–579.
16. Ben-Yoseph O., and Ross B. D. (1994). Oxidation therapy: the use of a reactive oxygen species-generating enzyme system for tumour treatment. *Br. J. Cancer*, **70**, pp. 1131–1135.

17. Yoshikawa T., Kokura S., Tanaka K., Naito Y., and Kondo M. (1995). A novel cancer therapy based on oxygen radicals. *Cancer Res.*, **55**, pp. 1617–1620.

18. Stegman L.D., Zheng H., Neal E. R., Ben-Yoseph O., Pollegioni L., Pilone M. S., and Ross B. D. (1998). Induction of cytotoxic oxidative stress by D-alanine in brain tumor cells expressing Rhodotorula gracilis D-amino acid oxidase: a cancer gene therapy strategy. *Hum. Gene. Ther.*, **9**, pp. 185–193.

19. Huang P., Feng L., Oldham E. A., Keating M. J., and Plunkett W. (2000). Superoxide dismutase as a target for the selective killing of cancer cells. *Nature*, **407**, pp. 390–395.

20. Fang J., Nakamura H., and Iyer A. K. (2007). Tumor-targeted induction of oxystress for cancer therapy. *J. Drug Targeting*, **15**, pp. 475–486.

21. Davies K. J. (1995). Oxidative stress: the paradox of aerobic life. *Biochem, Soc. Symp.*, **61**, pp. 1–31.

22. Sundaresan M., Yu Z. X., Ferrans V. J., Irani K., and Finkel T. (1995). Requirement for generation of H_2O_2 for platelet-derived growth factor signal transduction. *Science*, **270**, pp. 296–299.

23. Davies K. J. (1993). Protein modification by oxidants and the role of proteolytic enzymes. *Biochem. Soc. Transact.*, **21**, pp. 346–353.

24. Lindahl T. (1993). Instability and decay of the primary structure of DNA. *Nature*, **362**, pp. 709–751.

25. Wagner B. A., Buettner G. R., and Patrick Burns C. (1994). Free radical-mediated lipid peroxidation in cells: oxidizability is a function of cell lipid bis-allyic hydrogen content. *Biochemistry*, **33**, pp. 4449–4453.

26. Demple B., and Harrison L. (1994). Repair of oxidative damage to DNA: enzymology and biology. *Annu. Rev. Biochem.*, **63**, pp. 915–948.

27. Greenstein J. P. (ed.). (1954). *Biochemistry of Cancer*, 2nd edn. Academic Press, New York.

28. Hasegawa Y., Takano T., Miyauchi A., Matsuzuka F., Yoshida H., Kuma K., and Amino N. (2002). Decreased expression of glutathione peroxidase mRNA in thyroid anaplastic carcinoma. *Cancer Lett.*, **182**, pp. 69–74.

29. Yamanaka N., and Deamer D. (1974). Superoxide dismutase activity in WI-38 cell cultures: effect of age, trypsinization and SV-40 transformation. *Physiol. Chem. Phus.*, **6**, pp. 95–106.

30. Sato K., Ito K., Kohara H., Yamaguchi Y., Adachi K., and Endo H. (1992). Negative regulation of catalase gene expression in hepatoma cells. *Mol. Cell Biol.*, **12**, pp. 2525–2533.

31. Fang J., Nakamura H., Deng D. W., Akuta T., Greish K., Iyer A. K., and Maeda H. (2008). Oxystress inducing antitumor therapeutics via

targeted delivery of PEG-conjugated D-amino acid oxidase. *Int. J. Cancer*, **122**, pp. 1135–1144.

32. Simizu S., Takada M., Umezawa K., and Imoto M. (1998). Requirement of caspase-3 (-like) protease-mediated hydrogen peroxide production for apoptosis induced by various anticancer drugs. *J. Biol. Chem.*, **273**, pp. 26900–26907.

33. Sawa T., Wu J., Akaike T., and Maeda H. (2000). Tumor-targeting chemotherapy by a xanthine oxidase-polymer conjugate that generates oxygen-free radicals in tumor tissue. *Cancer Res.*, **60**, pp. 666–671.

34. Fang J., Sawa T., Akaike T., and Maeda H. (2002). Tumor-targeted delivery of polyethylene glycol-conjugated D-amino acid oxidase for antitumor therapy via enzymatic generation of hydrogen peroxide. *Cancer Res.*, **62**, pp. 3138–3143.

35. Fang J., Akaike T., and Maeda H. (2004). Antiapoptotic role of heme oxygenase (HO) and the potential of HO as a target in anticancer treatment. *Apoptosis*, **9**, pp. 27–35.

36. Maines M. D. (1988). Heme oxygenase: function, multiplicity, regulatory mechanisms, and clinical applications. *FASEB J.*, **2**, pp. 2557–2568.

37. Doi K., Akaike T., Fujii S., Tanaka S., Ikebe N., Beppu T., Shibahara S., Ogawa M., and Maeda H. (1999). Induction of haem oxygenase-1 by nitric oxide and ischaemia in experimental solid tumours and implications for tumour growth. *Br. J. Cancer*, **80**, pp. 1945–1951.

38. Tanaka S., Akaike T., Fang J., Beppu T., Ogawa M., Tamura F., Miyamoto Y., and Maeda H. (2003). Antiapoptotic effect of haem oxygenase-1 induced by nitric oxide in experimental solid tumours. *Br. J. Cancer*, **88**, pp. 902–909.

39. Balla G., Jacob H. S., Balla J., Rosenberg M., Nath K., Apple G., Eaton J. W., and Vercellotti G. M. (1992). Ferritin: a cytoprotective antioxidant strategem of endothelium. *J. Biol. Chem.*, **267**, pp. 18148–18153.

40. Sahoo S. K., Sawa T., Fang J., Tanaka S., Miyamoto Y., Akaike T., and Maeda H. (2002). Pegylated zinc portoporphyrin: a water-soluble heme oxygenase inhibitor with tumor-targeting capacity. *Bioconjug. Chem.*, **13**, pp. 1031–1038.

41. Fang J., Sawa T., Akaike T., Akuta T., Sahoo S. K., Greish K., Hamada A., and Maeda H. (2003). *In vivo* antitumor activity of pegylated zinc protoporphyrin: targeted inhibition of heme oxygenase in solid tumor. *Cancer Res.*, **63**, pp. 3567–3674.

42. Iyer A. K., Greish K., Seki T., Okazaki S., Fang J., Takeshita K., and Maeda H. (2007). Polymeric micelles of zinc protoporphyrin for tumor

targeted delivery based on EPR effect and singlet oxygen generation. *J. Drug Targeting*, **15**, pp. 496–506.

43. Falk J. E. (1964). Spectra. *Porphyrins and Metalloporphyrins, Their General, Physical and Coordination Chemistry, and Laboratory Methods*, Elsevier Publishing Company, Amsterdam, pp. 72–84.
44. Iyer A. K., Greish K., Fang J., Murakami R., and Maeda H. (2007). High-loading nanosized micelles of copoly(styrene-maleic acid)-zinc protoporphyrin for targeted delivery of a potent heme oxygenase inhibitor. *Biomaterials*, **28**, pp. 1871–1881.
45. Greish K., Nagamitsu A., Fang J., and Maeda H. (2005). Copoly(styrene-maleic acid)-pirarubicin micelles: high tumor-targeting efficiency with little toxicity. *Bioconjug. Chem.*, **16**, pp. 230–236.
46. Greish K., Sawa T., Fang J., Akaike T., and Maeda H. (2004). SMA-doxorubicin, a new polymeric micellar drug for effective targeting to solid tumours. *J. Control. Release,* **97**, pp. 219–230.
47. Nishide H., Mihayashi K., and Tsuchida E. (1977). Dissociation of aggregated ferroheme complexes and protoporphyrin IX by water soluble polymers. *Biochem. Biophys. Acta*, **498**, pp. 208–214.
48. Harada A. and Kataoka K. (1999). Chain length recognition: core-shell supramolecular assembly from oppositely charged block copolymers. *Science*, **283**, pp. 65–67.
49. Otsuka H., Nagasaki Y., and Kataoka K. (2003). PEGylated nanoparticles for biological and pharmaceutical applications. *Adv. Drug Deliv. Rev.*, **55**, pp. 403–419.
50. Ideta R., Tasaka F., Jang W.-D., Nashiyama N., Zhang G.-D., Harada A., Yanagi Y., Tamaki Y., Aida T., and Kataoka K. (2005). Nanotechnology-based photodynamic therapy for neovascular disease using a supramolecular nanocarrier loaded with a dendritic photosensitizer. *Nano Lett.*, **5**, pp. 2426–2431.
51. Veronese F. M., Schiavon O., Pasut G., Mendichi R., Andersson L., Tsirk A., Ford J., Wu G., Kneller S., Davies J., and Duncan R. (2005). PEG-doxorubicin conjugates: influence of polymer structure on drug release, *in vitro* cytotoxicity, biodistribution and antitumor activity. *Bioconjug. Chem.*, **16**, pp. 775–784.
52. Mohamed M. M., and Sloane B. F. (2006). Cysteine cathepsins: multifunctional enzymes in cancer. *Nat. Rev. Cancer*, **6**, pp. 764–775.
53. Miyamoto Y., Oda T., and Maeda H. (1990). Comparison of the cytotoxic effects of the high- and low-molecular-weight anticancer agents on multidrug-resistant Chinese hamster ovary cells *in vitro*. *Cancer Res.*, **50**, pp. 1571–1575.

54. Harush-Frenkel O., Altschuler Y., and Benita S. (2008). Nanoparticle-cell interactions: drug delivery implications. *Crit. Rev. Ther. Drug Carrier. Syst.*, **25**, pp. 485–544.

55. Mayerhofer M., Gleixner K. V., Mayerhofer J., Hoermann G., Jaeger E., Aichberger K. J., Ott R. G., Greish K., Nakamura H., Derdak S., Samorapoompichit P., Pickl W. F., Sexl V., Esterbauer H., Schwarzinger I., Sillaber C., Maeda H., and Valent P. (2008). Targeting of heat shock protein 32 (Hsp32)/heme oxygenase-1 (HO-1) in leukemic cells in chronic myeloid leukemia: a novel approach to overcome resistance against imatinib. *Blood*, **111**, pp. 2200–2210.

56. Fang J., Sawa T., Akaike T., Greish K., and Maeda H. (2004). Enhancement of chemotherapeutic response of tumor cells by a heme oxygenase inhibitor, pegylated zinc protoporphyrin. *Int. J. Cancer*, **109**, pp. 1–8.

57. Hirai K., Sasahira T., Ohmori H., Fujii K., and Kuniyasu H. (2007). Inhibition of heme oxygenase-1 by zinc protoporphyrin IX reduces tumor growth of LL/2 lung cancer in C57BL mice. *Int. J. Cancer*, **120**, pp. 500–505.

58. Nowis D., Bugajski M., Winiarska M., Bil J., Szokalska A., Salwa P., Issat T., Was H., Jozkowicz A., Dulak J., Stoklosa T., and Golab J. (2008). Zinc protoporphyrin IX, a heme oxygenase-1 inhibitor, demonstrates potent antitumor effects but is unable to potentiate antitumor effects of chemotherapeutics in mice. *BMC Cancer*, **8**, p. 197.

59. Ichijo H., Nishida E., Irie K., ten Dijke P., Saitoh M., Moriguchi T., Takagi M., Matsumoto K., Miyazono K., and Gotoh Y. (1997). Induction of apoptosis by ASK1, a mammalian MAPKKK that activates SAPK/JUK and p38 signaling pathways. *Science*, **275**, pp. 90–94.

60. Matsukawa J., Matsuzawa A., Takeda K., and Ichijo H. (2004). The ASK1-MAP kinase cascades in mammalian stress response, *J. Biochem.*, **136**, pp. 261–265.

61. Fujikawa T., Takeda K., and Ichijo H. (2007). ASK family proteins in stress response and disease. *Mol. Biotechnol.*, **37**, pp. 13–18.

62. Kondo R., Gleixner K. V., Mayerhofer M., Vales A., Gruze A., Samorapoompichit P., Greish K., Krauth M. T., Aichberger K. J., Pickl W. F., Esterbauer H., Sillaber C., Maeda H., and Valent P. (2007). Identification of heat shock protein 32 (Hsp32) as a novel survival factor and therapeutic target in neoplastic mast cells. *Blood*, **110**, pp. 661–669.

63. Hadzijusufovic E., Rebuzzi L., Gleixner K. V., Ferenc V., Peter B., Kondo R., Gruze A., Kneidinger M., Krauth M. T., Mayerhofer M., Samorapoompichit P., Greish K, Iyer A. K., Pickl W. F., Maeda H., Willmann M., and Valent P. (2008). Targeting of heat-shock protein 32/heme oxygenase-1

in canine mastocytoma cells is associated with reduced growth and induction of apoptosis. *Exp. Hematol.*, **36**, pp. 1461–1470.

64. Gleixner K. V., Mayerhofer M., Vales A., Gruze A., Pickl W. F., Lackner E., Sillaber C., Zielinski C. C., Maeda H., and Valent P. (2007). The Hsp32/HO-1-targeted drug SMA-ZnPP counteracts the proliferation and viability of neoplastic cells in solid tumors and hematologic neoplasms. *J. Clin. Oncol.* (meeting abstracts) **25**, p. 14122.
65. Murakami M., and Hirano T. (2008). Intracellular zinc homeostasis and zinc signaling. *Cancer Sci.*, **99**, pp. 1515–1522.
66. Regehly M., Greish K., Rancan F., Maeda H., Bohm F., and Roder B. (2007). Water-soluble polymer conjugates of ZnPP for photodynamic tumor therapy. *Bioconjugate. Chem.*, **18**, pp. 494–499.
67. Halliwell B., and Gutteridge J. M. C. (eds). (1999). *Free Radicals in Biology and Medicine*, Oxford University Press, NJ, US, pp. 617–859.
68. Nakamura H., Hoshino Y., Okuyama H., Matsuo Y., and Yodoi J. (2009). Thioredoxin 1 delivery as new therapeutics. *Adv. Drug Deliv. Rev.*, **61**, pp. 303–309.
69. Guyton K. Z., and Kensler T. W. (1993). Oxidative mechanisms in carcinogenesis. *Brit. Med. Bull.*, **49**, pp. 523–544.
70. Feig D. I., Reid T. M., and Loeb L. A. (1994). Reactive oxygen species in tumorigenesis. *Cancer Res.*, **54**, pp. 1890s–1894s.
71. Gerutti P. A. (1994). Oxy-radicals and cancer. *Lancet*, **344**, pp. 862–863.
72. Droge W. (2002). Free radicals in the physiological control of cell function. *Physiol. Rev.*, **82**, pp. 47–95.
73. Camhi S. L., Alam J., Wiegand G. W., Chin B. Y., and Choi A. M. K. (1998). Transcriptional activation of the HO-1 gene by lipopolysaccharide is mediated by 5′ distal enhancers: role of reactive oxygen intermediates and AP-1. *Am. J. Respir. Cell Mol. Biol.*, **18**, pp. 226–234.
74. Kurata S. I., Matsumoto M., Tsuji Y., and Nakajima H. (1996). Lipopolysaccharide activates transcription of the heme oxygenase gene in mouse M1 cells through oxidative activation of nuclear factor κB. *Eur. J. Biochem.*, **239**, pp. 566–571.
75. Rushworth S. A., and Macewan D. J. (2008). HO-1 underlies resistance of AML cells to TNF-induced apoptosis. *Blood*, **111**, pp. 3793–3801.
76. Kobayashi Y., Nishikawa M., Hyoudou K., Yamashita F., and Hashida M. (2008). Hydrogen peroxide-mediated nuclear factor kappaB activation in both liver and tumor cells during initial stages of hepatic metastasis. *Cancer Sci.*, **99**, pp. 1546–1552.

77. Sawa T., Zaki M. H., Okamoto T., Akuta Y., Tokutomi Y., Kim-Mitsuyama S., Ihara H., Kobayashi A., Yamamoto M., Fujii S., Arimoto H., and Akaike T. (2007). Protein S-guanylation by the biological signal 8-nitroguanosine 3′,5′-cyclic monophosphate. *Nat. Chem. Biol.*, **3**, pp. 727–735.

78. Hyoudou K., Nishikawa M., Kobayashi Y., Ikemura M., Yamashita F., and Hashida M. (2008). SOD derivatives prevent metastatic tumor growth aggravated by tumor removal. *Clin. Exp. Metastasis*, **25**, pp. 531–536.

79. Nishikawa M., Hashida M., and Takakura Y. (2009). Catalase delivery for inhibiting ROS-mediated tissue injury and tumor metastasis. *Adv. Drug Deliv. Rev.*, **61**, pp. 319–326.

80. Morikawa K., Shimokawa H., Matoba T., Kubota H., Akaike T., Talukder M. A., Hatanaka M., Fujiki T., Maeda H., Takahashi S., and Takeshita A. (2003). Pivotal role of Cu, Zn-superoxide dismutase in endothelium-dependent hyperpolarization. *J. Clin. Invest.*, **112**, pp. 1871–1819.

81. Okamoto T., Akaike T., Nagano T., Miyajima S., Suga M., Ando M., Ichimori K., and Maeda H. (1997). Activation of human neutrophil procollagenase by nitrogen dioxide and peroxynitrite: a novel mechanism for procollagenase activation involving nitric oxide. *Arch. Biochem. Biophys.*, **342**, pp. 261–274.

82. Okamoto T., Akaike T., Sawa T., Miyamoto Y., van der Vliet A., and Maeda H. (2001). Activation of matrix metalloproteinases by peroxynitrite-induced protein S-glutathiolation via disulfide S-oxide formation. *J. Biol. Chem.*, **276**, pp. 29596–29602.

Chapter 5

ORMOSIL Nanoparticles: Nanomedicine Approach for Drug/Gene Delivery to the Brain

Indrajit Roy

Department of Chemistry, University of Delhi, Delhi 110007, India
indrajitroy@rediffmail.com

Nanotechnology has immense potential in the delivery of various therapeutic molecules into the brain for treating brain-specific disorders. The brain is particularly amenable to gene therapy, where an exogenously administered transgene can stimulate neuronal stem/progenitor cells to differentiate into various neuronal cell types. Such induced neurogenesis can lead to the treatment of a number of neurodegenerative disorders. Organically modified silica (ORMOSIL) nanoparticles have shown a lot of promise for the delivery of genetic materials into the brain with high efficiency, without any sign of toxicity. In this chapter, I have discussed the effects of gene delivery using these nanoparticles in the brain. In addition, I have suggested various potential improvements in this technology that will drive its translation to the clinic. I have concluded with a brief discussion on the potential of these nanoparticles for the brain-specific delivery of other therapeutic molecules, such as short interfering RNA (siRNA) and small molecule drugs.

Nanotechnology in Health Care
Edited by Sanjeeb K. Sahoo

ISBN 978-981-4267-21-2 (Hardcover), 978-981-4267-35-9 (eBook)
www.panstanford.com

5.1 Nanotechnology in Medicine

Nanotechnology is playing a rapidly increasing role in diagnostics and therapeutics of human disease [1–3]. Over the last two decades, nanoparticles have revolutionized the field of drug and gene delivery [4]. Numerous therapeutic drugs and genes, though being highly efficacious, are limited in their *in vivo* applications owing to their poor solubility and stability in physiological medium. Nanoparticles not only enable the development of stable aqueous formulation of such therapeutic materials but also help in their enhanced bioavailability and site-specific delivery. In addition, nanoparticles also enable the sustained release of these therapeutic materials from the particle matrix within the target site of interest [5]. Externally triggered release of active molecules from nanoparticles is also a promising area of research. These enhanced drug-delivery properties, combined with the provision of coincorporation of diagnostic probes as well as easy access to hard-to-reach diseased sites, make nanoparticles ideal candidates for the cure of a number of diseases that are difficult to treat using standard chemo/radiotherapeutic and surgical approaches [6].

5.2 Brain

From the point of view of nanoparticle-mediated delivery of therapeutic drugs and genes, the brain is probably the most significant target organ. A variety of diseases are associated with this organ, including neurodegenerative diseases, stroke, obesity, neuro-AIDS, substance abuse, and brain cancer [7–9]. However, the development of effective therapies for these diseases is hampered by the poor understanding of the complex brain functions that lead to and sustain these diseases. Moreover, the effective delivery of diagnostic and therapeutic agents in the brain is severely impeded by the presence of the blood–brain barrier (BBB) [10, 11]. Recent studies show that more than 99% of large-molecule pharmaceutics, including peptides, recombinant proteins, monoclonal antibodies, and RNA interference (RNAi)-based drugs and gene therapies, do not cross the BBB [12]. A common misconception is that small molecules cross the BBB. Actually, small molecules readily penetrate the postvascular space of all organs of the body except for the brain and the spinal cord. There are >7,000 drugs in the Comprehensive Medicinal Chemistry (CMC) database, and only 5% of these drugs reach the central nervous system (CNS), and the drugs that do reach the CNS are limited to the treatment of just three conditions: depression, schizophrenia, and insomnia [13]. According to another study, 12% of all drugs are active in the CNS but only 1% of all drugs are active in the brain for diseases other than affective disorders [14].

5.3 BBB Permeability of Nanoparticles

The BBB is impermeable to nanoparticles owing to their large sizes. However, nanoparticles can be helped to "sneak" across the BBB following coating with specific biorecognition molecules. These include coating nanoparticles with transferrin and certain monoclonal antibodies whose corresponding receptors are overexpressed on the BBB [15, 16]. This method, popularly known as the Trojan horse approach, leads to receptor-mediated transcytosis across the BBB for drug delivery in the brain parenchyma with minimal damage to the BBB [17].

5.4 Gene Therapy in the Brain

There are more genes expressed in the brain than in any other tissues, reflecting the great diversity of the cell types and complexity of the function. With the advent of bioinformatics, the knowledge of the human genome has increased substantially, with a concomitant increase in the understanding of the roles that these genes play in normal as well as abnormal brain functions [18]. Therefore, several diseases of the brain are amenable to treatment using gene therapy following the brain-specific delivery of a suitable plasmid DNA [19]. Gene therapy of diseases of the CNS can be applied toward understanding the physiological roles of genes in development, homeostasis, and senescence, as well as toward the treatment of (a) inherited (mainly monogenic) and (b) acquired (both monogenic and multigenic) disorders [19, 20]. In recent years, a lot of promise has been shown toward the treatment of acquired CNS diseases such as spinal cord injury, stroke, and degenerative (Parkinson's and Alzheimer's) diseases [21–23]. This can be achieved by the introduction of transgene-encoding proteins, which bolster the natural survival and repair systems within the CNS, such as neurotransmitters, neurotrophic factors and their receptors, cytokines, and neuronal-survival (antiapoptotic) agents. [20]. Moreover, neuronal stem and progenitor cells (NSPCs) can be genetically induced to differentiate into various neuronal cell types, which have the potential to replenish areas developmentally impaired or undergoing neurodegeneration [24]. In essence, CNS gene therapy vectors should be able to carry out at least one of these three functions: (a) neuroprotection, (b) neuroregeneration, and (c) antiapoptosis [19].

However, despite the enormous promise of gene therapy in the brain, overall progress is stifled owing to the nonavailability of a suitable vector that would enable stable integration of an exogeneous transgene into target brain cells with no toxic side effects. Viral vectors, though effective in inducing therapeutically relevant gene expression, are considered unsafe for human use owing to their antigenicity, pathogenecity, and the risk of "insertional mutagenesis" [25–27]. Therefore, in recent years, a number of research activities have focused on the development of synthetic nonviral systems, which would enable efficient gene delivery, yet avoid the risk factors associated with their virus-based counterparts [25, 28]. Nanoparticulate carriers are particularly attractive in this regard owing to their ability to make target-specific delivery across the BBB [29]. In addition, these nanoparticles can contain other diagnostic agents, which would allow monitoring the effects of gene therapy in real time [1]. Therefore, a number of nanoparticles are currently being developed as CNS-specific carriers of therapeutic genetic materials.

5.5 Silica Nanoparticles

In the realm of nanomedicine, inorganic nanoparticles have a number of advantages over their polymeric and lipidic counterparts. These nanoparticles can be synthesized in the ultrafine size range (below 100 nm), which not only renders them suitable for unimpeded circulation in the bloodstream and extravasation into tumor tissues but also permits excretion through renal filtration without the need for their biodegradation [30]. Several such materials, including silica, gold nanoshells, and gold nanoparticles, are known for their nonantigenicity [31–35].

Among the various classes of inorganic nanomaterials, silica-based ones are probably the most widely known. In 1968, Stober *et al.* reported a stable method to produce highly monodispersed nanoparticles of silica by using a simple synthetic approach [36]. This report led to a burst of research activities in the field of synthesis and applications of silica nanoparticles of various sizes. Since silica nanoparticles are optically transparent, they can be doped with various fluorophores and used as efficient probes for optical bioimaging [37]. In addition, their chemically flexible surface can be exploited for the coincorporation of other diagnostic/therapeutic probes for multimodal imaging and therapy, as well as biorecognition molecules for their targeted delivery *in vitro* and *in vivo*. The combination of diagnostic and therapeutic properties within a single multifunctional nanosystem can also facilitate real-time monitoring of the drug action.

However, in spite of these advantages, the applications of silica-based nanoparticles in medicine have not been widely reported. One of the possible reasons for this is that they are not biodegradable and, therefore, are not deemed fit for potential translation into the clinic. This issue can be overcome by synthesizing silica nanoparticles with much smaller diameters (below 50 nm) so that they can be excreted from the body in the intact form via renal or hepatobiliary clearance [38]. Advances in synthetic techniques, coupled with better understanding of the pharmacokinetics of nanoparticles in the body, allow the development of such nanosystems. Their biomedical applications can be further bolstered by emerging therapeutic modalities such as gene therapy, whereby therapeutic genetic materials such as plasmid DNA and siRNA can be electrostatically condensed on the surface of these nanoparticles and delivered to appropriate cell types [39, 40].

Organically modified silica (ORMOSIL) nanoparticles are a class of silica-based nanoparticles that have recently shown enormous promise as diagnostic and therapeutic agents. These nanoparticles are generally synthesized by condensation-polymerization of their organosilane precursor molecules, where one or more of the alkoxy "arms" of the tetra-alkoxysilane precursor have been replaced by a hydrocarbon group. When this synthetic step is carried out in the confined dimensions of a microemulsion (either oil-in-water or water-in-oil), highly monodispersed and ultrafine (diameters less than 50 nm) nanoparticles are precipitated, which can be purified as an aqueous suspension through simple steps such as centrifugation or dialysis [41]. Since these particles are mesoporous, they can serve as sustained-release vehicles for encapsulated biomolecules. In addition, the rich chemistry of silica can be exploited in order to synthesize particles presenting a variety of active groups (carboxyl, thiol, or amino) on their surface, which can be further modified to incorporate imaging/diagnostic probes, genetic materials, and biorecognition molecules [42]. Thus, ORMOSIL can serve as an ideal nanoplatform for the assembly of "multimodal" nanoparticles for targeted diagnostics and therapeutics.

Our group has extensively demonstrated the utility of ORMOSIL nanoparticles in various applications in medicine, which includes the potential to serve as (a) targeted probes for optical bioimaging of cancer [37], (b) carriers of photosensitizing anticancer drugs for photodynamic therapy (PDT) in cancer [43], and (c) carriers of genetic materials for nonviral gene delivery [44, 45]. These studies strongly underline the need for further applied research in the field of these hybrid nanomaterials in order to fully exploit their diagnostic and therapeutic potential in various human diseases.

5.6 ORMOSIL Nanoparticles for Gene Delivery in the Brain

Amino-terminated ORMOSIL nanoparticles have been developed, which can form electrostatic complexes with negatively charged plasmid DNA, rendering stabilization of the DNA against enzymatic degradation. The resulting nanoplexes, with an average diameter of 30 nm, can also be fluorescently labeled in order to optically track their path *in vitro* and *in vivo* [45]. These nanoplexes were introduced *in vivo* in the CNS using direct stereotaxic injection into the brain of mice and rats [44]. The efficiency of gene expression using the plasmid encoding the enhanced green fluorescent protein (pEGFP) was investigated following delivery in the substantia nigra per compacta (SNc) region of the brain, which is an area richly populated with neuronal cells and of considerable interest for its role in Parkinson's disease and a number of other disorders [46, 47]. Robust EGFP expression of neuron-shaped cells in the SNc was detected following immunofluorescent staining using specific monoclonal antibodies to EGFP. Double-immunostaining studies using anti-EGFP and antityrosine hydroxylase (anti-TH) antibodies confirmed efficient *in vivo* transfection using the nanoplexes, since most of the SNc neurons are dopaminergic and can be specifically detected using antibodies to TH [48]. The efficiency of this nanoplex-mediated *in vivo* transfection was found to be equal to or greater than that obtained using herpes simplex virus (HSV), which has a natural tropism for the brain [44, 49]. Furthermore, this topical gene expression was observed in multiple areas of the brain (septum, cortex, hippocampus, etc.) surrounding the lateral ventricle (LV), following intraventricular injection of the nanoplex. Moreover, no marked toxic effects of the nanoparticles could be observed in the mouse even after two months of stereotaxic injection.

After confirming the robust expression of reporter genes using our nanoplexes in the CNS, we investigated the efficiency of nanoplex-mediated transfection of functional genes in the brain and their effects on the normal functioning of the transfected cells. Neurogenesis, the process of differentiation of neuronal stem/progenitor cells (NSPCs) into mature neurons, holds the key toward the treatment of various neurodegenerative disorders. A number of NSPCs are located in the subventricular zone (SVZ) of the LV, which can be made to differentiate into various cell types such as neurons, astrocytes, and oligodendrocytes. Therefore, this region represents an exciting target from the point of view of CNS gene therapy [50, 51]. Here, we used the nanoplex-mediated transfection of the functional gene nucleus-targeted fibroblast growth factor receptor type-1 (FGFR-1) [52]. Transfection with this gene is implicated in the modulation of the Integrative Nuclear FGF Receptor-1 Signaling (INFS) pathway, which is known to effectively control the development of NSPCs [52]. Stereotaxic injection of these nanoplexes into the SVZ resulted in significant modulation of the biology of the NSPCs, as evidenced by the marked reduction in the incorporation of bromodeoxiuridine (BrdU). Moreover, these nanoplexes were found to efficiently transfect recombinant nuclear forms of FGFR-1 and its ligand fibroblast growth factor 2 (FGF-2) into the brain SVZ, resulting in the INFS-mediated stimulation of the NSPCs to withdraw from the cell cycle and differentiate into doublecortin-expressing migratory neuroblasts and into mature neurons. These differentiated cells were then found to migrate to different regions of the brain, such as the olfactory bulb, subcortical brain regions, and in the brain cortex [53]. Therefore, the ability of these nanoplexes to induce the genetic manipulation of the NSPCs *in vivo* and their differentiation into neuronal cell types demonstrates their potential to be developed as a powerful tool for a number of CNS gene therapeutic approaches, including stimulation of neurogenesis, neutralization of growth inhibitory molecules, and repair of neuronal injury.

Recently, these nanoplexes have shown the potential for genetically inducing Huntington's disease in small animals. This approach, known as reverse engineering, can help create diseases in small animals whose pathology is more reflective of that in human diseases. This would facilitate better correlation between the outcome of a therapeutic regimen in small animals and humans, thus accelerating drug discovery research. Here, following stereotaxic injection of the abnormal plasmid encoding hemagglutinin-tagged polypeptides with extended (127)-glutamine repeats (Q127), complexed with the nanoparticles, treated mice have displayed pathological and behavioral abnormalities akin to Huntington's disease [54]. Characteristic nuclear and cytoplasmic Q127 aggregates in numerous striatal, septal, and neocortical cells have been observed following immunocytochemistry analyses. A marked increase in the reactive astrocytes positive for glial fibrillary acidic protein (GFAP) in striatum, septum, and brain cortex regions of the mouse indicated neurodegenerative changes and motor impairments. These characteristics were absent in the mice receiving injection of the nanoparticles, complexed with the corresponding plasmid with normal (20)-glutamine repeats (Q20). This demonstrates a direct application of these nanoparticles in gene transfer, leading to the engineering of a gene-based disease in small animals.

5.7 Future Perspectives

The above results show the enormous potential that ORMOSIL nanoparticle–mediated gene therapy has shown in the treatment of neurodegenerative disorders. It will be interesting to see whether such nanoparticle-mediated functional gene delivery translates into actual therapy of these and other diseases. However, presently the main drawback of these nanoparticles is the necessity for direct sterotaxic injection in the brain to achieve efficient transgene expression, which is a highly invasive procedure. Therefore, it is necessary to develop strategies that would allow similar levels of gene delivery in the brain following noninvasive systemic injection of the nanoplexes. This can be achieved by adapting the Trojan horse approach for the delivery of inorganic nanoparticles such as ORMOSIL across the BBB, which has already shown a lot of promise for the brain-specific delivery of liposomal and polymeric nanocarriers [17, 55]. Recently, such a delivery has been reported using rod-shaped nanocrystals of semiconductor materials (quantum rods) bioconjugated with the iron-transporting protein transferrin [56]. It will be interesting to observe whether ORMOSIL nanoparticles, complexed with suitable plasmid DNA, can also be similarly delivered into the brain.

In addition to the delivery of plasmid DNA, ORMOSIL nanoparticles can play a critical role in the delivery of small molecule therapeutics such as siRNA and other drugs in the brain for the treatment of several CNS disorders. Recently, gold nanorods, electrostatically complexed with the siRNA targeting the dopaminergic-signaling pathway in the brain, have shown the potential to modulate key proteins associated with this pathway [57]. Nanoparticle-mediated brain-specific delivery of such siRNA can play a critical role in the control and treatment of substance abuse, which is associated with this pathway. Owing to the mesoporous nature of ORMOSIL, they can host small molecule lipophilic drugs in their interior and release them in a sustained manner at the target of interest. The development of novel drug delivery strategies in the brain can lead to significant improvements toward the therapy of neuro-AIDS, via the delivery of antiretroviral drugs across the BBB [58]. A similar strategy can also be adapted for the ORMOSIL nanoparticle–mediated delivery of chemotherapeutics against various brain tumors. PDT of brain tumors using ORMOSIL nanoparticles is also a viable option.

In summary, nanoparticles are highly promising for the brain-specific delivery of therapeutic agents such as plasmid DNA, siRNA, and small molecule drugs, potentially allowing the treatment of a number of CNS disorders. Since so far no CNS toxicity of ORMOSIL nanoparticles has been reported, they can be considered to be a safer mode of drug delivery in the brain when compared to virus-based carriers. However, present challenges, such as delivery across an intact BBB and eventual excretion from the body, need to be properly addressed before these nanoparticles can find their way into the clinic for the treatment of various CNS disorders.

References

1. Prasad PN. *Nanophotonics*, New York: Wiley; 2004.
2. Farokhzad OC, Langer R. Impact of nanotechnology on drug delivery. *ACS Nano*, 2009 Jan 27; **3**(1): 16–20.
3. Whitesides GM. The "right" size in nanobiotechnology. *Nat. Biotechnol.*, 2003 Oct; **21**(10): 1161–1165.
4. Sanvicens N, Marco MP. Multifunctional nanoparticles–properties and prospects for their use in human medicine. *Trends Biotechnol.*, 2008 Aug; **26**(8): 425–433.
5. Uhrich KE, Cannizzaro SM, Langer RS, Shakesheff KM. Polymeric systems for controlled drug release. *Chem. Rev.*, 1999 Nov 10; **99**(11): 3181–3198.
6. Sahoo SK, Labhasetwar V. Nanotech approaches to drug delivery and imaging. *Drug Discov. Today*, 2003 Dec 15; **8**(24): 1112–1120.
7. Roy I, Stachowiak MK, Bergey EJ. Nonviral gene transfection nanoparticles: function and applications in the brain. *Nanomedicine*, 2008 Jun; **4**(2): 89–97.
8. Jain KK. Neuroprotection in traumatic brain injury. *Drug Discov. Today*, 2008 Dec; **13**(23–24): 1082–1089.
9. Solenski NJ. Emerging risk factors for cerebrovascular disease. *Curr. Drug Targets*, 2007 Jul; **8**(7): 802–816.
10. Eyal S, Hsiao P, Unadkat JD. Drug interactions at the blood–brain barrier: fact or fantasy? *Pharmacol Ther.*, 2009, **123**(1):80–104.
11. Brasnjevic I, Steinbusch HW, Schmitz C, Martinez-Martinez P. Delivery of peptide and protein drugs over the blood-brain barrier. *Prog. Neurobiol.*, 2009 Apr; **87**(4): 212–251.
12. Pardridge WM, Oldendorf WH, Cancilla P, Frank HJ. Blood–brain barrier: interface between internal medicine and the brain. *Ann. Intern. Med.*, 1986 Jul; **105**(1): 82–95.
13. Ghose AK, Viswanadhan VN, Wendoloski JJ. A knowledge-based approach in designing combinatorial or medicinal chemistry libraries for drug discovery. 1. A qualitative and quantitative characterization of known drug databases. *J. Comb. Chem.*, 1999 Jan; **1**(1): 55–68.

14. Lipinski CA. Drug-like properties and the causes of poor solubility and poor permeability. *J. Pharmacol. Toxicol. Methods*, 2000 Jul–Aug; **44**(1): 235–249.

15. Pardridge WM. The blood–brain barrier and neurotherapeutics. *NeuroRx*, 2005 Jan; **2**(1): 1–2.

16. Silva GA. Nanotechnology approaches to crossing the blood-brain barrier and drug delivery to the CNS. *BMC Neurosci.*, 2008; **9** Suppl 3:S4.

17. Pardridge WM. Molecular trojan horses for blood–brain barrier drug delivery. *Discov. Med.*, 2006 Aug; **6**(34): 139–143.

18. Austin CP. The impact of the completed human genome sequence on the development of novel therapeutics for human disease. *Annu. Rev. Med.*, 2004; **55:** 1–13.

19. Bowers WJ, Federoff HJ. Gene therapy for neurological diseases. In *Gene and Cell Therapy: Therapeutic Mechanisms and Strategies*, 2nd edn (ed. Templeton NS). New York: Mercel Dekker; 2004. pp. 601–627.

20. Karpati G, Lochmuller H, Nalbantoglu J, Durham H. The principles of gene therapy for the nervous system. *Trends Neurosci.*, 1996 Feb; **19**(2): 49–54.

21. Mochizuki H. Current status of gene therapy for Parkinson disease. *Brain Nerve*, 2009 Apr; **61**(4): 485–493.

22. Kennington E. Gene therapy delivers an alternative approach to Alzheimer's disease. *Nat. Rev. Drug Discov.*, 2009 Apr; **8**(4): 275.

23. Yamada Y, Ichihara S, Nishida T. Proinflammatory gene polymorphisms and ischemic stroke. *Curr. Pharm. Des.*, 2008; **14**(33): 3590–3600.

24. Gritti A, Bonfanti L. Neuronal-glial interactions in central nervous system neurogenesis: the neural stem cell perspective. *Neuron Glia Biol.*, 2007 Nov; **3**(4): 309–323.

25. Davis SS. Biomedical applications of nanotechnology–implications for drug targeting and gene therapy. *Trends Biotechnol.*, 1997 Jun; **15**(6): 217–224.

26. Deglon N, Hantraye P. Viral vectors as tools to model and treat neurodegenerative disorders. *J. Gene Med.*, 2005 May; **7**(5): 530–539.

27. Uren AG, Kool J, Berns A, van Lohuizen M. Retroviral insertional mutagenesis: past, present and future. *Oncogene*, 2005 Nov 21; **24**(52): 7656–7672.

28. Nishikawa M, Huang L. Nonviral vectors in the new millennium: delivery barriers in gene transfer. *Hum. Gene Ther.*, 2001 May 20; **12**(8): 861–870.

29. Agarwal A, Lariya N, Saraogi G, Dubey N, Agrawal H, Agrawal GP. Nanoparticles as novel carrier for brain delivery: a review. *Curr. Pharm. Des.*, 2009; **15**(8): 917–925.

30. Choi HS, Liu W, Misra P, Tanaka E, Zimmer JP, Itty Ipe B, Bawendi MG, Frangioni JV. Renal clearance of quantum dots. *Nat. Biotechnol.*, 2007 Oct; **25**(10): 1165–1170.

31. Liong M, Lu J, Kovochich M, Xia T, Ruehm SG, Nel AE, Tamanoi F, Zink JI. Multifunctional inorganic nanoparticles for imaging, targeting, and drug delivery. *ACS Nano*, 2008 May; **2**(5): 889–896.

32. Tallury P, Payton K, Santra S. Silica-based multimodal/multifunctional nanoparticles for bioimaging and biosensing applications. *Nanomedicine*, 2008 Aug; **3**(4): 579–592.

33. Wilson R. The use of gold nanoparticles in diagnostics and detection. *Chem. Soc. Rev.*, 2008 Sep; **37**(9): 2028–2045.

34. Hirsch LR, Gobin AM, Lowery AR, Tam F, Drezek RA, Halas NJ, West JL. Metal nanoshells. *Ann. Biomed. Eng.*, 2006 Jan; **34**(1): 15–22.

35. Huang X, Jain PK, El-Sayed IH, El-Sayed MA. Gold nanoparticles: interesting optical properties and recent applications in cancer diagnostics and therapy. *Nanomedicine*, 2007 Oct; **2**(5): 681–93.

36. Halas NJ. Nanoscience under glass: the versatile chemistry of silica nanostructures. *ACS Nano*, 2008 Feb; **2**(2): 179–183.

37. Kumar R, Roy I, Ohulchanskyy TY, Goswami LN, Bonoiu AC, Bergey EJ, Tramposch KM, Maitra A, Prasad PN. Covalently dye-linked, surface-controlled, and bioconjugated organically modified silica nanoparticles as targeted probes for optical imaging. *ACS Nano*, 2008 Mar; **2**(3): 449–456.

38. Longmire M, Choyke PL, Kobayashi H. Clearance properties of nano-sized particles and molecules as imaging agents: considerations and caveats. *Nanomedicine*, 2008 Oct; **3**(5): 703–717.

39. Slowing, II, Vivero-Escoto JL, Wu CW, Lin VS. Mesoporous silica nanoparticles as controlled release drug delivery and gene transfection carriers. *Adv. Drug Deliv. Rev.*, 2008 Aug 17; **60**(11): 1278–1288.

40. Juliano R, Alam MR, Dixit V, Kang H. Mechanisms and strategies for effective delivery of antisense and siRNA oligonucleotides. *Nucleic Acids Res.*, 2008 Jul; **36**(12): 4158–4171.

41. Das S, Jain TK, Maitra A. Inorganic- organic hybrid nanoparticles from *n*-octyl triethoxy silanes. *J. Colloid Interface Sci.*, 2002; 252: 82–88.

42. Sharma P, Brown S, Walter G, Santra S, Moudgil B. Nanoparticles for bioimaging. *Adv. Colloid Interface Sci.*, 2006 Nov 16; **123–126:** 471–485.

43. Roy I, Ohulchanskyy TY, Pudavar HE, Bergey EJ, Oseroff AR, Morgan J, Dougherty TJ, Prasad PN. Ceramic-based nanoparticles entrapping water-insoluble photosensitizing anticancer drugs: a novel drug-carrier system for photodynamic therapy. *J. Am. Chem. Soc.*, 2003 Jul 2; **125**(26): 7860–7865.

44. Bharali DJ, Klejbor I, Stachowiak EK, Dutta P, Roy I, Kaur N, Bergey EJ, Prasad PN, Stachowiak MK. Organically modified silica nanoparticles: a nonviral vector for *in vivo* gene delivery and expression in the brain. *Proc. Natl. Acad. Sci. USA*, 2005 Aug 9; **102**(32): 11539–11544.

45. Roy I, Ohulchanskyy TY, Bharali DJ, Pudavar HE, Mistretta RA, Kaur N, Prasad PN. Optical tracking of organically modified silica nanoparticles as DNA carriers: a nonviral, nanomedicine approach for gene delivery. *Proc. Natl. Acad. Sci. USA*, 2005 Jan 11; **102**(2): 279–284.

46. Fisher LJ, Gage FH. Radical directions in Parkinson's disease. *Nat. Med.*, 1995 Mar; **1**(3): 201–203.

47. Wong AH, Van Tol HH. Schizophrenia: from phenomenology to neurobiology. *Neurosci. Biobehav. Rev.*, 2003 May; **27**(3): 269–306.

48. Frielingsdorf H, Schwarz K, Brundin P, Mohapel P. No evidence for new dopaminergic neurons in the adult mammalian substantia nigra. *Proc. Natl. Acad. Sci. USA*, 2004 Jul 6; **101**(27): 10177–10182.

49. Corso TD, Torres G, Goulah C, Roy I, Gambino AS, Nayda J, Buckley T, Stachowiak EK, Bergey EJ, Pudavar H, Dutta P, Bloom DC, Bowers WJ, Stachowiak MK. Transfection of tyrosine kinase deleted FGF receptor-1 into rat brain substantia nigra reduces the number of tyrosine hydroxylase expressing neurons and decreases concentration levels of striatal dopamine. *Brain Res. Mol. Brain Res.*, 2005 Oct 3; **139**(2): 361–366.

50. Goldman J. Peripheral blood stem cells for allografting. *Blood*, 1995 Mar 15; **85**(6): 1413–1415.

51. Lois C, Alvarez-Buylla A. Proliferating subventricular zone cells in the adult mammalian forebrain can differentiate into neurons and glia. *Proc. Natl. Acad. Sci. USA*, 1993 Mar 1; **90**(5): 2074–2077.

52. Stachowiak MK, Fang X, Myers JM, Dunham SM, Berezney R, Maher PA, Stachowiak EK. Integrative nuclear FGFR1 signaling (INFS) as a part of a universal "feed-forward-and-gate" signaling module that controls

cell growth and differentiation. *J. Cell Biochem.*, 2003 Nov 1; **90**(4): 662–691.

53. Stachowiak EK, Roy I, Lee YW, Capacchietti M, Aletta JM, Prasad PN, Stachowiak MK. Targeting novel integrative nuclear FGFR1 signaling by nanoparticle-mediated gene transfer stimulates neurogenesis in the adult brain. *Integr. Biol. (Camb).*, 2009; **1**(5-6):394–403.

54. Klejbor I, Stachowiak EK, Bharali DJ, Roy I, Spodnik I, Morys J, Bergey EJ, Prasad PN, Stachowiak MK. ORMOSIL nanoparticles as a non-viral gene delivery vector for modeling polyglutamine induced brain pathology. *J. Neurosci. Methods*, 2007 Sep 30; **165**(2): 230–243.

55. Shi N, Pardridge WM. Noninvasive gene targeting to the brain. *Proc. Natl. Acad. Sci. USA*, 2000 Jun 20; **97**(13): 7567–8572.

56. Xu G, Yong KT, Roy I, Mahajan SD, Ding H, Schwartz SA, Prasad PN. Bioconjugated quantum rods as targeted probes for efficient transmigration across an *in vitro* blood–brain barrier. *Bioconjug. Chem.*, 2008 Jun; **19**(6): 1179–1185.

57. Bonoiu AC, Mahajan SD, Ding H, Roy I, Yong KT, Kumar R, Hu R, Bergey EJ, Schwartz SA, Prasad PN. Nanotechnology approach for drug addiction therapy: gene silencing using delivery of gold nanorod-siRNA nanoplex in dopaminergic neurons. *Proc. Natl. Acad. Sci. USA*, 2009 Apr 7; **106**(14): 5546–5550.

58. Arendt G, von Giesen HJ. Antiretroviral therapy regimens for neuro-AIDS. *Curr. Drug Targets Infect. Disord.*, 2002 Sep; **2**(3): 187–192.

Chapter 6

Magnetic Nanoparticles: A Versatile System for Therapeutics and Imaging

Fahima Dilnawaz, Abhalaxmi Singh, and Sanjeeb K. Sahoo

Laboratory of Nanomedicine, Institute of Life Sciences, Chandrasekharpur, Bhubaneswar-751023, Orissa, India

sanjeebsahoo2005@gmail.com

6.1 Introduction

The class of elements (iron, nickel, and cobalt) and their chemical compounds that can be manipulated using the magnetic field are called magnetic nanoparticles (MNPs).[1] Scaling down the material to the nano-scale range changes the fundamental structure of the material structure. This is because, when the grain size is reduced, the normal macroscopic domain structure transforms into a single domain state at a critical size that typically lies below 100 nm. Once this transformation occurs, the mechanism of magnetization reversal can only be via the rotation of the magnetization vector from one magnetic easy axis to another via a magnetically firm direction. This change of reversal mechanism and the basic underlying physical mechanism governing it was first discussed by E. C. Stoner.[2] These magnetic materials for their splendid features were used in applications of biology and medicine since 1960s. However, for

Nanotechnology in Health Care
Edited by Sanjeeb K. Sahoo

ISBN 978-981-4267-21-2 (Hardcover), 978-981-4267-35-9 (eBook)
www.panstanford.com

biomedical applications, magnetite is one of the most commonly used magnetic materials because it has strong magnetic property and low toxicity.[3,4] MNPs are of great interest and have been widely used in various disciplines, such as magnetic fluid[5] catalysis,[1] biotechnology/biomedicine,[3,6,7] and magnetic resonance imaging (MRI),[8] of medical fields with a multiskill approach (Fig. 6.1). A number of suitable methods have been deployed for the synthesis of MNPs of various compositions. However, the formed particles perform the best when the size of the nanoparticles is below the critical domain, which is dependent on the material typically around 10–20 nm. So each nanoparticle becomes a single domain and demonstrates superparamagnetic behavior. Superparamagnetism is a form of magnetism that appears in small ferromagnetic or ferrimagnetic nanoparticles. In nanoparticles, magnetization can randomly flip directions under the influence of temperature. The typical time between two flips is called the Neel relaxation time. In the absence of an external magnetic field, when the time used to measure the magnetization of the nanoparticles is much longer than the Neel relaxation time, their magnetization appears to be in average zero; hence, they are said to be in the superparamagnetic state. In this state, an external magnetic field is able to magnetize the nanoparticles, similarly to a paramagnet. However, their magnetic susceptibility is much larger than that of paramagnets. Such individual nanoparticle has a large constant magnetic moment and behaves like a giant paramagnetic atom with a fast response to the magnetic field with negligible remnance (residual magnetism) and coercivity (the field required to bring the magnetism to zero). These features make superparamagnetic nanoparticles very attractive for a broad range of biomedical applications because the risk of agglomeration becomes negligible at room temperature. Therefore, magnetic materials have their own advantages that provide many exciting opportunities in biomedical applications. First, their controllable sizes range in nanometers, and their optimization of sizes and properties that enable the site-specific delivery of the therapeutic agent. Second, nanoparticles can be manipulated by an external magnetic force. This "action at a distance" provides a tremendous advantage for many applications. Third, MNPs play an important role as MRI contrast-enhancement agents because the signal of the magnetic moment of a proton around MNPs can be captured by resonant absorption.

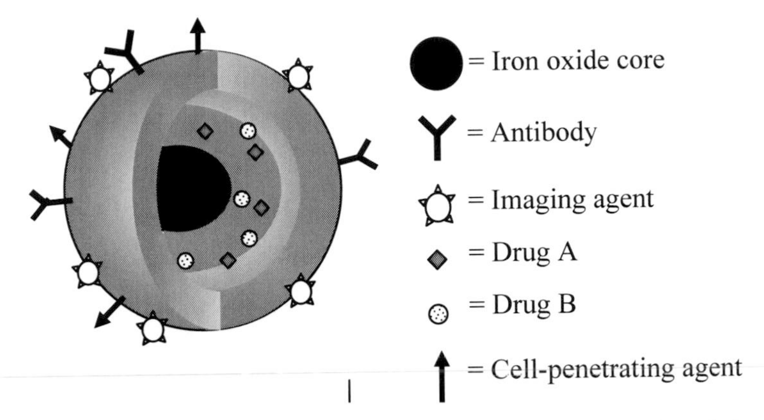

Figure 6.1 A schematic diagram of a multifunctional MNP-based drug delivery vehicle.

The most unavoidable problem associated with the particles size is their intrinsic instability over a longer period of time. Therefore, such particles tend to have the aggregation to reduce the energy associated with a high surface area to have a high surface-area-to-volume ratio of the nanosized particles. Furthermore, the metallic nanoparticles are chemically highly active and easily oxidized in air, resulting generally in loss of magnetism and dispersibility. For various applications, therefore it is crucial to develop protection against degradation during and after synthesis. Mostly, this has been achieved by grafting or coating with organic species, including surfactants, polymers, or coating with inorganic layers such as silica or carbon. These protective coverings further can also be used for attaching various ligands depending upon the application. Furthermore, additional magnetic dipole-dipole attractive forces between the nanoparticles enhance agglomeration.[9] Considering the above mentioned, facts the nature of the "coat" of superparamagnetic iron oxide nanoparticles (SPIONs) is of paramount significance.[6] Primarily, it influences the stability and surface properties of their colloidal dispersions. For their stabilization in aqueous media, electrostatic and steric stabilizing agents such as organic surfactants and polymers have been incorporated into inorganic colloidal dispersions.[10–12] Major parameters considered in the selection and design of coating materials for superparamagnetic nanoparticles include (a) their *in vivo* kinetics and biodistribution behavior and (b) the potential to target them to specific tissues or molecules of interest by conjugation with affinity probes (peptides, antibodies, aptamers, and small molecules).[6,13–15] As a result, these coatings provide a means to tailor the surface properties and chemical functionality of the superparamagnetic nanoparticles.

6.2 Role of Superparamagnetic Nanoparticles in Therapeutics and Imaging

MNPs are emerging as an ideal probe for the imaging of soft tissues, cell tracking, and tracking of drug delivery vehicles *in vivo*. Because of its high resolution and lack of ionizing radiation, MRI is a powerful tool for noninvasive *in vivo* monitoring. The ability of MNPs to enhance the proton relaxation of specific tissues helps MNPs to serve as MRI contrast agents. MRI relies on the counterbalance between the exceedingly small magnetic moment on a proton and the exceedingly large number of protons present in biological tissue. This leads to a measurable effect in the presence of large magnetic fields.[16,17] MNPs have magnetic moment, which gets hindered by lattice orientation due to the small crystal size. Therefore, these particles do not exhibit hysteresis and, hence, are called superparamagnetic.[18] When an external magnetic field is applied, the individual moments align themselves along the field. This creates large microscopic field gradients for dephasing nearby protons.[19] This, in turn, dramatically shortens the nuclear magnetic resonance T_2 (transverse) relaxation time far beyond the usual dipole-dipole interaction mechanism affecting both T_1 (longitudinal) and T_2 relaxations.[18]

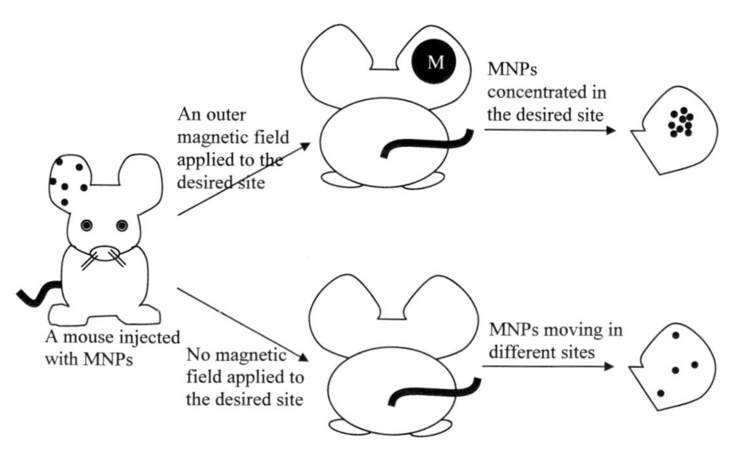

Figure 6.2 A schematic illustration of the localization of MNPs at the target site by the application of an external magnetic field.

Due to the greater sensitivity for MRI, superparamagnetic nanoparticles are the choice contrast agents in cell labeling and tracking systems. MNPs have been extensively examined as MRI contrast agents to improve the detection, diagnosis, and therapeutic management of solid tumors. Regarding therapeutics, the primary shortcoming related to chemotherapeutic agents is the nonspecificity and side effects on the healthy tissues. MNPs play a major role in solving this problem. By applying an external magnetic field, MNP drug carriers can be targeted to specific sites, helping in site-specific delivery of drugs and reduction in the side effects on the healthy tissues (Fig. 6.2). Due to these versatility features, MNPs are playing a wide role in therapeutics.[20,21]

6.3 Functionalization of the Superparamagnetic Nanoparticles

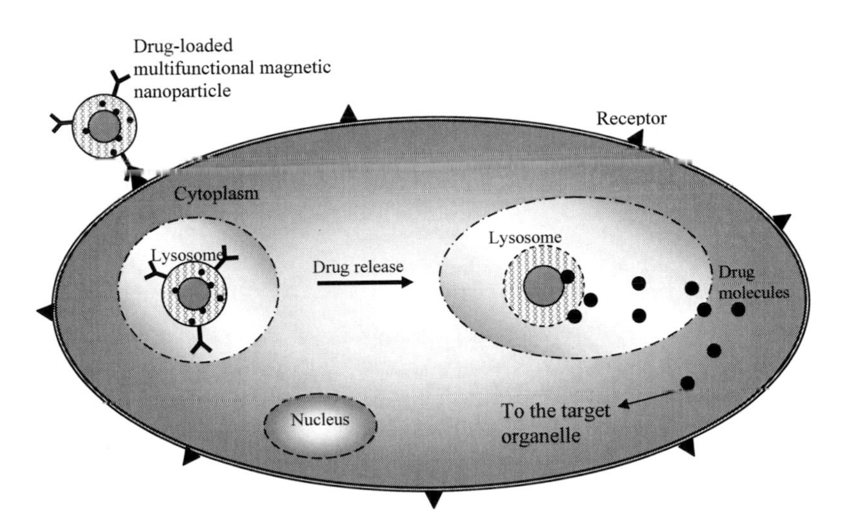

Figure 6.3 A schematic illustration of the specific uptake of an MNP drug carrier into a target cancer cell through receptor-mediated endocytosis.

The use of diverse nanostructured materials allows the development of novel multifunctional nanomedical platforms for multimodal imaging and simultaneous diagnosis and therapy. For example, the combination of an MRI contrast agent and a fluorescent organic dye can allow the detection of cancer through noninvasive MRI and the optical guide of surgery. The encapsulation of an MRI contrast agent and an anticancer drug in a nanostructured matrix has the potential to allow for simultaneous diagnosis and targeted chemotherapy. There are many possible combinations of the various imaging and therapeutic modalities. In the following section, we discuss the recent developments of multifunctional nanoplatforms for biomedical applications in the form of multimodal-imaging probes and simultaneous diagnostic and drug delivery (Fig. 6.3).

6.3.1 Surface Functionalized Superparamagnetic Nanoparticles for MRI

MRI is a noninvasive imaging technique used in clinics for diagnostic purposes for a diverse range of diseases such as cardiovascular, neurological disorders, and cancer. In order to impart stability, biocompatibility, and functionality for targeting, MNPs require surface coating or conjugation of various materials.[22] Commonly, the coating materials include lipids,[23] proteins,[24] dendrimers,[13] polyethylene glycol (PEG),[25] and polysaccharides.[26] Till now, most of the clinical MNPs (Ferridex, Combidex, Resovist, and AMI-288/gerumoxytrol) are based on dextran or a similar type of carbohydrate coating. However, these MNPs were quite nonspecific and their signal enhancement was still unsatisfactory because these dextran-based agents are readily and nonspecifically taken up by phagocytic cells and accumulate in the reticuloendothelial system (RES) such as lymph nodes, spleen, and the Kupffer cells of the liver. Thus they are commonly used as contrast agents for liver MRI.[27] Furthermore, such dextran-based SPIONs are used in clinical MRI to assist in accurate cancer imaging, nodal staging, and detection of metastases.[28,29] A significant drawback of polysaccharide coatings is that they present structural instability in highly acidic environments.[30] Furthermore, in dextran-coated nanoparticles, dextran is not strongly associated with the iron oxide core and can be easily detached from the surface of the iron oxide particles, leading to their aggregation and eventually their precipitation under physiological conditions.[14]

Recently, there has been a growing interest in the development of targeted MNP-based probes for tumor diagnostics to improve specificity and signal enhancement. In addition, MNPs have served as drug carriers, delivering and releasing the drugs.[31] The multifunctional MNPs with targeted moieties and/or therapeutic drugs can recognize tumors or other lesions at molecular or cellular events[13,32–35] and further allow the simultaneous diagnosis and treatment of the diseased tissues with more efficient targeting, precise diagnosis, and therapeutic applications. Targeted MRI contrast agents are thought to offer this possibility. The nontargeted commercially available negative MRI contrast agents such as Feridex consist of multiple iron oxide cores embedded in a macromolecular matrix such as dextran. This results in clusters with a hydrodynamic diameter, which is a multiple of the iron oxide core diameter and has a broad size distribution.

An alternative to the reversibly binding dextran is PEG-gallol. The latter molecule has a considerably higher binding affinity toward iron oxide nanoparticles compared to dextran, leading to enhanced particle stability and smaller particle diameters. SPIONs have been synthesized by aqueous precipitation reaction and were stabilized individually using PEG-gallol. To functionalize the former particles, iron oxide cores were coated with a mixture of biotinylated PEG (3400)-gallol and nonbiotinylated PEG(550)-gallol. Neutravidin, a biotin-binding protein, served as a linker between the PEGylated particles bearing biotin sites and biotinylated functional groups. In a first approach, these neutravidin-coated PEGylated nanoparticles were used to target atherosclerotic sites by attaching a custom-synthesized biotinylated peptide sequence known to bind to E-selectin to them.[36] E-selectin is a transmembrane protein expressed on inflamed endothelial cells.[37] It thus is an early marker for atherosclerosis. The stabilization of a single SPION with PEG-gallol results in high particle stability under physiological conditions and allows further functionalization of these negative MRI contrast agents. Due to the smaller hydrodynamic diameter, narrower particle size distribution, enhanced particle stability, and similar r2-values of PEGylated particles compared to Feridex-IV, the former particles are suited as versatile and easy-to-handle research tool for comparing binding efficiencies of ligands immobilized on these negative MRI contrast agents.

MNP surface coating with dextran or citrate facilitates monodispersed particles, colloidal stability, and biocompatibility, which are crucial requirements for clinical application.[38,39] Furthermore, coating the particles with oleic acid can create a hydrophobic surface that reduces particle oxidation.[38] The subsequent replacement of oleic acid with alternative compounds, such as silane, allows greater flexibility with regard to surface chemistry modification and biocompatibility.[40–42] Commercially available end-labeled silane derivatives allow for the introduction of different chemical moieties such as amine groups or PEG onto the surface of MNPs.[8] Hydrophilic PEG molecules have been used to reduce the phagocytic capture of nanoparticles by cellular components of the immune system, leading to extended circulation and subsequent accumulation in tumors as a consequence of the enhanced permeability and retention (EPR) effect due to leaky vasculature and poor lymphatic drainage in tumors.[43–47] The EPR effect occurs because the newly formed vessels in the tumor are irregular in shape and leaky with large openings and have poor lymphatic drainage. The EPR effect can be utilized for passive targeting of nanoparticles in areas with increased angiogenesis, where there is enhanced permeability of the nanoparticles out of the blood vessels and a longer retention time in the tumor. This approach has been utilized in the development of the commercial PEGylated liposomal Doxil as an anticancer treatment.[48] The application and characterization of PEGylated approaches for silated PEG MNP-mediated imaging of tumors is unexplored. In the following section, we describe the preparation and characterization of silane-PEGcoated MNPs using a simple synthesis method based on the use of biocompatible silane-PEG as a coating agent. The effect of size on the phagocytic capture of PEGylated MNPs *in vitro* and tumor accumulation *in vivo* using MRI is determined for the optimal design of diagnostic nanoparticles.

6.4 Multimodal-Imaging Approach

The utilization of multimodal-imaging probes comprising both MRI and optical-imaging modalities are popular because they can offer spatial resolution and simultaneously give physiological and anatomical information. Optical imaging is used for rapid screening. The dual-imaging modalities offer the combination of MRI and optical imaging probes. However, with trimodal-imaging probes, an additional component — positron emission tomography (PET) isotopes such as 111In or 64Cu — emitting gamma rays from the decay is used as a third probe, along with dual MRI and optical-imaging probes. MRI is one of the most powerful and noninvasive diagnostic techniques for living organisms based on the interaction of protons with the surrounding molecules of tissues. Currently, either paramagnetic complexes (usually gadolinium [Gd^{3+}] or manganese [Mn^{2+}] chelates)[49] or SPIONs are being used as MRI agents.

The paramagnetic complexes accelerate the T_1 relaxation of water protons and, therefore, exhibit bright contrast where they are localized. The most widely used T_1 contrast agent is Gadolinium diethylenetriaminepentaacetate (Gd-DTPA). On the other hand, the SPIONs accelerate the T_2 relaxation of water protons and exhibit dark contrast. Commercially used T_2 contrast agents of iron oxide nanoparticles are coated with hydrophilic polymer dextran. For the additional qualities of optical imaging, various dye molecules, dye-doped silica materials, quantum dots, lanthanide compounds with up- or down-conversion properties, and near-infrared (NIR) emitting nanostructures can be incorporated. All optical-imaging modalities can be coupled with MRI contrast agents. Based on the component of the MRI contrast agent, the multimodal-imaging probes can be categorized into (1) SPION-based multifunctional nanoplatforms and (2) paramagnetic gadolinium (Gd) complex–based multifunctional nanoplatforms. Here, we will focus on the development of the multimodal-imaging aspects of the SPIONs.

6.4.1 Superparamagnetic-Based Multimodal-Imaging Probes

The multimodal-imaging probe of SPIONs is coupled with fluorescent organic dyes. Josephson *et al.* developed multimodal-imaging probes composed of cross-linked iron oxide nanoparticles (CLIO) conjugated with NIR fluorescent dyes.[50] Optical imaging in the NIR region between 700 to 900 nm has low absorption by intrinsic photoactive biomolecules, allows light to penetrate several centimeters into the tissue, and has minimal tissue autofluorescence. To achieve this, arginyl peptides were conjugated to CLIO, followed by the attachment of the indocyanine dye (Cy5.5). With the subcutaneous injection of this probe into nude mice, the lymph nodes were darkened on the MRI images and simultaneously detectable by NIR fluorescent imaging. For probing the brain tumor model, Kircher *et al.* conjugated Cy5.5 directly with aminated CLIO to prepare the multimodal probe. They injected CLIO-Cy5.5 via the tail vein into rats in which a brain tumor was developed by the xenograft of 9L gliosarcoma cells with green fluorescent protein (GFP) expression.[31] In T_2-weighted MRI images, a reduction of the signal intensity in the tumor region indicates that the brain tumor could be diagnosed and the tumor site was specified by preoperative MRI. This demarcation of the brain tumor in intraoperative fluorescent imaging was examined after craniotomy. Using the multimodal-imaging probe, the brain tumor was clearly visualized by Cy5.5 NIR fluorescence (NIRF) and the imaged region was correlated with the actual tumor extent that was determined by GFP fluorescence. Therefore, multimodal MRI and NIR fluorescent probes permitted the preoperative visualization of brain tumors by serving as T_2 MRI contrast agents and allowing the intraoperative discrimination of tumors from the brain tissue using their NIRF.

Active cancer targeting with a multimodal-imaging probe (CLIO-Cy5.5) can be done by conjugating a targeting molecule, including peptides and small molecules. Moore *et al.* synthesized cancer-targeted multimodal-imaging probes, consisting of CLIO-Cy5.5 attached to synthetic EPPT (YCAREPPTRTFAYWG) peptides on a dextran coating, to target the underglycosylated mucin-1 (uMUC-1) antigen of various cancer cells.[51] An *in vivo* MRI was performed on animals bearing bilateral uMUC-1-positive and uMUC-1-negative tumors in their legs before and 24 h after the intravenous injection of the probe. On administration of the probe, there was a significant signal reduction in T_2 MRI and brighter NIR emission was observed in the uMUC-1-positive tumors compared to those in the uMUC-1-negative tumors. The Weissleder group designed the trimodality-imaging probes having MRI, NIR fluorescent imaging, and PET functionalities using CLIO as a platform.[52] To the aminated dextran CLIO platform, DTPA was conjugated to chelate PET tracer 64 Cu, forming a PET, MRI, and optically detectable imaging agent. The advantage of PET imaging is that it provides a highly sensible high detection magnitude unlike MRI. With the trimodality nanoprobe, there was a higher level of *in vivo* detection of atherosclerotic plaques. Because the macrophages in atherosclerosis have an affinity for polysaccharide-containing supramolecular structures, the dextran-coated nanoparticles could target the macrophages. As an alternative to dextran coating, PEG represents a biocompatible coating material for iron oxide nanoparticles used in biomedical applications.

Zhang and coworkers modified the surface of iron oxide nanoparticles with trifluoroethylester-terminal-PEG-silane, which was then converted to an amine-terminated PEG.[53] The terminal amine groups were used for the conjugation of Cy5.5 and chlorotoxin, a targeting peptide for glioma tumors. *In vitro* MRI and confocal fluorescence microscopy showed the strong preferential uptake of the multimodal probes by glioma cells as compared to the control nanoparticles. With this, a significantly higher degree of internalization of the probes by glioma cells was observed as compared to the control noncancerous cells, indicating the cancer-targeting abilities of the probes for gliomas.

Lee *et al.* reported multimodal probes consisting of iron oxide nanoparticles with thermally cross-linked polymer shells,[54] They synthesized triblock polymers having $-Si(OCH_3)_3$ groups for the purpose of bonding to iron oxide and the cross-linking of the polymer shells, PEG for biocompatibility, and N-hydrosuccinimide-activated carboxylic acid for the further conjugation of fluorescent dyes. The *in vivo* T_2 MR and NIR fluorescent imaging of tumor-bearing mice after the intravenous injection of the Cy5.5 conjugated multimodal probes revealed that the probes were accumulated at the tumor site via the EPR effect, which made it possible to detect tumors by MRI and optical imaging. The *ex vivo* NIR fluorescent images of several organs and tumors indicated that the highest fluorescence intensity was observed in the tumor. Compared to the Cy5.5-conjugated multimodal probes, when the free Cy5.5 dye was intravenously injected into a tumor-bearing mouse as a control experiment, only a faint fluorescence signal was observed in the tumor.

The bifunctional nanoparticles were shown to act as simultaneous T_2 MRI and optical cell labeling agents. The Hyeon group reported that PEG-derivatized phosphine oxide ligands can make water-dispersible metal oxide nanoparticles.[55] The ligands were synthesized from a simple reaction between $POCl_3$ and PEG. The phosphine group can be exchanged with the stabilizing ligands of various hydrophobic metal oxide nanoparticles of Fe_3O_4, NiO, MnO, and TiO_2. A fluorescent dye, fluorescein isothiocyanate (FITC), was attached to the activated PEG terminal group of Fe_3O_4 nanoparticles to synthesize fluorescent MNPs. Generally, fluorescent dyes show a low fluorescence quantum yield and severe photobleaching. To overcome these problems, the dye molecules were incorporated in a protective silica matrix.[56] Silica is known to be biocompatible, and its surface can be easily modified with various organic functional groups, allowing the conjugation of targeting molecules. On the basis of these advantages, the silica nanomatrix was embedded with dye molecules that exhibited more intense fluorescence and better photostability than conventional molecular dyes. A stronger fluorescence signal was observed than that was obtained with a single dye molecule under the same excitation conditions, because a large number of dye molecules were confined in the relatively small volume of a single silica nanoparticle. Also, the silica nanomatrix serves as a shield to protect the dyes from quenching. In a combinational form, iron oxide nanoparticles are assembled with fluorescent silica to make multimodal-imaging probes. Various silica nanostructures, including nanoshells, mesoporous silicas, and silica nanoparticles, have been employed for multimodal probes using dye-doped silica.

Combinational nanoparticles composed of iron oxide nanoparticles and dye-doped silica particles offer a multimodality mode of action. Lee *et al.* designed hybrid nanoparticles composed of dye-doped silica as the core and multiple iron oxide nanoparticles as the satellite.[57] Interestingly, these probes exhibited superior T_2 MRI capabilities due to the synergistic magnetism of the multiple Fe_3O_4 satellites surrounding the core silica nanoparticles as compared to free water-soluble iron oxide nanoparticles of the same size.

6.5 Superparamagnetic Nanoparticles for Synchronized MRI and Therapeutic Drug Delivery

For an effective method for diagnosis and therapeutic application, it is desirable to conjugate MNPs with therapeutic drugs and targeting moieties so that MNPs can serve both as contrast enhancement agents in MRI and as a drug carrier in controlled drug delivery and targeted cancer diagnosis and therapy.[58,59] Kohler *et al.* fabricated MNPs with a therapeutic drug methotrexate (MTX), targeting folate receptor overexpressing cancer cells.[60,61] After 2 h of incubation, MTX-conjugated MNPs showed higher internalization (approximately tenfold) in Hela cells and (approximately twentyfold) in MCF-7 cells compared to other normal cells. Similarly, in another approach, Dilnawaz *et al.* developed aqueous dispersible glyceryl monooleate MNPs capable of carrying a high payload of hydrophobic anticancer drug (paclitaxel and rapamycin) either single or in combination. For the targeted therapy, Herceptin-2 antibody was conjugated to drug-loaded MNPs, which demonstrated enhanced antiproliferative activity in breast cancer cell line (MCF-7).[3]

To enhance the stability and biocompatibility of the MNPs *in vivo*, polymers can be coated on to the surface; however, these coated polymers are lost under harsh *in vivo* conditions, resulting in aggregation.[62,63] To prevent the aggregation of polymers, thermally cross-linked SPIONs (TCL-SPIONs) have been developed by using an antibiofouling PEG polymer containing Si–OH, poly(3-(trime thoxysilyl)propylmethacrylate-r-PEGmethylethermethacrylate-r-N-acryloxysuccinimide). The COOH of TCL-SPIONs was further converted to amine-modified TCL-SPIONs and then finally conjugate Cy5.5 to obtain Cy5.5 dye-labeled TCL-SPIONs for use as a multimodal (MR/fluorescence)-imaging probe.[33] MRI and fluorescence images demonstrated that TCL-SPIONs showed higher tumor accumulation without any targeting moieties. With this, a drug doxorubicin has been conjugated to perform the dual function of a drug carrier and an MRI agent, that is, DOX@TCL-SPIONs.[64] The DOX has been incorporated in the polymeric shell of TCL-SPIONs via electrostatic interactions between positively charged DOX and the negatively charged polymer, showing a faster release pattern of drug at the mildly acidic pH of tumor areas than at the neutral pH of vascular compartments. Thus, systemically administered DOX@TCL-SPIONs displayed a much lower toxicity in normal cells but exerted a therapeutic response to cancer cells. The DOX@TCL-SPIONs could efficiently detect Lewis lung carcinoma (LLC) and efficiently deliver DOX to the tumor tissue, thereby showing excellent anticancer activity along with the *in vivo* MRI. Jain *et al.* developed combined drug delivery and imaging properties of MNPs coated with oleic acid and stabilized with pluronic F-127, which demonstrated sustained release of the drug molecule along with enhanced contrast in the whole tumor, whereas the behavior of the commercial contrast agent, Feridex IV, was transient and confined to the tumor periphery. The prolonged presence of nanovehicles in tumors is an advantage not only for MRI but also for the delivery of anticancer drugs. In addition to drug delivery and MRI, MNPs can also be targeted to the tumors by conjugating antibodies to the MNPs for the receptors overexpressed on the tumor cell surfaces. The conjugation of a targeting ligand can enhance the efficiency and specificity of the MNPs. Therefore, targeted nanocarriers with simultaneous imaging and drug delivery capabilities are clinically important, allowing the detection of pathology and delivery of the therapeutics.[7]

Papahadjopoulos *et al.* have developed a hybrid micelle using poly(ethylene glycol) methyl ether methacrylate (PEGMA) and 2-(Acetoacetoxy) ethyl methacrylate (AEMA).[48] PEGMA was chosen to be the repeating unit constituting the hydrophilic block within the block copolymer because of its biocompatibility and improved blood circulation times as well as its thermoresponsive properties.[65] AEMA was chosen to be the repeating unit for the second block because of its well-known ability to act as a strong bidentate ligand and bind effectively onto metal ions of different geometries and oxidation states, aiming at improving stabilization upon binding onto the inorganic iron oxide surfaces.[66] PEGMA*x*-*b*-AEMA*y* diblock copolymers enable the stabilization of iron oxide MNPs in water via encapsulation within the AEMA ligating core, resulting in novel biocompatible superparamagnetic hybrid micelles. These hybrid micelles exhibit macrophage exclusion, superior to those of the tested dextran-based magnetic contrast agent (Resovit). By lowering the uptake of SPIONs by RES, such as macrophages, the MNPs circulate long enough and accumulate in the tumor by the EPR effect for the *in vivo* use of SPIONs as well as the imaging of cancer. The novel superparamagnetic hybrid self-assemblies with distinct and valuable biodistribution characteristics enable their potential application as magnetic contrast agents.

6.5.1 Superparamagnetic Nanoparticles for MRI and Gene Delivery

Antisense oligonucleotides have been applied for effective antisense therapy. Gene therapy is associated with problems of rapid degradation by exonuclease or endonuclease and poor diffusion across the cell membrane during the clinical use. However, the related problems should be solved for the effective clinical use of antisense therapy.[67] Nanovehicles such as dendrimers are excellent nonviral vectors since they are safer, simpler to use, and more easily mass-produced than other viral vectors.[68,69] To solve the problems in antisense therapy, Pan *et al.* fabricated polyamidoamine (PAMAM) dendrimer-conjugated MNPs as a gene transfection vector.[70] The surface of MNPs was coated with 3-aminopropyl-trimethoxysilane (APTS) to make generation zero dendrimer MNPs (G0 dMNP) and then further excessive methacrylate was added. By the excessive use of ethylenediamine, the methacrylate group of G0 dMNP was further converted to amine-modified G0 dMNP. Stepwise growth was formed by repeating methacryalte and ehtylenediamine until the desired number of generations from 1.0 to 5.0 (G1.0–G5.0) was achieved. As the generation of the dendrimer increased, the amount of antisense survivin oligonuelcotide (asODN) absorbed by dMNPs also increased via electrostatic interactions, leading to the accumulation of positive charges on the surfaces. The antisense survivin–loaded dendrimer conjugated MNP (asODNG 5.0dMNP) with more positive charges were highly internalized to cross tumor cell membranes, inhibiting the growth of tumor cells and showing a strong inhibition effect on the expression of the survivin gene and protein. This study showed that dMNPs as a high-efficiency gene-delivery system are helpful to protect asODN from degradation by enzymes inside cells.

Small interfering RNA (siRNA) molecules are short double-stranded nucleic acid molecules that can act as mediators of RNA interference (RNAi) within the cytoplasm of cells. The therapeutic application of siRNAs requires the effective delivery of siRNAs in to the target cells since naked siRNAs cannot enter cells on their own. Various delivery methods have been developed and deployed such as the use of lipid-based agents,[71] antibody-protein fusion proteins,[72] liposomes,[73] and nanoparticles.[74] For the clinical trials, a noninvasive approach of siRNA delivery to target tissues is needed to optimize experimental treatment strategies. The *in vivo* imaging of siRNA is currently confined to the bioluminescence imaging of siRNA-mediated silencing.[75] Recently, noninvasive dual-modality imaging was accomplished using multifunctional MNPs for the simultaneous *in vivo* transfer of siRNA and imaging of siRNA accumulation in tumors by both MRI and NIRF optical imaging.[76] For this, Cy5.5-labeled MNPs are covalently linked to siRNA molecules as therapeutic target genes and further modified with membrane translocation peptides, that is, myristoylated polyarginine peptides (MPAP), for intracellular delivery.[77] The results of the *in vivo* tracking of these multifunctional MNPs in the tumor by MR and NIRF imaging demonstrated that they could simultaneously deliver and detect siRNA-based therapeutic agents *in vivo*. However, a detailed investigation is further needed to clearly understand the precise mechanisms mediating efficient gene silencing *in vivo*.[78]

6.5.2 Multifunctional Superparamagnetic Hybrid Nanosystem for Cancer Imaging and Therapy

Biocompatible polymers are suitable for targeted drug delivery.[79–81] The use of a multifunctional hybrid nanosystem, that is, multifunctional magnetopolymeric nanohybrids (MMPNs) that combine MNPs as MR, anticancer drugs, antibodies, and biodegradable amphiphilic block copolymers in one system can be an effective mode of therapy.[82] With the use of the nanoemulsion method, hydrophobic magnetic nanocrystals ($MnFe_2O_4$) and doxorubicin (DOX) were simultaneously incorporated into poly(lactic-co-glycolic acid) — polyethylene glycol, (PLGA)-PEG-COOH, and then further human epidermal growth factor receptor 2 (HER) was conjugated with (HER-MMPNs).[82] The HER-MMPNs have excellent colloidal stability at a high concentration in a wide range of salt concentrations and within various pH ranges, showing sustained drug-release profiles due to polymer degradation. *In vitro* MR images demonstrated that multifunctional MMPNs were the efficient targeted system for the HER2/neu receptor by showing efficient R2 values in cells treated with HER-MMPNs compared to those of irrelevant antibody-conjugated MMPNs (IRR-MMPNs). Indeed, HER-MMPNs displayed ultrasensitive targeted detection by MRI in NIH3T6.7 *in vivo*. The HER-MMPNs after internalization by endocytosis could efficiently release DOX, showing an enhanced inhibitory effect of HER-MMPNs on cell proliferation, demonstrating promising tumor-growth inhibition. The Brian Ross group has developed a light-activated theragnostic nanosystem. These MMPNs have a polyacrylamide (PAA) core containing a photoactive agent, Photofrin (PDTagent), iron oxide (MRI agent), F3-peptide (tumor vascular homing peptide), and PEG for increased circulation time.[83] To study the behavior of cellular uptake, the particles were also fluorescently labeled with Alexa Fluor 594. After an appropriate time of incubation, F3-targeted nanoparticles were significantly internalized into MDA-MB435, a breast cancer cell line, and 90% of the cells receiving the targeted particles were dead after the light irradiation. In an MRI study, the tumor localization of targeted and nontargeted particles was similar within 10 min after injection. After 2 h, the nontargeted particles were removed from the glioma (9L) tumor, whereas the F3-targeted particles showed continuous accumulation. The analysis by dynamic scanning MRI data suggested that the F3-targeted nanoparticles increased the tumor half-life from 39 to 123 min. Also, therapeutically, the F3-targeted nanoparticles produced massive regional necrosis with a significant decrease in the tumor volume with a much longer survival time than that of either nontargeted nanoparticles or just free Photofrin or laser irradiation. Notably, there was a complete eradication of brain cancers in three out of five animals within 60 days posttreatment.[78]

6.6 Conclusions and Future Perspective

Superparamagnetic nanoparticles have been used as clinical tools in the MRI of numerous diseases. In the near future, the new generation of multifunctional and multimodal MNPs combined with therapeutic drugs, targeting moieties, MRI contrast agents, and optical imaging probe will allow for the investigation of diseases across a number of platforms, thereby enabling the accumulation of a vast amount of information in clinics. The ultimate goal in creating these multifunctional and multimodal nanomaterials is for the efficient and specific treatment as well as diagnosis of diseases. Clinically, in the futuristic approach, many issues, including the biocompatibility, toxicity, *in vivo* targeting efficacy, and long term stability of the multifunctional nanoparticles, need to be addressed. The development of novel multifunctional nanomaterials and the exact investigation of their characteristics in a living organism will open the way to the diagnosis and therapy of diseases in the future.

References

1. Lu, A.-H., Schmidt, W., Matoussevitch, N., Bönnemann, H., Spliethoff, B., Tesche, B., Bill, E., Kiefer, W., and Schüth, F., *Angew. Chem. Int. Ed.*, **2004**, 43(33), 4303–4306.
2. Stoner, E. C., and Rhodes, P., **1949**, vol. 62, p. 481.
3. Dilnawaz, F., Singh, A., Mohanty, C., and Sahoo, S., *Biomaterials*, **2010**, 31, 3694–3706.
4. Huang, S., Liao, M., and Chen, D., *Biotechnol. Prog.*, **2003**, 19, 1095–1100.

5. Albrecht, T., Bührer, R., Fahnle, M., Maier, K., Platzek, D., and Reske, J., First observation of ferromagnetism and ferromagnetic domains in a liquid metal. *Appl. Phys. A Mater. Sci. & Process*, **1997**, 65, 215–220.
6. Gupta, A. K., and Gupta, M., *Biomaterials*, **2005**, 26(18), 3995–4021.
7. Jain, T. K., Morales, M. A., Sahoo, S. K., Leslie-Pelecky, D. L., and Labhasetwar, V., *Mol. Pharm.*, **2005**, 2(3), 194–205.
8. Mornet, S. P. J., and Duguet, E., *J. Magn. Magn. Mater.*, **2005**, 293, 127–134.
9. Vekas, L., Avdeev, M. V., and Bica, D., in *Nanoscience in Biomedicine.*, **2009**, Springer, New York.
10. Harris, L. A., Goff, J. D., Carmichael, A. Y., Riffle, J. S., Harburn, J. J., St. Pierre, T. G., and Sauders, M., *Chem. Mater.*, **2003**, 15, 1367–1377.
11. Shen, L., Laibinis, P., and Hatton, T., *Langmuir*, **1999**, 15, 447–453.
12. Wormuth, K., *J. Colloid Interf. Sci.*, **2001**, 241, 366–377.
13. Bulte, J. W., Douglas, T., Witwer, B., Zhang, S. C., Strable, E., Lewis, B. K., Zywicke, H., Miller, B., van Gelderen, P., Moskowitz, B. M., Duncan, I. D., and Frank, J. A., *Nat. Biotechnol.*, **2001**, 19, 1141–1147.
14. Mc Carthy, J., and Weissleder, R., *Adv. Drug Deliv. Rev.*, **2008**, 60, 1241–1251.
15. Neves, A., and Brindle, K., *Biochem. Biophys. Acta*, **2006**, 1766, 242–261.
16. Elster, A. D., Challa, V. R., Gilbert, T. H., Richardson, D. N., and Contento, J. C., *Radiology*, **1989**, 170, 857–862.
17. Trohidou, K. N., *Monte Carlo Studies of Surface and Interface Effects in Magnetic Nanoparticles*, **2005**, Springer, US, 45–74.
18. Bulte, J. W., Duncan I. D., and Frank, J. A., *J. Cereb. Blood Flow Metab.*, **2002**, 22, 899–907.
19. Bulte, J., Brooks, R., Moskowitz, B., Bryant, L. J., and Frank, J., *Magn. Reson. Med.*, **1999a**, 42, 379–384.
20. Dobson, J., *Drug. Devel. Res.*, **2006a**, 67, 55–60.
21. Pankhurst, Q. A., Connolly, J., Jones, S. K., and Dobson, J., *J. Phys. D: Appl. Phys.*, **2003**, 36, R167–R181.
22. Kim, D., Mikhaylova, M., and Wang, F., *Chem. Mater.*, **2003**, 15, 4343–4351.
23. Nitin, N., LaConte, L., Zurkiya, O., Hu, X., and Bao, G., *J. Biol. Inorg. Chem.*, **2004**, 9, 706–712.
24. Wilhelm, C., Billotey, C., Roger, J., Pons, J. N., Bacri, J. C., and Gazeau, F., *Biomaterials*, **2003**, 24, 1001–1011.
25. Illium, L., Church, A. E., Butterworth, M. D., Arien, A., Whetstone, J., and Davis, S. S., *Pharm. Res.* **2001**, 18, 640–645.

26. Kellar, K. E., Fujii, D. K., Gunther, W. H. H., Briley-Sæbø, K., Bjørnerud, A., Spiller, M., and Koenig, S. H., *J. Magn. Reson. Imaging*, **2000**, 11, 488.
27. Reimer, P., and Tombach, B., *Eur. Radiol.*, **1998**, 8, 1198–1204.
28. Harisinghani, M. G., Barentsz, J., Hahn, P. F., Deserno, W. M., Tabatabaei, S., Van de Kaa, C. H., De la Rosette, J., and Weissleder, R., *N. Engl. J. Med.*, **2003**, 348(25), 2491–2499.
29. Tanimoto, A., and Kuribayashi, S., *Eur. J. Radiol.*, **2006**, 58, 200–216.
30. Leslie-Pelecky, D., Labhasetwar, V., and Kraus, R. H., Jr., Biomagnetics, in *Advanced Magnetic Nanostructures.*, **2006**, Springer, New York, pp. 461–482.
31. Kircher, M. F., Mahmood, U., King, R. S., Weissleder, R., and Josephson, L., *Cancer Res.*, **2003**, 63, 8122–8125.
32. Huh, Y. M., Jun, Y. W., Song, H. T., Kim, S., Choi, J. S., Lee, J. H., Yoon, S., Kim, K. S., Shin, J. S., Suh, J. S., and Cheon, J., *J. Am. Chem. Soc.*, **2005**, 127(35), 12387–12391.
33. Lee, J. H., Huh, Y. M., Jun, Y. W., Seo, J. W., Jang, J. T., Song, H. T., Kim, S., Cho, E. J., Yoon, H. G., Suh, J. S., and Cheon, J., *Nat. Med.*, **2006**, 13, 95–99.
34. Weissleder, R., Moore, A., Mahmood, U., Bhorade, R., Benveniste, H., Chiocca, E. A., and Basilion, J. P., *Nat. Med.*, **2000**, 6, 351–354.
35. Zhao, M., Beauregard, D. A., Loizou, L., Davletov, B., and Brindle, K. M., *Nat. Med.*, **2001**, 7, 1241–1244.
36. Martens, C. L., Cwirla, S. E., Lee, R. Y., Whitehorn, E., Chen, E. Y., Bakker, A., Martin, E. L., Wagstrom, C., Gopalan, P., Smith, C. W., *et al.*, *J. Biol. Chem.*, **1995**, 270(36), 21129–21136.
37. Choudhury, R. P., Fuster, V., and Fayad, Z. A., *Nat. Rev. Drug Discov.*, **2004**, 3(11), 913–925.
38. Maity, D., and Agrawal, D. C., *J. Magn. Magn. Mater.*, **2007**, 308(46).
39. Wang, Y. X., Hussain, S. M., and Krestin, G. P., *Eur. Radiol.*, **2001**, 11(11), 2319–2331.
40. De Palma, R., Peeters, S., Van Bael, M. J., Van den Rul, H., Bonroy, K., Laureyn, W., Mullens, J., Borghs, G., and Maes, G., *Chem. Mater.*, **2007**, 19, 1821–1831.
41. Fan, Q.-L., Neoh, K.-G., Kang, E.-T., Shuter, B., and Wang, S.-C., *Biomaterials*, **2007**, 28, 5426–5436.
42. Sun, Y., Ding, X., Zheng, Z., Cheng, X., Hua, X., and Peng, Y., *Chem. Commun.*, **2006**, 26, 2765–2767.

43. Allen, T. M., *Adv. Drug Delivery Rev.*, **1994**, 13, 285–309.

44. Brigger, I., Dubernet, C., and Couvreur, P., *Adv. Drug Delivery Rev.*, **2002**, 54, 631–651.

45. Folkman, J., *J. Natl. Cancer Inst.*, **1990**, 82, 4–7.

46. Iyer, A. K., Khaled, G., Fang, J., and Maeda, H., *Drug Discov. Today*, **2006**, 11, 812–818.

47. Miller, J. C., Pien, H. H., Sahani, D., Sorensen, G. A., and Thrall, J. H., *J. Natl. Cancer Inst.*, **2005**, 97, 172–187.

48. Papahadjopoulos, D., Allen, T. M., Gabizon, A., Mayhew, E., Matthay, K., and Huang, S. K., *Proc. Natl. Acad. Sci. USA*, **1991**, 88, 11460–11464

49. Caravan, P., *Chem. Soc. Rev.*, **2006**, 35, 512–523.

50. Josephson, L., Kircher, M. F., Mahmood, U., Tang, Y., and Weissleder, R., *Bioconjugate Chem.*, **2002**, 13(3), 554–560.

51. Moore, A., Medarova, Z., and Potthast, A., *Cancer Res.*, **2004**, 64, 1821–1827.

52. Weissleder, R., Kelly, K., Sun, E. Y., Shtatland, T., and Josephson, L., *Nat. Biotechnol.*, **2005**, 23, 1418–1423.

53. Veiseh, O., Sun, C., Gunn, J., Kohler, N., Gabikian, P., Lee, D., Bhattarai, N., Ellenbogen, R., Sze, R., Hallahan, A., Olson, J., and Zhang, M., *Nano Lett.*, **2005**, 5(6), 1003–1008.

54. Lee, H., Yu, M. K., Park, S., Moon, S., Min, J. J., Jeong, Y. Y., Kang, H. W., and Jon, S., *J. Am. Chem. Soc.*, **2007**, 129, 12739–12745.

55. Na, H. B., Lee, I. S., Seo, H., Park, Y. I., Lee, J. H., Kim, S.-W., and Hyeon, T., *Chem. Commun.*, **2007**, 5167–5169.

56. Burns, A., Ow, H., and Wiesner, U., *Chem. Soc. Rev.*, **2006**, 35, 1028–1042.

57. Lee, J., Young-wook Jun, Y., Yeon, S., Shin, J., and Cheon, J., *Angew. Chem. Int. Ed. Engl.*, **2006**, 45(48), 8160–8162.

58. Alexiou, C., Arnold, W., Klein, R. J., Parak, F. G., Hulin, P., Bergemann, C., Erhardt, W., Wagenpfeil, S., and Lubbe, A. S., *Cancer Res.*, **2000**, 60(23), 6641–6648.

59. Bulte, J., Hoekstra, Y., Kamman, R. L., Magin, R. L., Webb, A. G., Briggs, R. W., Go, K. G., Hulstaert, C. E., Miltenyi, S., The TH., *et al.*, *Magn. Reson. Med.*, **1992**, 25(1), 148–157.

60. Kohler, N., Sun, C., Fichtenholtz, A., Gunn, J., Fang, C., and Zhang, M., *Small*, **2006**, 2(6), 785–792.

61. Kohler, N., Sun, C., Wang, J., and Zhang, M., *Langmuir*, **2005**, 21(19), 8858–8864.

62. Moghimi, S. M., Hunter, A. C., and Murray, J. C., *Pharmacol. Rev.*, **2001**, 53(2), 283–318.

63. Zhang, Y., Kohler, N., and Zhang, M., *Biomaterials*, **2002**, 23(7), 1553–1561.

64. Yu, M. K., Jeong, Y. Y., Park, J., Park, S., Kim, J. W., Min, J. J., Kim, K., and Jon, S., **2008**, 47(29), 5362–5365.

65. Lutz, J. F., *J. Polym. Sci., Part A: Polym. Chem.*, **2008**, 46, 3459–3470.

66. Mehrotra, R. C., Bohra, B., and Gaur, D. P., *Metal [Beta]-Diketonates and Allied Derivatives*, **1978**, Academic Press, New York.

67. Tarkanyi, I., Horváth, A., Szatmari, I., Eizert, H., Vámosi, G., Damjanovich, S., Ségal-Bendirdjian, E., and Aradi, J., *FEBS Lett.*, **2005**, 579(6), 1411–1416.

68. Majoros, I. J., Myc, A., Thomas, T., Mehta, C. B., and Baker, J. R., Jr., *Biomacromolecules*, **2006**, 7(2), 572–579.

69. Radu, D. R., Lai, C. Y., Jeftinija, K., Rowe, E. W., Jeftinija, S., and Lin, V. S., *J. Am. Chem. Soc.*, **2004**, 126(41), 13216–13217.

70. Pan, B., Cui, D., Sheng, Y., Ozkan, C., Gao, F., He, R., Li, Q., Xu, P., and Huang, T., *Cancer Res.*, **2007**, 67(17), 8156–8163.

71. Landen, C. N., Jr., Chavez-Reyes, A., Bucana, C., Schmandt, R., Deavers, M. T., Lopez-Berestein, G., and Sood, A. K., *Cancer Res.*, **2005**, 65(15), 6910–6918.

72. Song, E., Zhu, P., Lee, S. K., Chowdhury, D., Kussman, S., Dykxhoorn, D. M., Feng, Y., Palliser, D., Weiner, D. B., Shankar, P., Marasco, W. A., and Lieberman, J., *Nat. Biotechnol.*, **2005**, 23(6), 709–717.

73. Zimmermann, T. S., Lee, A. C., Akinc, A., Bramlage, B., Bumcrot, D., Fedoruk, M. N., Harborth, J., Heyes, J. A., Jeffs, L. B., John, M., Judge, A. D., Lam, K., McClintock, K., Nechev, L. V., Palmer, L. R., Racie, T., Rohl, I., Seiffert, S., Shanmugam, S., Sood, V., Soutschek, J., Toudjarska, I., Wheat, A. J., Yaworski, E., Zedalis, W., Koteliansky, V., Manoharan, M., Vornlocher, H. P., and MacLachlan, I., *Nature*, **2006**, 441(7089), 111–114.

74. Bartlett, D. W., and Davis, M. E., *Bioconjugate Chem.*, **2007**, 18(2), 456–468.

75. Takeshita, F., Minakuchi, Y., Nagahara, S., Honma, K., Sasaki, H., Hirai, K., Teratani, T., Namatame, N., Yamamoto, Y., Hanai, K., Kato, T., Sano, A., and Ochiya, T., *Proc. Natl. Acad. Sci. USA*, **2005**, 102(34), 12177–12182.

76. Medarova, Z., Pham, W., Farrar, C., Petkova, V., and Moore, A., *Nat. Med.*, **2007**, 13(3), 372–377.

77. Mae, M., and Langel, U., *Curr. Opin. Pharmacol.*, **2006**, 6(5), 509–514.

78. Park, K., Lee, S., Kang, E., Kim, K., Choi, K., and Kwon, I. C., *Adv. Func. Mater.*, **2009**.

79. Farokhzad, O., Cheng, J., Teply, B. A., Sherifi, I., Jon, S., Kantoff, P. W., Richie, J. P., and Langer, R., *Proc. Natl. Acad. Sci.*, **2006**, 103(16), 6315–6320.

80. Michalet, X., Pinaud, F. F., Bentolila, L. A., Tsay, J. M., Doose, S., Li, J. J., Sundaresan, G., Wu, A. M., Gambhir, S. S., and Weiss, S., *Science*, **2005**, 307(5709), 538–544.

81. Sengupta, S., Eavarone, D., Capila, I., Zhao, G., Watson, N., Kiziltepe, T., and Sasisekharan, R., *Nature*, **2005**, 436(7050), 568–572.

82. Yang, J., Lee, C. H., Ko, H. J., Suh, J. S., Yoon, H. G., Lee, K., Huh, Y. M., and Haam, S., *Angew. Chem. Int. Ed.*, **2007**, 46, 8836–8839.

83. Reddy, G. R., Bhojani, M. S., McConville, P., Moody, J., Moffat, B. A., Hall, D. E., Kim, G., Koo, Y. E., Woolliscroft, M. J., Sugai, J. V., Johnson, T. D., Philbert, M. A., Kopelman, R., Rehemtulla, A., and Ross, B. D., *Clin. Cancer Res.*, **2006**, 12, 6677–6686.

Chapter 7

Nanobiotechnology: A New Generation of Biomedicine — Innovative Nanotechnology in Key Areas of Biomedical Engineering and Cancer Therapy

Prasanna Vidyasekar, Pavithra Shyamsunder, and Rama S. Verma

Stem Cell and Molecular Biology Laboratory, Department of Biotechnology, Indian Institute of Technology Madras, Chennai, India

vermars@iitm.ac.in

The convergence of medical science and nanotechnology has created many new and promising fields, prominent among them the merger of biotechnology and nanotechnology. "Nanobiotechnology," as this chapter describes it, has tremendously successful potential applications in the field of biomedical engineering, especially in regenerative medicine. The use of nanotechnology to create growth- and differentiation-enhancing surfaces, scaffolds, or patterns and the problems in designing such submicron structures are discussed in this chapter's section on regenerative therapy. Cancer therapy has, of course, already seen much progress and advances in that this nascent technology is one of the forerunners in embracing "nanotech." The nanoparticle formulations that are in current use to combat cancer in its various manifestations are discussed in the chapter's section on cancer therapy. Nanotechnology is a new generation of medicine, and its wide spread application in varied fields demonstrates its immense potential.

Nanotechnology in Health Care
Edited by Sanjeeb K. Sahoo

ISBN 978-981-4267-21-2 (Hardcover), 978-981-4267-35-9 (eBook)
www.panstanford.com

7.1 Introduction

There is plenty of room at the bottom. Many of the cells are very tiny, but they are active: they manufacture substance; they walk around; they wiggle: and they do all kinds of marvelous things all on a very small scale. Also they store information. Consider the possibility that we too can make things very small which does what we want when we want-and that we can manufacture an object that maneuvers at that level.

— Nobel Laureate **Richard P. Feynman**, in a 1959 lecture at the California Institute of Technology

There's plenty of room at the bottom was one of the first insights into nanotechnology — a sprawling field in the present day having pervaded many aspects of science and technology. It has entered many disciplines, including medicine, revolutionizing the traditional discipline in the process. In time, it will hopefully provide a cure for diseases like cancer and Alzheimer's. It is unlikely that Richard Feynman imagined 50 years ago during the annual meeting of the American Physical Society that nanotechnology would one day transform traditional science or garner the kind of funding it does today. The United States invested $1.3 billion in 2006 in the National Nanotechnology Initiative (NNI) and proposed a budget of $1.45 billion for 2008. By the end of 2008, the United States was supposed to have invested an estimated $3.7 billion in nanoscience and nanotechnology. The National Cancer Institute of the United States had announced that it would spend $144.3 million to fund cancer-related nanotechnology research for a five-year period. Japan has supposedly invested $3 billion toward this emerging field of research. These are big numbers, and they suggest that medicine's newest tool might actually have some potential amid all the hype.

7.1.1 A New Tool

Nanos is Greek for dwarf. A nanoparticle is only nanometers big, and a nanometer (nm) is a billionth of a meter (10^{-9} m). In relative terms, that would be about 1/80,000 times the thickness of a human hair. Diameters of atoms are in the tenths of a nanometer, and a DNA strand is a few nanometers wide. But chemistry, biology, and the material sciences deal with atoms, molecules, and small entities just the same as nanotechnology does. So what qualifies nanotechnology as an individual field? Nanotech differs from the traditional disciplines in the sense that it does not deal with these molecules in "bulk." It actually manipulates individual atoms and molecules in very specific ways, creating new materials and particles having novel properties and functions. The assembly and organization of molecules (which includes atoms) within a size range of 1–100+ nm is *nanotechnology* and these *nanoparticles* usually have none of the behavioral characteristics of their larger fundamental solid, liquid, or gaseous counterparts. These nanoparticles are versatile and varied and will find excellent application in many aspects of medicine. "Nanotech" has immense potential for the simple reason that this technology is at the scale of molecules, making it possible to develop devices and systems smaller and much more efficient than the gear currently available.

Biology might just benefit the most by embracing nanotechnology. It can turn out to be an essential ally because many biological species have basic molecular structures such as proteins, carbohydrates, and lipids — each and every one a molecule of nanoscale dimensions. These have a wide array of chemical, physical, and functional properties, all of which can exhibit utterly different characteristics (such as structure and properties) when individual molecules are introduced into a defined and controlled *nanosystem*.

BOX 1 Nanosystems

It is not within the scope of this chapter to detail what a nanosystem is. However, we will still describe it in brief because the concept will help in understanding some topics later. The technical term "nanosystem" is used to describe, in a wider sense, technical arrangements with the following properties:

- An independent function that is usable externally
- A defined geometric correlation with an external technical arrangement
- An integration into an external functional environment with appropriate interfaces
- The use of at least one unit with nanometer dimensions that is essential for the functioning of the device

Simply put, technical arrangements with the above features, drawing or receiving signals from the environment and transforming them into actions with the provision that one or more vital elements have definite nanometer dimensions, are nanosystems. But *how is this relevant to biologists?*

"Productive nanosystems" have been defined as functional nanometer-scale systems that make atomically specified structures and devices that are under programmatic control, that is, they manufacture to atomic precision. However, present-day technologies are limited in various ways and, therefore, large atomically precise structures that exist in nature such as crystals or complex three-dimensional (3-D) structures such as polymers like DNA and proteins cannot be, *as of yet*, mimicked. While it is possible to build very small atomically precise structures using techniques like scanning probe microscopy to manipulate individual atoms or small groups of atoms, it is not yet possible to combine components in a systematic way to build larger, more complex systems. But technology continues to progress, and it's only a matter of time before we have such incredible machines, and in the meantime, concepts and prototypes of these technologies that are *under construction* have prompted offshoots that are being used for many fabrication processes in areas such as biomedical engineering and biomedicine.

7.1.2 The New Tool in Medicine

Nanotechnology has benefited each field it merged with. One such field of medicine that has profited from its "marriage" to nanomedicine is biomedical engineering. Biomedical engineering, in simple terms, is the application of engineering to solve problems in medicine and biomedical sciences. So we have biomedical engineers specializing in biomaterials to develop materials that can be safely implanted in the body, and biomechanical engineers who apply principles from physics to biological systems and develop artificial organs (such as the artificial heart). Bioinstrumentation engineers use computers or other electronic devices to diagnose or treat diseases. Rehabilitation engineers improve the quality of life for people with disabilities by designing prosthetic limbs or man-made devices for mobility. Tissue and cellular engineers grow cells outside of the body to be implanted *in vivo* and serve some particular function and so on. The merger of nanotechnology and medicine has given rise to an entirely new field of its own — *nanomedicine*. Nanomedicine can be described as the application of nanotechnology and nanoparticles for the treatment, diagnosis, and monitoring of disease. Nanomedicine and biomedical engineering are promising fields, and together they can provide many breakthroughs for medical science. A good example is biological mimetics — materials that have been fabricated and synthesized using principles of biological systems. These include materials such as nanofibers and polymeric nanoparticles often used as biomaterials and biosensors and for laboratory diagnostics.

7.2 Nanotechnology Rejuvenates Regenerative Medicine

Cells (mammalian cells, as far as this chapter is concerned) behave *in vivo* in response to the biological signals they receive from the surrounding environment, which is an edifice of nanometer-scaled components. Therefore, any material we use to repair the human body will have to reproduce, if not all the correct signals, at least the ones that have a bearing in guiding the cells toward a particular behavior. Producing material structures that mimic the biological ones is a considerably complex task, because there are so many factors that influence the fate of a cell. A material that has factored in and incorporated all the signals and cues of an actual *in vivo* biological microenvironment is yet to be discovered or invented, but a good material that possesses a few but vital features mimicking the real structure is possible and it can be produced by nanotechnology. Nanotechnology not only is an excellent tool to produce such material structures but also holds the promise of providing efficient delivery systems [1].

What are the typical scenarios that warrant mimicking a biological entity like a tissue or a cellular microenvironment?

When tissue cannot self-renew, for example, following trauma, an age-related disease, degenerative conditions, or end-stage organ failure, tissue regeneration is required. Regenerating tissue is not an easy task, but it is the ultimate therapy for diseases and the only actual treatment for many incapacitating diseases. Doctors have so far been only *managing* such diseases, treating the symptoms without being able to cure the patient. The possibility of a defective, traumatized tissue being regenerated to its full, original potential makes for a rather appealing goal. Therefore, we have a promising new field known as regenerative medicine, which can be defined as technologies that provide substitute tissues (both synthetic and natural) and/or cells for implantation into the body or promote tissue remodeling for the purpose of replacing, repairing, regenerating, reconstructing, or enhancing function. It is currently an emerging multidisciplinary field that studies the restoration, maintenance, or enhancement of tissues and by extension of organ functions. The ideal that researchers seek is to regenerate damaged or nonfunctional tissues by using a readily available off-the-shelf synthetic or completely biological product. The regeneration of tissues can be achieved by the combination of live cells and materials. The cells will provide biological functionality (be the seed or source in most cases), while the materials will act as scaffolds to support cell proliferation. Diseases like Parkinson's, Alzheimer's, osteoporosis, and cancer and trauma like spine injuries can then be treated by regenerating the diseased or damaged tissue [1].

It being a very vast and developing field, covering all its aspects is beyond the scope of this chapter. We will instead focus on a few innovative and emerging aspects of biomaterials that have utilized nanotechnology such as the fabrication of materials, nanoparticles, and scaffolds for tissue engineering (TE) and nanopatterning of surfaces aimed at eliciting specific biological responses from the host tissue.

Cells have micrometer dimensions, and most mammalian cells being adherent evolve *in vivo* by attaching to and spreading on an underlying matrix comprising a collection of insoluble proteins and glycoaminoglycans known as an extracellular matrix (ECM) — a substratum with topographical and structural features of nanometer size. This adherence is vital for carrying out normal metabolism, proliferation, and differentiation. This ECM, in addition to maintaining the organization and mechanical properties of tissue, also presents many peptide and carbohydrate ligands that are recognized by cellular receptors. These signaling interactions are crucial for maintaining cell function, making it possible for cells to react suitably to their situation. The chief role of the ECM is to act as a go-between for the adhesion of cells, usually between the substrata of tissues or layers of cells where a mediating plane for cell adhesion is required. Without adhesion, most cells initiate a program of apoptosis (programmed cell death), which, as the definition suggests, is fatal, while the loss of adhesion-related signal transduction pathways will lead to cancer. Adhesion, thus, plays a key role in determining cell fate besides being important for cell differentiation, a fundamental feature of regenerative medicine. Differentiation is basically a progenitor (an origin) cell giving rise to a new cell type (or cell types depending on the pluri/multipotency of the progenitor cell). An example of differentiation in humans is hematopoiesis, in which pluripotent stem cells (in the bone marrow) divide and differentiate, passing through many recognizable intermediate steps to form red blood cells, platelets, white blood cells, etc.

Nanotechnology is used to produce the surface, structure, and material with nano-scale features that can mimic the natural environment of cells, to promote certain functions, especially cell adhesion and cell differentiation. These materials can also be used to enhance cell mobility and migration. Ideally, the *in vivo* regeneration or the *in vitro* generation of a complex functional organ consisting of a scaffold made out of synthetic or natural materials, loaded with living cells, is required. Therefore, most often, stem cells are used to seed the scaffold.

BOX 2

Stem cells, as we know, have the potential to develop into many different cell types in the body during early life and growth. A stem cell divides into two cells, and each new cell has the potential either to remain a stem cell or become another type of cell with a more specialized function. They are unspecialized cells capable of renewing themselves through cell division, sometimes after long periods of inactivity. In some organs, such as the bone marrow, stem cells regularly divide to repair and replace worn out or damaged tissues. In other organs, such as the pancreas and the heart, stem cells divide only under special conditions. The more interesting (and relevant) fact is that under certain physiologic or experimental conditions, they can be induced to become tissue- or organ-specific cells with special function and it is this feature that is exploited in regenerative medicine.

The scaffold used must ideally be porous because it has to accommodate molecules and nanoparticles besides keeping the topography nonplanar for a true 3-D version of the actual cellular environment. The biomaterial can then be functionalized, that is, impregnated with different biomolecules that have some function depending on the targeted cells (they will target and act specifically on those particular cells). The material can also be loaded or enmeshed with nanoparticles carrying growth factors, drugs, or genes.

While the process appears straightforward, there are major issues such as stem cell isolation from the patient and their proliferation, the culturing process *in vitro*, and the time delay before the engineered hybrid construct is implanted back into the patient. Multiple invasive procedures on an already traumatized patient (which will be the case usually) for sourcing or implanting are not advisable either. There is also the problem of immune rejection; even though it is the patient's own cells (ideally), the scaffold can, sometimes, cause rejection. So a nonimmunogenic, inert scaffold has to be developed. There can be no one universal scaffold for every cell type or tissue. Every cell line may differ in its preference for a scaffold [1].

7.2.1 Biomaterial Surfaces and Nano-scale Features

The behavior of most cells largely depends on their interactions with the environment. As a result, the interactions between cells and implantable materials will control the success of a restorative patch; a delivery system, cell orientation pattern, or whatever is the intended use of the hybrid construct. Cellular reactions are influenced by the physicochemical factors of the biomaterial surface, like surface energy, surface charges, and chemical composition. Topography is one of the most crucial physical signals for cells. Microtopography influences cell adhesion, proliferation, and differentiation, and, more recently, it has become evident that nanotopography also guides cell behavior significantly. Attaining functional tissues like nerves or tendons requires precise direction of cell orientation. In applications where corneal stroma or intervertebral-disc regeneration is required, contact guidance of cells by such micro- and nanotopographical patterns is a viable prospect. Chemical cues in the form of various different nanometer-scale biomolecules, such as adhesive protein or growth factors, also influence cell behavior significantly. For example, fibronectin and laminin are able to augment the adhesion of different cell types. Hence, extensive work has gone into modifying biomaterial surfaces chemically by immobilization of these biomolecules [2–8].

7.2.2 Surface Patterning: Creating Nano-scale Features on Growth Surfaces

As we have already seen, the topography of the surface on which cells grow obviously influences cell behaviour. A common observation has been that, *in vitro,* cells generally tend to prefer flat featureless surfaces (like tissue culture flask surfaces) even when provided a seemingly better incentive for growth or differentiation in the form of micro- or nanostructures. For some reason that is not yet clear, for cells growing in a two-dimensional (2-D) culture flask to go against gravity and scale edifices or pillars, even though they are only nanometers in height, does not appear to be an entirely easy task. Conversely, growth within an organism is never 2-D; therefore, *in vitro* culture of cells under such (–3D) conditions will perhaps lead to tissue differentiation or more ordered growth resembling actual tissues or tumors (in the case of cancer cells). Nanoparticles offer suitably sized functional components for developing in-plane patterns and offer an extremely convenient route to developing nanofeatures over large areas. A variety of methods have been employed to fabricate nanotopography on biomaterial surfaces. Techniques for creating an ordered topography with a consistent controlled pattern and methods for constructing unordered topography with random orientation and organization are being developed. For acquiring randomly ordered patterns, colloidal lithography, polymer demixing, and chemical etching are used. Soft-lithography techniques or different sources of radiation like electrons, ions, or photons to etch the substrate are the most commonly used procedures to produce regular, ordered geometries. Finally, dip-pen lithography (DPL) is a simple method to create chemical patterns at the nano-scale [1].

Molecular self-assembly is a strategy for nanofabrication that involves designing molecules using the principle of shape complementarity, which causes them to aggregate into desired structures. Self-assembly has a lot of advantages: primarily, it carries out many of the most difficult steps in nanofabrication, critically the ones involving atomic-level modification of structure. Self-assembly is actually a naturally occurring process for the development of many (especially biological) complex, functional structures. Therefore, when *we* use self-assembly, incorporating biological structures directly as components in the final system is convenient. Since it requires that the final end products or structures be thermodynamically the most stable ones open to the system, it tends to produce structures that are relatively defect free and self-healing. Most techniques to create *nanostructuration*, including the ones discussed, here can be used to functionalize a surface, often using self-assembly. A further note on self-assembly in biomometics is provided elsewhere in this chapter.

Nanostructuration using self-assembly is often used to functionalize and create nonfouling surfaces. Fouling is the accumulation of unwanted material on solid surfaces, most often in aquatic environments. The fouling material can be either inorganic or organic. Fouling is usually distinguished from other surface-growth phenomena in that this phenomenon occurs on a surface of a component carrying out a defined and useful function and the fouling process impedes or interferes with this function. Nonfouling surfaces created using nanostructuring can be useful in ophthalmological and cardiovascular application. This can be accomplished by the functionalization of metal surfaces like gold with alkanethiol self-assembled molecules, which can bind polyethylene glycol molecules.

In brief, nanolithography or nanostructuration can be phased into a few steps. Master print or primary pattern writing is the first stage in nanofabrication. This is carried out using direct writing on a base substrate using techniques like laser ablation, scanning probe lithography, or e-beam lithography. Self-assembly techniques as described earlier can also be used to mask a base substrate. These patterns can then be transferred to a suitable material substrate to create a master stamp, die, or mold. The next step is to successively transfer the inverse of the original pattern onto final impressionable polymer surfaces using replication technologies like molding, embossing, casting, or printing.

Soft lithography, as the name suggests, uses a soft, elastomeric stamp to produce structures on a given material surface. Many techniques come under the category of soft lithography, which includes replica molding, micromolding (in capillaries and solvent assisted), microcontact printing, microtransfer molding, and soft embossing. The elastomeric stamp that is used in soft lithography techniques is most commonly silicone — polydimethylsiloxane (PDMS) — also known as Sylgard 184, which is its commercial name. A master with the desired features is created (often virtually designed with CAD software like Autocad® or other computer-assisted design tools) using common lithography methods like photolithography, and EBL, which is then successively used to reproduce the pattern on a substrate. In replica molding, the PDMS pattern is used as a mold for casting another polymer, which, after curing, will give a negative replica of the PDMS. Micromolding in capillaries, sometimes referred to as MIMIC, is often used to create high, sharp features. This involves a PDMS stamp being placed on the substrate to be patterned to form a network of empty channels between the substrate and the stamp. A drop of polymer is placed at one end of the channels, and then the channels are filled by capillarity. The PDMS stamp is removed after curing. Another micromolding technique is solvent-assisted micromolding, where a solvent is used to wet the PDMS stamp, which is then placed against the substrate. The substrate is dissolved by the solvent, and the resulting fluid is molded in the PDMS pattern. After evaporation of the solvent and solidification of the substrate, a complementary structure to that of PDMS is obtained. Microcontact printing is used to transfer molecules from the stamp to a substrate in a controlled geometry [1, 9]. Solvent-assisted micromolding (SAMIM) uses volatile solvents that are essential to dissolve the polymer substrate and wet the PDMS mold but without altering or damaging the pattern being transferred. Such issues of reproducibility of the original pattern are common in soft lithography techniques. Other issues, such as inappropriate surface energy for producing high-fidelity patterns or maintenance of structural integrity, have had researchers looking for better alternatives such as photocurable perfluropolyethers (PFPEs). Although these have not been used in biological applications yet, PFPE may turn out to be a stable and consistent nanopatterning solution.

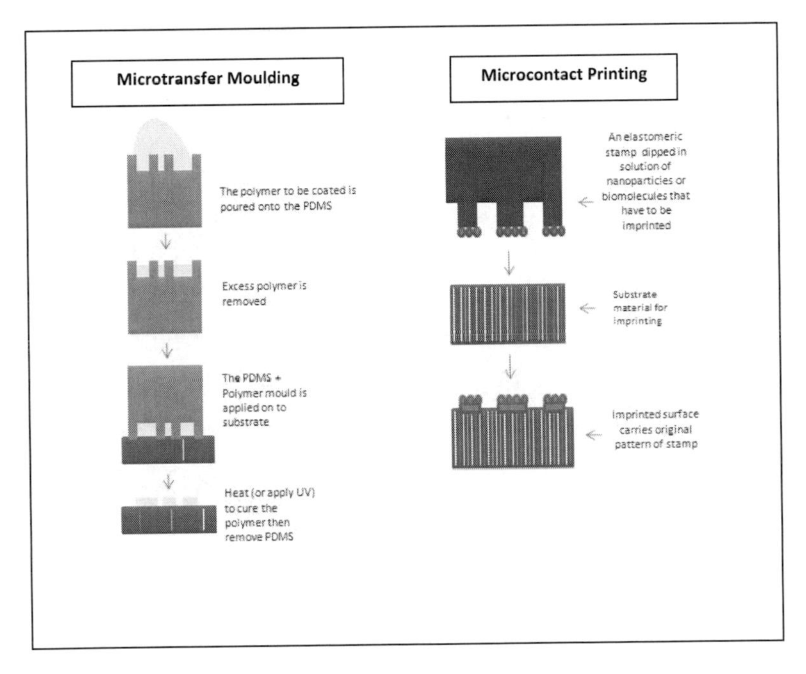

Figure 7.1 Lithography techniques.

Using reactive ion or chemical etching, colloids can be employed as a mask to produce a master die with nanometric features. Colloidal lithography basically uses a nanocolloidal solution that will act as an etch mask (an etch mask refers to material blocking etching in selected areas of the surface). It is dispersed as a monolayer on a substrate, which then self-assembles electrostatically. This is followed by etching using a reactive ion-beam bombardment that etches the entire area, including and surrounding the nanocolloid particles, creating a pattern on the substrate (because the particles acted as an etch mask) [1]. Colloids per se can be used to produce surfaces with heterogeneous chemistry. For example, particles can be attached to a titanium-coated silica base substrate and used as an etch mask to produce titanium pillars on a silica substrate, allowing the selective adsorption of proteins relative to the underlying template. An advantage of using colloids is that they are very "adjustable" — many factors can be altered such as colloidal and substrate materials, colloidal shape, size, and monolayer distribution. In addition, simple electrostatic repulsion occurring between individual colloids results in irregular monolayer patterning in the absence of charge-shielding materials, which is a much easier alternative considering that the irregular patterning of substrates utilizing other nanofabrication techniques like e-beam lithography is time consuming and difficult. Thus, colloids are a great tool for irregular in-plane nanopattern production.

Nanoimprint lithography, or hot embossing lithography (HEL), is an uncomplicated, low-cost, high-resolution patterning technique. Hot embossing is essentially stamping a pattern using a rigid stamp made of silicone into a thermoplastic polymer softened by raising the temperature of the polymer just above its glass transition temperature. The stamp used to impress the pattern onto the polymer is made using LIGA, or the pattern can be etched using techniques like electron-beam lithography (EBL) and reactive-ion etching (RIE). LIGA (X-ray lithography electroforming and molding) is a technology used to define high aspect ratio structures in nickel. A sheet of polymethylmethacrylate (PMMA) bonded to a wafer is exposed to X-ray lithography. After the PMMA sheet is developed, the exposed regions are replaced by electroplating nickel. The nickel covering is subsequently removed by polishing. After the PMMA is removed, the high aspect ratio nickel remains anchored to the substrate.

The thermoplastic polymer (substrate) is prepared as a thick slice or spin-coated onto a stiff or flexible substrate. HEL makes it possible to perform high-fidelity surface alteration or design of plastic materials where standard lithographic strategies are not possible owing to the common incompatibility of plastics with the solutions involved in conventional nanofabrication processes such as developers and organic solvents [1].

BOX 3

A small note on the development of these lithographic techniques is relevant here. The amazing progress of these fabrication processes in biology in recent years is due to the convergence of semiconductor manufacturing technology in the electronics industry and bioanalytical/mimetic devices. The technologies that were originally developed for fabricating electronics such as processors with transistors 45 nm or 90 nm apart (typical distances and sizes of entities found within cellular environments) are being applied with an increasing rate of success in the field of nanofabrication of biological surfaces such as the ones we are seeing in this chapter. Since the micro/nanolithographic materials and techniques are expressly designed for high-resolution patterning, their straightforward application to the fabrication of biomicro/nanodevices requires a minimal reengineering effort.

E-beam or ion-beam lithography uses particle exposure of a sensitive resist (a particle-sensitive coating on a substrate) to produce a pattern that can be revealed chemically in a second step or used directly to initiate polymer grafting. Extreme ultraviolet (EUV) lithography uses a wavelength range between 5 and 0.2 nm.

Three lithographic techniques using ions have been developed: The focused ion beam (FIB) technique, where a slow, focused, heavy ion beam (with energies typically around 30 keV) is written over a surface to create a pattern through modification, deposition, or sputtering; proton beam writing, where fast (typically MeV) protons are used to direct-write deep precise 3-D patterns into resist; and ion projection lithography (IPL), where medium energy ions (typically 100 keV) are projected through a patterned mask for rapid fabrication [1].

DPL can be used to produce the primary pattern or the master die as well as impress onto the final polymer substrate because it is a direct write technique. DPL uses an atomic force microscope's tip in the tapping mode to transfer molecules like proteins or polymers to a target region of the substrate directly [10].

BOX 4

The atomic force microscope (AFM) has established itself as one of the foremost tools for imaging, measuring, and manipulating matter at the nano-scale. The AFM uses a micro-scale cantilever with a sharp tip known as probe at its end used to scan a specimen's surface. AFM tips and cantilevers are micro-fabricated from Si or Si_3N_4. The typical tip radius is from a few to 10s of nanometers. When the tip is brought into proximity of a sample surface, forces between the tip and the sample lead to a deflection of the cantilever. A laser beam deflection system is used, where a laser is reflected from the back of the reflective AFM lever and onto a position-sensitive detector (usually photo diodes). Depending on the state, forces that are measured in AFM include Van der Waals forces, mechanical contact force, chemical bonding, electrostatic forces, and magnetic forces. In addition to force, additional quantities may simultaneously be measured through the use of specialized probes [11, 12].

There are many modes of operation of the AFM, but for the most part, we are interested in the "tapping mode," given that it is used for DPL. In the contact mode, the first and foremost mode of operation, the tip is raster-scanned across the surface and it deflects as it moves over the surface corrugation. The noncontact mode uses an oscillating cantilever — a stiff cantilever is oscillated in the attractive regime, implying that the tip is quite close to the sample, but not touching it. In DPL, the tapping mode, a more common reference to the dynamic force mode (DFM) of the operation of the AFM, is used. A stiff cantilever is oscillated closer to the sample than in the noncontact mode. Part of the oscillation extends into the repulsive regime, so the tip intermittently touches, or taps, the surface. This principle is used to transfer biomolecules or nanoparticles straight onto a targeted region of the substrate directly, allowing patterning much more fidelity [11, 12].

Polymer demixing is based on the spontaneous phase separation of a polymer mixture under the spin-casting process onto a substrate like silicon or glass. Polymer demixing depends upon the spontaneous phase separation of polymer blends. Polymer demixing allows the production of islands with controlled heights from 10 to 100 nm depending on the polymer blend used.

Island fabrication, a polymer mixture or a solid amorphous polymer, has a level and featureless surface. Even so, a well-defined topography is possible to achieve. The spontaneous demixing of the components of a binary (dual) blend under certain circumstances on special substrates provides a marked topography. The mutual compatibility of the polymers controls the generation of topography in thin films of the blend. For example, poly(styrene) (PS) is blended with a series of brominated polymers- poly(p-bromo$_{\mathbf{x}}$-styrene), or PBrS (**x** is the fraction of aromatic rings that are brominated). The compatibility of the brominated polymer with PS depends on the extent of bromination. The polymers are incompatible at higher fractions, and the compatibility increases as the fractions decrease. The thickness of the edge/separating boundary layer between the PS film and a PBrS overlayer is measured as the index of compatibility. Thin films have smooth surfaces when the fraction of aromatic rings is low. As the fraction increases, the topography becomes more and more distinct, directly proportional to the decreasing compatibility. The nature of the topography varies according to the relative amounts of polymer components of the blend. Islands of brominated polymer can be made to protrude from a sea of PS or link up to form a sheet with holes that expose the underlying PS based on the weight fraction. The topography can be controlled by changing the overall thickness of the polymer film, which results in islands that are higher and wider. More subtle control of the topography can be achieved using polymer components of varying molecular weights [1].

7.2.3 Nanocoatings and Nanophase Materials

Nanophase materials (i.e., materials with nanometer-scaled grains) can be used to produce nanometer features on biomaterial surfaces to guide cell behavior along a desired biological response. In bone-regeneration applications, promising results have been obtained with the nanophase materials, ceramics, and metals, with which increased osteoblast adhesion, proliferation, and calcium deposition have been observed compared with conventional materials (i.e., with micrometer-scaled grains). Nanophase materials can also be deposited on a biomaterial surface to improve its bioactivity and/or biocompatibility. For example, nanocrystalline apatite coatings, produced by sol-gel methods or pulse electrodeposition, are used commonly to enhance the osteointegration of an orthopedic device. Other techniques, such as layer-by-layer (LBL) assembly deposition, lead to nanocoatings (a few nanometers thick) with a controlled structure by the sequential adsorption of oppositely charged polyelectrolytes. LBL can be useful for drug-delivery systems and surface functionalization of biomaterial surfaces [13, 14].

7.2.4 Materials for Nanoparticles

Nanoparticle research within regenerative medicine has been addressed mainly toward the development of entrapment and delivery systems for genetic material, biomolecules, such as growth and differentiation factors, and bone morphogenetic proteins and also as reinforcing- or bioactivity- enhancement phase for polymeric matrices in 3-D scaffolds for TE. The controlled delivery of biomolecules is crucial in the support and enhancement of tissue growth in TE applications. Nanotechnology approaches in delivery systems can enhance the success of specific therapeutic agents, such as growth factors and DNA among others, which are of paramount importance for tissue regeneration. Carriers in the nano-scale enable the intracellular delivery of molecules and the possibility of reaching targets that are inaccessible normally, such as the blood-brain barrier, tight junctions, and capillaries, whereas the control over biomolecule dosage and delivery period is increased. The ultimate challenge is to develop artificial nanocarriers that can target cells with efficiency and specificity similar to that of viruses. Examples of nanoparticles for delivery systems include currently microspheres, microcapsules, liposomes, micelles, and also dendrimers. Different types of nanoparticles have been developed, such as, solid, hollow, and porous. The most common development methods are molecular self-assembly, nanomanipulation, bioaggregation, and photochemical patterning. We discuss these in more detail in the following section on cancer therapy in this chapter, but just as a primer and in relevance to regenerative medicine, we briefly mention here a few important delivery systems and materials.

Biodegradable polymers are the most commonly used materials in drug delivery. Polylactic acid (PLA), polyglycolic acid (PGA), and polyethylene glycol (PEG) and its copolymers have been used widely in combination with hydrogels to attain nanocarriers that exhibit different release properties. Particularly important for the development of nanoparticles for delivery purposes are "smart" or "stimuli-responsive" polymers that can undergo conformational changes, such as swelling or shrinkage, on variations in temperature, pH, and magnetic field. The most widely studied temperature-sensitive polymer is poly (N-isopropylacrylamide) (PNIPAAm). Polyelectrolytes, such as polymethacrylic acid (PMAA) and polyacrylic acid (PAA), that are able to ionize under acidic or alkaline pH present interesting characteristics for drug carriers in applications in which pH changes occur, such as in the delivery of genetic material. In the case of genetic-material delivery, nano-scale DNA carriers must overcome enzymatic degradation of endosomes to reach the cell nucleus and trigger specific cascades involved in tissue regeneration. Nanocarriers made of pH-sensitive polymers facilitate endosomal escape and enable the development of new nonviral genetic-material delivery systems with high transfection efficiencies. In addition to biomolecule encapsulation and delivery, solid surface-modified nanoparticles might also be used for regenerative. Although polymers are the most-used nanoparticles in the delivery area, the use of ceramics has also been investigated [14–17]. Hydroxyapatite nanoparticles functionalized with biomolecules could enhance osteoblast adhesion and bone regeneration. Ceramic nanoparticles and nanofibers are also suitable in the elaboration of bioinspired nanocomposites for bone TE applications, acting as the reinforcing phase of a polymer matrix and improving scaffold bioactivity [18]. Although the development of nanoparticles seems to have great potential for several biomedical fields, there has been little progress in the attainment of effective results in current human therapy. However, it must be said that the use of nanoparticles also raises the need of a comprehensive understanding of their secondary effects and cytotoxicity once they enter the body. The large surface area of nanoparticles makes them very reactive in the cellular environment. Their dimensions enable them to penetrate the lungs, skin, or intestinal tract, and they might get deposited in several organs, causing adverse biological reactions. Moreover, the fact that these particles are able to penetrate the cell membrane and reach the cell nucleus might raise some concern about possible unknown risks attributed to the particle's nature.

7.2.5 Nanofiber Scaffolds

We have been trying, since TE developed into what it is today, to design and fabricate 3-D constructions that could mimic the structure of the tissue that required repair. These constructions, or scaffolds as we better know them now, were made using biodegradable materials and had a porous structure that would ensure growth of the tissue cell type over it or within it as required. Among the possible structures that could replace the natural ECM, the use of nanofibers as scaffolds has several advantages compared with other techniques. Nanofibers show a high surface area and a highly interconnected porous architecture, which facilitate the colonization of cells in the scaffold and the efficient exchange of nutrients and metabolic waste between the scaffold and its environment. These nanofibers can be made of synthetic or natural material or a combination of both types of material. A few representative but relevant methods for the production of nanofibers that are used in TE applications are described.

Electrospinning is a simple and cost-effective fabrication process that uses an electric field to control the deposition of polymer fibers onto a target substrate. This system can produce fibers with diameters ranging from several microns down to 100 nm or less. The generated fibers can mimic the structural profile of the proteins found in the native ECM. Different synthetic and natural polymers have been used as materials to create 3-D matrices for tissue repair. Some of these polymers have been studied in terms of fiber fabrication, diameter of the fibers, and potential applications. The possibility of aligning these fibers is of interest in terms of mimicking the ECM. Different materials have been used to generate such fibers: synthetic biodegradable polymers, such as poly-L-lactic acid (PLLA) [19, 20], e-caprolactone (PCL) [21], PGA [22], and also natural polymers, such as collagen, silk, and DNA. The combination of natural and synthetic fibers has been achieved as well. In addition, electrospinning is able to produce both random and aligned networks. This prospect of controlling the orientation of fibers is a prerequirement for the biomimicking of natural tissues.

Phase separation is another method for producing 3-D scaffolds of fibers in the submicron range. Current cutting-edge techniques use a thermally induced phase separation process to produce a nanofibrous foamed material. However, this method involves several steps, such as raw-material dissolution, gelation, solvent extraction, freezing, and drying, which make this process time consuming. The advantages of this method are that it does not require any sophisticated equipment and that the resulting pore sizes and morphology can be controlled by changing the processing parameters [23, 24]. The most widely used material for phase-separation foams is biodegradable PLLA, which is sometimes combined with collagen. The potential of PLLA nanofibrous scaffolds prepared by phase separation for nerve TE applications was investigated. The resulting scaffold supported cell differentiation and neurite outgrowth. Although this technique is a good approach to mimic the ECM, it has so far failed to control fiber orientation. The distribution and arrangement of the ECM has a crucial role in controlling cell shape, regulating physiological function, and defining organ architecture and it is believed that controlling the fiber orientation will increase [25].

Self-assembly is a process in which molecules and supramolecular aggregates organize and arrange themselves into an ordered structure through weak and noncovalent bonds [26]. The use of self-assembly to generate hierarchical supramolecular structures is a biomimetic strategy to produce synthetic materials that resemble biological ECMs, which are able to interact with cells at the molecular level to control the processes of tissue regeneration effectively. With this technique, nanofibers can be produced using natural or synthetic macromolecules. Several studies report promising results of this strategy. For example, a peptide amphiphile (chemical compound possessing both hydrophilic and hydrophobic properties) nanofiber network could be mineralized with hydroxyapatite to recreate the nano-scale structure of bone [27]. These amphiphile nanofibers have been designed to mimic the collagen structure-building protein-like structural motifs that incorporate sequences of biological interest [28]. These nanofibers have been also applied to promote rapid and selective differentiation of neural progenitor cells into neurons [29]. Self-assembly was also used successfully to encapsulate chondrocytes within a self-assembled peptidehydrogel scaffold for cartilage repair [30].

Carbon nanotubes (CNTs), though not strictly nanofibers, are another type of nanomaterial that can be used as scaffolds for TE applications. The discovery that carbon could form stable, ordered structures other than graphite and diamond guided researchers to fullerene-related CNTs by using an arc-evaporation apparatus [31]. The tubes contained at least two layers (often many more) and ranged in outer diameter from approximately 3 to 30 nm. Since their discovery, they have been proposed for many TE applications owing to their exceptional physical properties. These nanomaterials consist of graphite, either in a single layer (single-walled nanotubes) or in concentric layers (multiwalled CNTs). The unique properties of CNTs, such as the fine electronic, mechanical properties, and the high specific surface, might provide a 3-D microenvironment to facilitate the use of stem cells in tissue regeneration [32].

CNTs can be prepared by different methods, but chemical-vapor deposition (CVD) is most commonly used. This process involves the reaction of a metal catalyst with a hydrocarbon feedstock at high temperatures (>700°C) [33]. The common use of Ni as a catalyst has raised serious concern about their subsequent use in biomedical applications. In addition, the lack of a scalable production technique for high-purity CNTs has impeded their use in practical applications. However, it has been possible to remove the metal catalyst and to avoid microstructural defects by using CVD at higher temperatures (1,800–3,000°C) [32]. Another important issue is that CNTs are not biodegradable and they have to be removed once the tissue has been replaced. CNTs have the potential to be used in clinical applications, such as scaffolds for neural implants, because they are highly conductive and are, hence, an ideal template for transmitting electrical signals to neurons [31]. Moreover, studies on bone engineering have shown that CN scaffolds are good candidates for supporting the differentiation of stem cells into mature osteoblasts and the production of bone tissue. Related to health safety, some concerns about using CNTs as scaffolds for TE have been raised. There are reports that demonstrate that nanotubes could be used to separate DNA because DNA strands wrap around CNTs. A potential application seems to be separation purposes, although the potential consequences of CNTs' entering the human body raise a reasonable worry among the scientific community about their safe use in humans.

7.2.6 Nanodevices

An interesting development during the growing progress of nanotech is nanodevices — devices that can act or detect at the nano-scale. This technological advance has been made possible through advances in microfabrication technology, which was developed initially for microelectronic applications. More recently, the fabrication of biomicroelectromechanical systems (BioMEMS) [34] has enabled the application of nanodevices in biomedicine [35]. For the purpose of this review, only BioMEMS with potential uses in regenerative medicine, such as biocapsules, bioreactors, biosensors, and laboratory-on-a-chip, will be discussed and evaluated. Biocapsules are nanodevices in the form of a shell structure that enable the storage and transport of drugs or molecules to be delivered or collected in a controlled manner. Biocapsules can be fabricated to isolate specific molecules. For example, microfabricated biocapsules with a uniform pore-size distribution that enables the passage of molecules smaller than 6 nm but excludes molecules larger than 15 nm have been engineered [36]. Such a device has a wide range of applications owing to its versatility and simplicity in concept. Thus, further development of biocapsules can have a tremendous impact on the future of regenerative medicine. Biocapsules could be used as an accurate and locally sensitive diagnostic tool, for example, when another nanodevice is placed inside the biocapsule, which would be able to analyse entrapped molecules. Such a "smart" biocapsule could, therefore, be used as a real-time diagnostic tool and could also be used for the prevention or treatment of a disease when combined with a drug-release system. Bioreactors are devices used *in vitro* in which regenerative cells and tissues are grown under controlled monitoring and operating conditions (e.g., pH, temperature, pressure, fluidic and mechanical environment, nutrient supply, and waste control). These devices integrate several types of BioMEMS into a single device to optimize tissue regeneration and to provide specific conditions for large-scale industrial applications [37]. Biosensors and laboratory-on-a-chip are integrated inside bioreactors to monitor and detect specific cellular processes. Most biosensors available currently are based on microtechnology, but advances in nanotechnology foresee the potential for many applications for nanobiosensors. A nanobiosensor is a nanostructure that reacts to the local environment by providing an optical or electrical response. This response is a result of biological, chemical, mechanical, or electrical reactions occurring on the sensor. Examples of nanobiosensors are quantum dots, fluorescent nanoparticles, metallic nanoparticles, CNTs [33], pH sensors, and oxygen sensors that use nanotechnology for locally discrete measurements or a molecule-release sensor (such as the release of calcium or potassium) [38]. Nanosensors can be supplied energy through the integration of motor proteins that function through adenosine triphosphate (ATP) [39]. Once nanobiosensors are integrated into bioreactors, they would in theory be able to regulate culture conditions automatically by feedback loops and this would improve tissue regeneration considerably.

As a final point, the prospect of replacing damaged tissue with regenerated tissue would impact and change medical science definitely and rather radically at that. Today's interest in applying nanotechnology to regenerative medicine is growing owing to its capacity for producing nanostructures that are able to mimic natural tissues as well as nanoparticles for use in delivery systems. Regenerative medicine aspects that focus on TE have evolved into two main strategies. The first strategy consists of an elegant approach in which stem cells harvested from the patient are expanded and seeded on 3-D scaffolds within a bioreactor. The resulting hybrid construct is then implanted into the patient (together with growth factors) as a tissue matrix. However, the need to harvest and expand stem cells poses great efficacy and efficiency problems that define the success of the entire process. The second strategy relies on the development of intelligent materials that would be able to send signals to the stem cells already present in the diseased or damaged tissue niches that would then trigger the regeneration process. Nanotechnology is a powerful tool for creating these "smart" materials. This approach is challenging and is still far from being achieved. But still, counting among other advantages, it would raise the possibility to have such cell-free materials ready and available for use as and when required [1].

7.3 Nanotechnology in Cancer Therapy

Cancer is one of the most widespread and damaging diseases on the planet, recording over 10 million new cases yearly. Still, there has been a substantial drop in the mortality rate as a result of noteworthy advances in diagnostic devices that allow cancer to be diagnosed at an earlier (and therefore, sometimes, curable) stage, better treatment options, and improved knowledge of cancer biology. Cancer therapy is at present by and large chemotherapy, and a general chart of the therapy is initial chemotherapy to reduce the tumor, followed by invasive surgery to remove all traces of the cancer, which is more often than not, a very challenging task. Postoperative treatment includes, once again, chemotherapy and radiation to make sure that the cancer does not return. However, complete remission is rare because chemotherapy (or radiation therapy) is neither efficient nor targeted. Tumor cells are much more vulnerable to the effects of chemotherapy (or radiation therapy) than healthy cells because they grow at a much higher rate than normal, healthy cells do. So the treatment's effectiveness can only be judged by its ability to precisely target and kill cancer cells alone, affecting as few healthy cells as possible in the process. Chemotherapy (or radiation therapy) is selectively more intensive and efficient on particular cancers and, therefore, the patient's postoperative quality of life or life expectancy is directly related to this targeting ability of the treatment. The actual downside to this treatment, however, is the large dosage of administration of chemo (or radiation), which causes side effects, sometimes so intense that the treatment is discontinued before it can even get rid of the tumor. As is obvious, new therapy is needed or current therapies need to be tweaked with new technology to treat cancer successfully. We will discuss a few relevant, promising therapy models with a focus on nanoparticle formulations that are being developed.

BOX 5 Growth of Tumors

A single cancerous cell surrounded by healthy tissue will replicate at a rate higher than the other cells, placing a strain on the nutrient supply and elimination of metabolic waste products. Once a small tumor mass has formed, the healthy tissue will not be able to compete with the cancer cells for the nutrients from the bloodstream. Tumor cells will displace healthy cells until the tumor reaches a diffusion-limited maximal size. While tumor cells will typically not initiate apoptosis in a low-nutrient environment, they do require the normal building blocks of cell function like oxygen, glucose, and amino acids. The vasculature was, however, designed to supply the now-extinct healthy tissue that did not place as high a demand for nutrients due to its slower growth rate. Tumor cells continue dividing because they do so without regard to the nutrient supply; many tumor cells perish because the amount of nutrients is insufficient. The tumor cells at the outer edge of a mass have the best access to nutrients while the cells on the inside die, creating a necrotic core within tumors that rely on diffusion to deliver nutrients and eliminate waste products. In essence, a steady-state tumor size forms because the rate of proliferation is equal to the rate of cell death until a better connection with the circulatory system is created. This diffusion-limited maximal size of most tumors is around 2 mm^3. To grow beyond this size, the tumor must recruit the formation of blood vessels to provide the nutrients necessary to fuel its continued expansion. It is thought that there could be numerous tumors at this diffusion-limited maximal size throughout the body. Until the tumor can gain that access to the circulation, it will remain at this size and the process can take years. The exact molecular mechanisms that initiate angiogenesis at a tumor site are not known and could be unique to the site of origin, but more information about what factors play a role in this process is being discovered.

7.3.1 Characteristics of Typical Nanoparticles

A common hurdle any drug or delivery system faces is its elimination from the blood stream after a point of time, and nanoparticles are no exception. To effectively deliver a drug to the targeted tumor tissue, nanoparticles must have the ability to remain in the bloodstream for a considerable time without being eliminated. Conventional nanoparticles are often caught in the circulation by the liver or spleen because of their size and shape. So, it is possible to control the timespan of retention within the blood if we could adjust the size and surface characteristics of the particle. Fortunately, an advantage of nanoparticles is that their size is tunable and they can be created to be just large enough to not be rapidly released into the blood capillaries and yet small enough to evade macrophages in the liver and spleen. Studies have shown that the typical size of such nanoparticles must be up to 100 nm to effectively reach tumor tissues. A modified surface such as a hydrophilic one will also let nanoparticles evade macrophages by preventing a process known as opsonization, where either antibodies or plasma proteins called complement proteins blanket the foreign body completely, acting as a beacon for macrophages and consequent phagocytosis. Therefore, a 100 nm nanoparticle coated with PEG (a hydrophilic polymer) or entirely created from block copolymers with hydrophilic and hydrophobic domains will repel plasma proteins and serve as a good delivery system that is retained in the blood long enough.

These particles have fared well in theory and research; however, when clinically translated, they must, in order to be efficient delivery systems, be made from a material that is biocompatible so there are no immunogenic or rejection issues, and have a lengthy circulating half-life, no aggregation, and importantly a long shelf life. The target cell must have a preference for these particles, that is, the tumor cells must have higher differential uptake efficiency relative to normal cells. Solubility (or a colloidal nature) can be useful to increase efficiency especially under aqueous conditions, but it is not a vital feature. Nanocarriers can be specifically tailored to suit particular tumors and tissues, increasing their efficiency in terms of intracellular penetration or enhanced absorption of the drugs into selective tissue, even protecting the drug from premature degradation or premature interaction with tissue (target or environmental). It is possible to control the pharmacokinetic and drug tissue distribution profile using nanocarriers.

7.3.2 Nanocarriers are Nanoparticles Used as Drug Delivery Systems

Submicron-sized particles, devices, or systems ranging in size from 3 to 200 nm, can be made using materials like polymers (polymeric nanoparticles, micelles, or dendrimers), lipids (liposomes), viruses (viral nanoparticles), and even organometallic compounds.

Depending on the method of preparation, in polymer-based preparations, the drug is usually physically entrapped within or, in certain cases, covalently bound to the polymer matrix, creating a capsulelike structure (polymeric nanoparticles), an amphiphilic core/shell (polymeric micelles), or hyperbranched macromolecules like dendrimers [39]. Polymers used as drug conjugates can be broadly divided into two groups — natural polymers and synthetic polymers. Polymers such as albumin, chitosan, and heparin occur naturally and have been a material of choice for the delivery of oligonucleotides, DNA, and protein, as well as drugs for a long time. Paclitaxel is a compound with antineoplastic activity that binds to tubulin and inhibits the disassembly of microtubules, resulting in the inhibition of cell division. In addition, paclitaxel induces apoptosis by binding to and blocking the function of the apoptosis inhibitor protein Bcl-2 (B-cell Leukemia- 2). A nanoparticle formulation of serum albumin carrying paclitaxel (nanometer-sized albumin bound to paclitaxel)] called Abraxane has been applied in the clinic for the treatment of metastatic breast cancer and also evaluated in clinical trials involving many other cancers, including non-small cell lung cancer and advanced nonhematologic malignancies [40–43]. Synthetic polymers include N-(2-hydroxypropyl)-methacrylamide copolymer (HPMA), PEG, and poly-L-glutamic acid (PGA). HPMA and PEG are the most widely used nonbiodegradable synthetic polymers [44, 45].

Typically, micelles have hydrophobic and hydrophilic regions that result in self-assembly in an aqueous environment, creating a hydrophobic core and a hydrophilic exterior or shell. Amphiphilic block copolymers assemble to form nanosized core/shell structured in aqueous media. The hydrophobicity of the core region serves as a reservoir for hydrophobic drugs, while the hydrophilic shell region stabilizes the hydrophobic core. The polymeric micelle is still water soluble and, therefore, can be administered *intravenously*. The drug can be inserted into a polymeric micelle through encapsulation or covalent attachment. See Tables 7.1 and 7.2 for examples [46–48].

Polyamidoamine dendrimer is a dendrimer that has been widely used as a scaffold. This dendrimer is conjugated with cisplatin. Dendrimers have nanometer dimensions and are synthetic polymeric macromolecules composed of multiple highly branched monomers that emerge radially from a central core. These are very modifiable and have attractive properties that qualify them as excellent scaffolds — properties such as multivalency, solubility, a surface that can be functionalized, and, most importantly, a central cavity that can house a drug moiety. The multivalency of a dendrimer is especially useful because it can be simultaneously conjugated with several molecules such as imaging contrast agents, targeting ligands, and therapeutic drugs, providing a multifunctional delivery system [49–51].

Table 7.1 Some representative drug carriers in commercial use

Compound	Nanocarrier	Type of cancer
Styrene maleic anhydride-neocarzinostatin	Polymer–protein conjugate	Hepatocellular carcinoma
Peg-l-asparaginase	Polymer–protein conjugate	Acute lymphoblastic leukemia
Peg-granulocyte colony-stimulating factor	Polymer–protein conjugate	Prevention of chemotherapy-associated
IL-2 fused to diphtheria toxin	Immunotoxin (fusion protein)	Cutaneous t-cell lymphoma
Anti-CD33 antibody conjugated to Calicheamicin	Chemo-immunoconjugate	Acute myelogenous leukemia
Anti-CD20 conjugated to yttrium-90 or indium-111	Radio-immunoconjugate	Relapsed or refractory, low-grade, follicular, or transformed non-Hodgkin's lymphoma
Anti-CD20 conjugated to iodine-131	Radio-immunoconjugate	Relapsed or refractory, low-grade, follicular, or transformed non-Hodgkin's lymphoma Kaposi's sarcoma
Daunorubicin	Liposomes	Kaposi's sarcoma
Doxorubicin	Liposomes	Combinational therapy of recurrent breast cancer, ovarian cancer, Kaposi's sarcoma
Doxorubicin vincristine	Peg-liposomes Liposome	Refractory Kaposi's sarcoma, recurrent breast cancer, ovarian cancer relapsed aggressive non- Hodgkin's lymphoma (nHl)
Paclitaxel	Albumin-bound paclitaxel nanoparticles	Metastatic breast cancer

Table 7.2 Examples of nanocarriers and drugs bound to them

Type of carrier and mean diameter (nm)	Drug entrapped or linked	Type of cancer (for clinical trials)
Immunotoxins, Immunopolymers	Various drugs, toxins	Various types of cancer fusion proteins (3–15)
Immunoliposomes (100–150)	Doxorubicin, platinum-based drugs, Vinblastin, Vincristin	Metastatic stomach cancer Topotecan, Paclitaxel
Immuno-PEG-liposomes (100)	Doxorubicin	
Dendrimers (~5)	Methotrexate	
Nanoshells (gold-silica) (~130)	No drug (for photothermal therapy	
Gold nanoparticles (10–40)	No drug (for photothermal ablation)	
Nanocages (30–40)	No drug	
Micelles (lipid based and polymeric) (5–100)	Doxorubicin	Metastatic or recurrent solid tumors refractory to conventional chemotherapy
	Paclitaxel	Pancreatic, bile duct, gastric
Polymersomes (~100)	Doxorubicin, Paclitaxel	
Polymeric nanoparticles	Doxorubicin, Paclitaxel, platinum based drugs, Docetaxel	A Denocarcinoma of the esophagus metastatic breast cancer and acute lymphoblastic leukemia
Liposomes (both PEG and non-PEG coated) (85–100)	Lurtotecan, Annamycin	Solid tumors, renal cell carcinoma, mesothelioma, ovarian, and acute lymphoblastic leukemia
Polymer-drug conjugates (6–15)	Doxorubicin, Paclitaxel, Camptothecin, Platinate	Various tumors

Perhaps one of the most used because of their relative success as a drug and molecule delivery system, liposomes can self-assemble into compact, closed colloidal structures composed of lipid bilayers and have a spherical shape in which an outer lipid bilayer surrounds a central aqueous space [52–54].

Viruses target cells and tissues specifically; besides, even if they do not, they can be engineered to do so. Functional tissue targeting ligands and peptides can be engineered onto the capsid surface of the virus through genetic recombination. For example, antibodies, folic acid, and transferrin have been engineered onto capsid surfaces and used *in vivo* for specific tumor targeting. Besides, many viruses naturally have ligands that can bind to many cell surface receptors, such as transferrin receptors often found up regulated on tumors. Coupled with their innate ability to escape or avoid cell surveillance systems, viruses are excellent delivery particles. The cowpea mosaic virus, cowpea chlorotic mottle virus, canine parvovirus, and several bacteriophages have been developed for biomedical and nanotechnology applications, including tissue targeting and drug delivery. A virus is, however, still a virus, and typical concerns always abound when considering a virus for any application in therapy, including drug delivery [55–58].

Often, technology carryover (nanotechnology in medicine in itself is a technology carryover) results in amazing advances in the field it adopts. CNTs were initially applied as biological sensors for detecting DNA and protein, as diagnostic devices (we also discussed their use as nanoscaffold fibers). They were used in discriminating different proteins from serum. Presently, they are also applied as delivery systems for vaccines and peptides. CNTs are basically carbon cylinders composed of benzene rings and completely insoluble in all solvents. The insolubility is a drawback, and concerns over its toxicity are common. Chemical modification rendering them water soluble removes these concerns, and by functional attachments to molecules like peptides, proteins, DNA/RNA, or therapeutic drugs, CNTs become a very viable option for drug delivery. Amphotericin B and methotrexate have been successfully linked to CNTs covalently. Drugs bound to CNTs have been shown to be more effectively internalized into cells relative to free drugs. In addition, the tips and sidewalls of CNTs can be used as further attachment sites for covalent modification. We, therefore, have a multitasking drug delivery system, a useful feature, especially in the treatment of cancer [59–63].

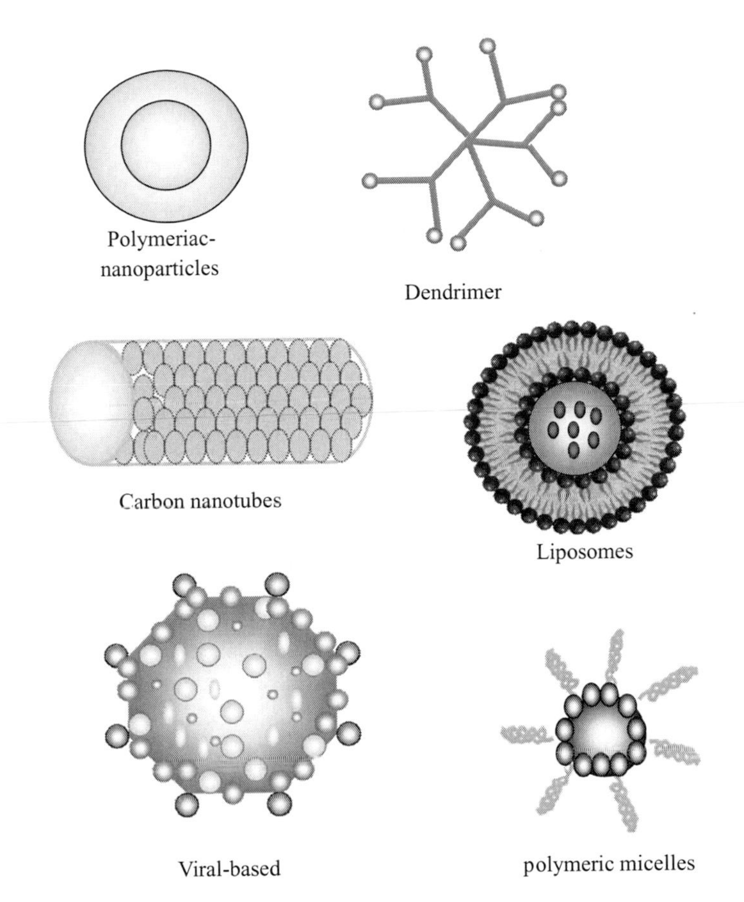

Figure 7.2 Types of nanocarriers for drug delivery: (Clockwise from the left) *Liposomes*: Self-assembling structures composed of lipid bilayers in which an aqueous volume is entirely enclosed by a membranous lipid bilayer. *Dendrimers*: A synthetic polymeric macromolecule of nanometer dimensions, which is composed of multiple highly branched monomers that emerge radially from the central core. *Viral-based nanoparticles*: Protein cages that are multivalent, self-assembles structures. *Polymeric nanoparticles*: Polymeric nanoparticles in which drugs are conjugated to or encapsulated in polymers. *Polymeric micelles*: Amphiphilic block copolymers that form to nanosized core/shell structure in an aqueous solution. The hydrophobic core region serves as a reservoir for hydrophobic drugs, whereas the hydrophilic shell region stabilizes the hydrophobic core and renders the polymer to be water soluble. *Carbon nanotubes*: Carbon cylinders composed of benzene rings. See also Color Insert.

Most of the popular nanocarriers fall into the categories described in brief above; others include unconventional but equally successful approaches such as the more-recent nanoshells and gold nanoparticles. Nanoshells are inorganic compositions composed of a silica core and a metallic outer layer, ranging in size from100 to 200 nm. These are used for imaging in addition to drug delivery, often serving both purposes at once. Novel ways are being developed to kill tumors, an interesting mode of therapy being hyperthermia-based therapy. As the name suggests, it uses heat to kill tumor cells. Nanoshells are excellent mediators for this novel therapy. Possessing optical resonances that can be adjusted to absorb or scatter any wavelength of light within the electromagnetic spectrum, these shells can be used to absorb near-infrared (NIR — 820 nm — an optimal wavelength for the transmission of light through tissue) radiation and heat up the surrounding cancer tissue, killing it. Scattering nanoshells are similarly used as contrast agents for imaging applications. Reports of successful administration of therapy based on NIR absorption by nanoshells in mice have boosted confidence in these novel approaches. The NIR-nanoshell treatment was reported to have resulted in rapid localized heating that selectively killed tumors implanted in the mice. Tissues that were heated above the thermal damage threshold displayed coagulation, cell shrinkage, and loss of nuclear staining (indicators of irreversible thermal damage), whereas control tissues appeared undamaged [64–66].

Gold nanocages are smaller (<50 nm) than nanoshells, but these too can be constructed to produce and use heat to kill tumors from NIR light. A possible advantage is that compared to nanoshells and nanocages, pure gold nanoparticles are relatively easy to synthesize and manipulate [65, 67].

In the end, despite their potential as good delivery systems, inorganic particles are not favored over their contemporaries because of certain drawbacks. They are not biodegradable, and because of their relatively larger size, they are not cleared from the system easily, which causes long-term toxicity. Mucus linings and the surrounding mucosa often hinder nanocarriers in their transport toward the targeted tissue or tumor. Similarly, nonspecific uptake by nontarget tissues, cells, or linings is also a problem.

Like we described in brief earlier, a tumor generally has angiogenesis (formation of new blood vessels from existing ones) going on and, therefore, will have imperfect blood vessels with increased permeability, a characteristic feature of rapid and defective angiogenesis. They will also have a poor lymphatic drainage system. Free drugs will just diffuse nonspecifically through these leaky vessels, but a nanocarrier will extravasate into the tumor through the same vessels by the enhanced permeability and retention (EPR) effect [65, 68]. Due to the EPR effect, molecules such as carriers or other biologically compatible material accumulate at much higher concentrations in tumor tissues than in normal tissues or organs. The EPR effect has been observed with macromolecules of sizes larger than 50 kDa in most human solid tumors and other model organisms. On average, the accumulation of polymeric drugs in tumor tissue is 5 to 10 times higher than plasma concentrations after a period of 24 hours and 10 times higher than in noncancerous muscle. The impaired lymphatic drainage will retain the accumulated nanocarriers or molecules, allowing them to release drugs into the vicinity of the tumour cells.

Studies so far have shown that the maximum size of a typical nanocarrier that can extravasate in and around the tumor is 400 nm, but an average size of less than 200 nm produces better results and is more effective. While the above concept is true for most drugs, it is not so for all drugs because some drugs just cannot diffuse efficiently. This random approach also produces a new problem — multiple drug resistance (MDR), a condition where cancer cells develop resistance to one or more drugs. MDR is attributed to the overexpression of transporter proteins on the surface of tumor cells that expel drugs from within the cells [69, 70]. These drawbacks can be addressed by engineering the nanocarriers to carry a specific ligand or attachment molecule for a cell type so that the carriers attach to specific cells immediately following extravasation. This will ensure that the carrier is internalized before it delivers the drug. Receptor-mediated internalization is often necessary if nanocarriers are to release drugs inside the cell. Selecting a ligand for a receptor that is specifically and highly overexpressed on the tumor cells will improve the odds of a successful delivery. For example, in comparison to nontargeted nanocarriers, the most efficient delivery of liposomes to B-cell receptors using anti-CD19 monoclonal antibodies requires a receptor density of 104–105 receptors on the surface of the cell, as shown by studies, while yet another study showed an improved therapeutic outcome in addition to successful delivery using a ligand for an internalizing receptor like CD19 over a noninternalizing receptor like CD20 in B-cell lymphoma cells [71].

This does not necessarily mean that internalizing receptors comprise the better strategy, because noninternalizing receptors can be used to treat solid tumors through the by-stander effect where neighboring cells receive the drug even though they lack the specific receptor. There is also evidence that too strong a binding by certain nanocarriers to their receptors prevents penetration into the tissue, defeating the original purpose and proving that noninternalizing receptors are a better strategy for delivery and therapy in such cases.

7.4 Conclusion

Nanoparticles and their use in cancer therapy and regenerative medicine will increase the life span or improve the quality of life of patients before it cures diseases or provides remedies for debilitating conditions. However, from what we have seen, nanotechnology does have the potential to replace conventional therapies entirely and given time, provide comprehensive solutions. It is necessary that we increase research around the world in this field while supporting and encouraging existing research. Of course, as with every upcoming field, there is a lot of hype that often hides the drawbacks that the field comes along with, nanotechnology being no exception. Over a period of time, we will be able to measure the potential of therapy using nanotechnology and whether it can deliver on all accounts as it promises, but as of now, it seems like a good answer.

References

1. Engel, E., Michiardi, A., Navarro, M., Lacroix, D., and Planell, J. A. (2008). Nanotechnology in regenerative medicine: the materials side. *Trends Biotechnol.*, **26**(1), 39–47.
2. Zinger, O. *et al.* (2005). Differential regulation of osteoblasts by substrate microstructural features. *Biomaterials*, **26**, 1837–1847.
3. Boyan, B. D. *et al.* (2002). Osteoblast-mediated mineral deposition in culture is dependent on surface microtopography. *Calcif. Tissue Int.*, **71**, 519–529.

4. Hasirci, V. *et al.* (2006). Nanobiomaterials: a review of the existing science and technology, and new approaches. *J. Biomater. Sci. Polym. Ed.*, **17**, 1241–1268.

5. Wilkinson, C. D. W. *et al.* (2002). The use of materials patterned on a nano- and micro-metric scale in cellular engineering. *Mater. Sci. Eng.*, **C19**, 263–269.

6. Teixeira, A. I. *et al.* (2006). The effect of environmental factors on the response of human corneal epithelial cells to nanoscale substrate topography. *Biomaterials*, **27**, 3945–3954.

7. Gomez, N. *et al.* (2007). Immobilized nerve growth factor and microtopography have distinct effects on polarization versus axon elongation in hippocampal cells in culture. *Biomaterials*, **28**, 271–284.

8. Massia, S. P., and Stark, J. (2001). Immobilized RGD peptides on surface-grafted dextran promote biospecific cell attachment. *J. Biomed. Mater. Res.*, **56**, 390–399.

9. Li, P. (2003). Biomimetic nano-apatite coating capable of promoting bone in growth. *J. Biomed. Mater. Res. A*, **66**, 79–85.

10. Salaita, K., Wang, Y., and Mirkin, C. A. (2007). Applications of dip-pen nanolithography. *Nat. Nanotechnol.*, **2**(3), 145–155.

11. Kuwahara, S., Akita, S., Shirakihara, M., Sugai, T., Nakayama, Y., and Shinohara, H. (2006). Fabrication and characterization of high-resolution AFM tips with high-quality double-wall carbon nanotubes. *Chem. Phys. Lett.*, (429), 581–585.

12. Müller, D. J., and Dufrêne, Y. F. (2008). Atomic force microscopy as a multifunctional molecular toolbox in nanobiotechnology. *Nat. Nanotechnol.*, **3**(5). 261–269.

13. Rudra, J. S. *et al.* (2006). Antimicrobial polypeptide multilayer nanocoatings. *J. Biomater. Sci. Polym. Ed.*, **17**, 1301–1315.

14. Ai, H. *et al.* (2002). Electrostatic layer-by-layer nanoassembly on biological microtemplates: platelets. *Biomacromolecules*, **3**, 560–564.

15. Gil, E. S., and Hudson, S. M. (2004). Stimuli responsive polymers and their conjugates. *Prog. Polym. Sci.*, **29**, 1173–1222.

16. Murthy, N. *et al.* (2003). Design and synthesis of pH responsive polymeric carriers that target uptake and enhance the intracellular delivery of oligonucleotides. *J. Control. Release*, **89**, 365–374.

17. Langer, R., and Tirrel, D. A. (2004). Designing materials for biology and medicine. *Nature*, **428**, 487–492.

18. Liu, H., and Webster, T. J. (2007). Nanomedicine for implants: a review of studies and necessary experimental tools. *Biomaterials*, **28**, 354–369.
19. Bognitzki, M. *et al.* (2002). Nanostructured fibers via electrospinning. *Adv. Mater.*, **13**, 70–72.
20. Yang, F. *et al.* (2005). Electrospinning of nano/micro scale poly(L-lacticacid) aligned fibers and their potential in neural tissue engineering. *Biomaterials*, **26**, 2603–2610.
21. Li, W-J. *et al.* (2005). A three-dimensional nanofibrous scaffold for cartilage tissue engineering using human mesenchymal stem cells. *Biomaterials*, **26**, 599–609.
22. Li, W-J. *et al.* (2002). Electrospun nanofibrous structure: a novel scaffold for tissue engineering. *J. Biomed. Mater. Res.*, **60**, 613–621.
23. Yang, F. *et al.* (2004). Fabrication of nano-structured porous PLLA scaffold intended for nerve tissue engineering. *Biomaterials*, **25**, 1891–1900.
24. Wei, G., and Ma, P. X. (2004). Structure and properties of nanohydroxiapatite/polymer composite scaffolds for bone tissue engineering. *Biomaterials*, **25**, 4749–4757.
25. Matthews, J. A. *et al.* (2002). Electrospinning of collagen nanofibers. *Biomacromolecules*, **3**, 232–238.
26. Murugan, R., and Ramakrishna, S. (2007). Design strategies of tissue engineering scaffolds with controlled fiber orientation. *Tissue Eng.*, **13**, 1845–1866.
27. Hartgerink, J. D. *et al.* (2001). Self assembly and mineralization of peptide-amphibile nanofibers. *Science*, **294**, 1684–1688.
28. Fields, G. *et al.* (1998). Proteinlike molecular architecture: biomaterial applications for inducing cellular receptor binding and signal transduction. *Peptide Sci.*, **47**, 143–151.
29. Silva, G. A. *et al.* (2004). Selective differentiation of neural progenitor cells by high-epitope density nanofibers. *Science*, **303**, 1352–1355.
30. Kisiday, J. *et al.* (2002). Self-assembling peptide hydrogel fosters chondrocyte extracellular matrix production and cell division: implications for cartilage tissue repair. *Proc. Natl. Acad. Sci. USA*, **99**, 9996–10001.
31. Iijima, S. (1991). Helical microtubules of graphitic carbon. *Nature*, **354**, 56–58.
32. Andrews, R. *et al.* (2001). Purification and structural annealing of multiwalled carbon nanotubes at graphitization temperatures. *Carbon*, **39**, 1681–1687.

33. Harrison, B. S., and Atala, A. (2007). Carbon nanotube applications for tissue engineering. *Biomaterials*, **28**, 344–353.

34. Bashir, R. (2004). BioMEMS: state-of-the-art in detection, opportunities and prospects. *Adv. Drug Deliv. Rev.*, **56**, 1565–1586.

35. Khademhosseini, A. *et al.* (2006). Interplay of biomaterials and microscale technologies for advancing biomedical applications. *J. Biomater. Sci. Polym. Ed.*, **17**, 1221–1240.

36. Desai, T. A. (2000). Micro- and nanoscale structures for tissue engineering constructs. *Med. Eng. Phys.*, **22**, 595–606.

37. Martin, I. *et al.* (2004). The role of bioreactors in tissue engineering. *Trends Biotechnol.*, **22**, 80–86.

38. Bishnoi, S. W. *et al.* (2006). All-optical nanoscale pH meter. *Nano Lett.*, **6**, 1687–1692.

39. Cho, K., Wang, X., Nie, S., Chen, Z. G., and Shin, D. M. (2008). Therapeutic nanoparticles for drug delivery in cancer. *Clin. Cancer Res.*, **14**(5), 1310–1316.

40. Danson, S. *et al.* (2004). Phase I dose escalation and pharmacokinetic study of pluronic polymer-bound doxorubicin (SP 1049C) in patients with advanced cancer. *Brit. J. Cancer*, **90**, 2085–2091.

41. Moghimi, S. M. (2006). Recent developments in polymeric nanoparticle engineering and their applications in experimental and clinical oncology. *Anticancer Agents Med. Chem.*, **6**, 553–561.

42. Lee, K. S. *et al.* (2007). Multicenter phase II trial of Genexol-PM, a cremophor-free, polymeric micelle formulation of paclitaxel, in patients with metastatic breast cancer. *Breast Cancer Res. Treat.*, **108**, 241–250.

43. Gradishar, W. J., Tjulandin, S., Davidson, N., *et al.* (2005). Phase III trial of nanoparticle albumin-bound paclitaxel compared with polyethylated castor oil-based paclitaxel in women with breast cancer. *J. Clin. Oncol.*, **23**, 7794–7803.

44. Duncan, R. (2006). Polymer conjugates as anticancer nanomedicines. *Nat. Rev. Cancer*, **6**, 688–701.

45. Satchi-Fainaro, R., Duncan, R., and Barnes, C. M. (2006). *Polymer Therapeutics II: Polymers as Drugs, Conjugates and Gene Delivery Systems*, vol. 193 (ed. Satchi-Fainaro, R., and Duncan, R.) Springer-Verlag, Berlin, 1–65.

46. Torchilin, V. P. (2007). Micellar nanocarriers: pharmaceutical perspectives. *Pharm. Res.*, **24**, 1–16.

47. Batrakova, E. V. *et al.* (1996). Anthracycline antibiotics non-covalently incorporated into the block copolymer micelles: *In vivo* evaluation of anti-cancer activity. *Brit. J. Cancer*, **74**, 1545–1552.

48. Nakanishi, T. *et al.* (2001). Development of the polymer micelle carrier system for doxorubicin. *J. Control. Release*, **74**, 295–302.

49. Kukowska-Latallo, J. F. *et al.* (2005). Nanoparticle targeting of anticancer drug improves therapeutic response in animal model of human epithelial cancer. *Cancer Res.*, **65**, 5317–5324.

50. Kato, K. *et al.* (2006). Phase I study of NK105, a paclitaxel-incorporating micellar nanoparticle, in patients with advanced cancer. *J. Clin. Oncol.*, **24**(suppl.), 2018.

51. Gillies, E. R., and Frechet, J. M. J. (2005). Dendrimers and dendritic polymers in drug delivery. *Drug Discov. Today*, 10, 35–43. Torchilin, V. P. (2005) Recent advances with liposomes as pharmaceutical carriers. *Nat. Rev. Drug Discov.*, **4**, 145–160.

52. Gabizon, A. A. (2001). Pegylated liposomal doxorubicin: metamorphosis of an old drug into a new form of chemotherapy. *Cancer Invest.*, **19**, 424–436.

53. Gabizon, A. A. (2001). Stealth liposomes and tumor targeting: one step further in the quest for the magic bullet. *Clin. Cancer Res.*, **7**, 223–225.

54. Safra, T. *et al.* (2000). Pegylated liposomal doxorubicin (doxil): reduced clinical cardiotoxicity in patients reaching or exceeding cumulative doses of 500 mg/m^2. *Ann. Oncol.*, **11**, 1029–1033.

55. Manchester, M., and Singh, P. (2006). Virus-based nanoparticles (Vnanoparticles): platform technologies for diagnostic imaging. *Adv. Drug Deliv. Rev.*, **58**, 1505–1522.

56. Singh, P., Destito, G., Schneemann, A., and Manchester, M. (2006). Canine parvovirus-like particles, a novel nanomaterial for tumor targeting. *J. Nanobiotechnology*, **4**, 2.

57. Flenniken, M. L., Willits, D. A., Harmsen, A. L. *et al.* (2006). Melanoma and lymphocyte cell-specific targeting incorporated into a heat shock protein cage architecture. *Chem. Biol.*, **13**, 161–170.

58. Flenniken, M. L., Liepold, L. O., Crowley, B. E., Willits, D. A., Young, M. J., and Douglas, T. (2005). Selective attachment and release of a chemotherapeutic agent from the interior of a protein cage architecture. *Chem. Commun. (Camb.)*, **4**, 447–449.

59. Hersam, M. C. (2008). Progress towards monodisperse single-walled carbon nanotubes. *Nat. Nanotechnol.*, **3**(7), 387–394.

60. Bianco, A., Kostarelos, K., Partidos, C. D., and Prato, M. (2005). Biomedical applications of functionalised carbon nanotubes. *Chem. Commun.*, **5**, 571–577.

61. Bianco, A., Kostarelos, K., and Prato, M. (2005). Applications of carbon nanotubes in drug delivery. *Curr. Opin. Chem. Biol.*, **9**, 674–679.

62. Wu, W., Wieckowski, S., Pastorin, G., *et al.* (2005). Targeted delivery of amphotericin B to cells by using functionalized carbon nanotubes. *Angew. Chem. Int. Ed. Engl.*, **44**, 6358–6362.

63. Pastorin, G., Wu, W., Wieckowski, S., *et al.* (2006). Double functionalisation of carbon nanotubes for multimodal drug delivery. *Chem. Commun.*, **11**, 1182–1184.

64. Peer, D., Karp, J. M., Hong, S., Farokhzad, O. C., Margalit, R., and Langer, R. (2007). Nanocarriers as an emerging platform for cancer therapy. *Nat. Nanotechnol.*, **2**(12), 751–760.

65. Hirsch, L. R. *et al.* (2003). Nanoshell-mediated near-infrared thermal therapy of tumors under magnetic resonance guidance. *Proc. Natl. Acad. Sci. USA*, **100**, 13549–13554.

66. Loo, C., Lowery, A., Halas, N., West, J., and Drezek, R. (2005). Immunotargeted nanoshells for integrated cancer imaging and therapy. *Nano Lett.*, **5**, 709–711.

67. Chen, J. *et al.* (2005). Gold nanocages: bioconjugation and their potential use as optical imaging contrast agents. *Nano Lett.*, **5**, 473–477.

68. Matsumura, Y., and Maeda, H. (1986). A new concept for macromolecular therapeutics in cancerchemotherapy — mechanism of tumoritropic accumulation of proteins and the antitumor agent smancs. *Cancer Res.*, **46**, 6387–6392.

69. Gottesman, M. M., Fojo, T., and Bates, S. E. (2002). Multidrug resistance in cancer: role of ATP-dependent transporters. *Nat. Rev. Cancer*, **2**, 48–58.

70. Peer, D., and Margalit, R. (2006). Fluoxetine and reversal of multidrug resistance. *Cancer Lett.*, **237**, 180–187.

71. Sapra, P., and Allen, T. M. (2002). Internalizing antibodies are necessary for improved therapeutic efficacy of antibody-targeted liposomal drugs. *Cancer Res.*, **62**, 7190–7194.

Chapter 8

Aptamers and Nanomedicine

Sarah Shigdar, Adam Smith, and Wei Duan

School of Medicine, Deakin University,
Pigdons Road, Victoria, Australia
wduan@deakin.edu.au

Aptamers, also known as chemical antibodies, are short single-stranded DNA, RNA, or peptide molecules that can fold into complex three-dimensional structures and bind to target molecules with high affinity and specificity.[1] In this chapter, we discuss the applications of nucleic acid aptamers in medicine.

The term "aptamers" was derived from the Latin *aptus* (to fit) and the Greek *meros* (part or region).[2] In 1990, the laboratories of Gold and Ellington independently pioneered the selection procedures of nucleic acid aptamers from combinatorial libraries by an iterative *in vitro* selection procedure known as the systematic evolution of ligands through exponential enrichment (SELEX).[2,3] It is now well established that aptamers bind to their ligands via adaptive recognition involving conformational alteration of either the target or the aptamer, precise stacking of flat moieties, specific hydrogen bonding, and molecular shape complementarity. The multiple, highly specific, spatially distinct contacts across the target are formed without the involvement of covalent bonds.[4]

Nanotechnology in Health Care
Edited by Sanjeeb K. Sahoo

ISBN 978-981-4267-21-2 (Hardcover), 978-981-4267-35-9 (eBook)
www.panstanford.com

Unmodified nucleic acids are very susceptible to nuclease attack and are, therefore, lacking the desired stability required for therapeutic agents. However, a number of chemical modifications of nucleic acids have been shown to confer nuclease resistance. For example, modifications at the 5′-end or 3′-end of the nucleic aptamer can increase the half-life of the molecule from minutes to hours. Aptamers containing 2′-O-methyl pyrimidines, 2′-deoxy purines, as well as 2′-fluorine-pyrimidines have been shown to possess extended *in vivo* stability. In fact, the first aptamer approved by the US Food and Drug Administration (FDA) in 2004 for treating age-related macular degeneration, Pegaptanib sodium (Macugen), contains 2′-O-methylated purines and 2′-fluorine-modified pyrimidines.[5] One can tailor various chemical modifications into nucleic acid aptamers to achieve desired pharmacokinetics and biodistribution of an aptamer for a given clinical application.

Aptamers have several advantages that offer the possibility of overcoming limitations of antibodies: (1) they can be selected against toxic or nonimmunogenic targets; (2) aptamers can be chemically modified by using modified nucleotides to enhance their stability in biological fluids or by incorporating reporter molecules, radioisotopes, and functional groups for their detection and immobilization; (3) they have very low immunogenicity; (4) they display high stability at room temperature, in extreme pH, or solvent; (5) once selected, they can be chemically synthesized free from cell-culture-derived contaminants, and they can be manufactured at any time, in large amounts, at relatively low cost and reproducibly; (6) they are smaller and thus can diffuse more rapidly into tissues and organs, leading to faster targeting in drug delivery; (7) and they have lower molecular weights, which can lead to faster body clearance, resulting in a low background noise for imaging and minimizing the radiation dose to the patient in diagnostic imaging. Thus, the versatility, high selectivity and sensitivity, and ease of screening and production make aptamers a class of highly attractive agents for both *in vitro* diagnostics and *in vivo* molecular imaging, targeted drug delivery, and novel therapeutics.

8.1 SELEX: Methodology and Variations

8.1.1 Methodology

SELEX is the method by which aptamers are selected to bind to a particular target from a combinatorial library of synthetic oligonucleotides consisting of a pool of single-stranded DNA fragments with enormous repertoire and functionality. The random oligonucleotide library consists of a randomized central region with fixed terminal regions to allow primer binding. Typical aptamer sequences are between 20 and 60 nucleotides in length, although aptamers have been selected at 220 nucleotides long. Randomization of the central sequence provides diversity within the library, typically within the range of 1×10^{15} independent aptamers, which allows for the high probability of a binding sequence being presented within the library.

Aptamer selection is characterized by the completion of successive steps of binding between the random oligonucleotide library and a target molecule, the separation of bound aptamers from unbound sequences, the elution of bound aptamers from the target, and the amplification of bound aptamers via polymerase chain reaction (PCR) to form a new, more refined aptamer library.[6,7] Following a number of SELEX cycles (usually around 10–15) that continue to enrich the binding species, the library can be cloned and sequenced, followed by the confirmation of binding, resulting in an aptamer with high specificity and affinity for its target molecule. When designing a random oligonucleotide library, certain factors have to be taken into consideration. As the library is subjected to a high number of PCR cycles, the dominance of PCR artifacts becomes an issue. As such, terminal primer binding regions should be designed to avoid amplification artifacts, through AT-rich termini, and by avoiding primer dimer-susceptible sequences. When considering the length of the random sequence to be incorporated, it should be based on a balance between the structural complexities of longer fragments versus the efficient amplification of shorter fragments, as determined by the purpose of the aptamer.

In order to separate unbound aptamers from bound ones, the target is typically immobilized to a solid support matrix, which allows unbound species to be washed off while retaining bound species. Matrix-binding species must also be taken into account as they will bind to the matrix rather than to the target. As the nontarget-binding species are retained and amplified, they can eventually dominate instead of target-binding species within the library. Traditional solid support binding methods include nitrocellulose filtration, agarose immobilization, and microtitre plates.[8] As the SELEX cycles progress, binding stringency is typically increased to select for species with high affinity. The aptamer pool:target ratio is the base determinant for stringency conditions, with a higher ratio of 10:1 → 100:1 suitable for initial rounds of binding.

The elution of bound aptamers from their target is usually determined by the nature of the target and solid support. Traditional elution methods involve the use of heat or the addition of reagents such as urea, sodium dodecyl sulfate, and ethylenediaminetetraacetic acid. Following elution, the aptamers are amplified via PCR.[7] To aid in high throughput and other labor-intensive SELEX procedures, a number of research teams have implemented the use of automated robot systems, also known as automated SELEX.[9,10]

8.1.2 Variation of SELEX

Since the inception of SELEX, a number of variations of the standard method have been designed. A variety of partition techniques have been devised to provide a solid support for the target molecules.[7] Affinity chromatography involves the binding of target protein via an affinity tag or antibody and includes immobilization on magnetic beads,[11] agarose beads,[12] and agarose.[13] Capillary electrophoresis is an exception to the rule as it is based on the mobility shift variation between bound complexes and unbound aptamers rather than the partition of the aptamer to the immobilized target.[10,13,14]

Complex-target SELEX involves the use of a nonpurified target.[15] Cell fragments/membrane preparations, whole parasites/bacteria, viral capsids, and whole cell binding are common examples of complex environments used in SELEX.[12,15] This target-rich environment can lead to significant nonspecific binding, and often counter selection is incorporated into the modified SELEX protocol.

Counter selection (negative selection) involves aptamers binding to a target-free but otherwise identical environment, and bound, non-specific species are eliminated before another binding step with the target present to select specific binding species.[15] Another selection variation is parallel selection, where a multitarget environment is presented, allowing for the coselection of multiple aptamers specific to multiple targets.[15] In addition, there is sequential target selection (X-SELEX), where the target presented to the aptamer pool is changed between SELEX cycles, thereby selecting for individual aptamers that specifically bind to multiple targets.[15]

There are a number of methods used for amplification of the initial random aptamer library that vary from traditional PCR. Tailored

SELEX involves the ligation and cleavage of primer sites before and after amplification, preventing the impact of the fixed sequence on aptamer-target binding interactions.[10] Expression cassette SELEX incorporates a chimeric $tRNA^{Met}$/RNA construct into an expression vector to allow the amplification of the aptamer *in vivo* to target intracellular targets (classically demonstrated by the intramer construct against HIV-1 RT).[10,16] Non-SELEX incorporates rounds of partitioning without any amplification via capillary electrophoresis separation of aptamer-target complex into the purified target for further refinement.[17]

It can be advantageous to utilize the inherent properties across a variety of SELEX methodologies, and in such a situation, variation across SELEX cycles facilitates the selection. Alternating binding conditions can provide the benefits of purified protein to minimize nonspecific binding, followed by the native protein in complex SELEX for example.[12]

In later SELEX cycles, it may be beneficial to incorporate DNA evolution to enrich the library and refine binding species.[18] Standard PCR confers little to no evolution of aptamer DNA, whereas error-prone PCR introduces random point mutations that may increase affinity for the target. Homologous recombination introduces crossovers at homologous regions between aptamers, whereas nonhomologous random recombination introduces a number of variations from the initial library, such as random crossovers and reordering/deletion of sequences.

Nucleic acid aptamers have the benefit of being easily modified to confer desirable properties, typically in respect to their application following SELEX (Fig. 8.1). Modified nucleotides, such as 2′-deoxypurines, 2′-O-methyl pyrimidines, and 2′- fluoro pyrimidines confer nuclease resistance *in vivo*. However, the modification often affects tertiary folding. Therefore, it is necessary to use the modified nucleotides during SELEX rather than modifying after selection.[19,20]

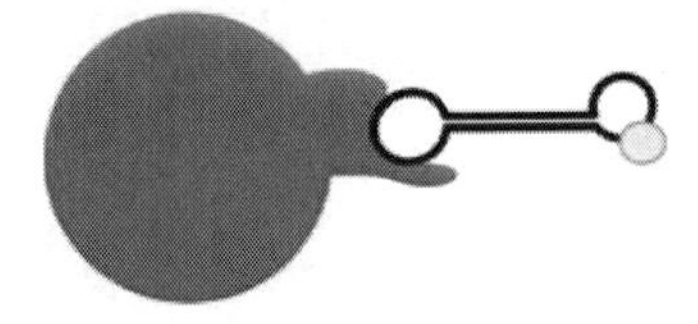

Figure 8.1 Modification of aptamers. A cell-target-aptamer complex showing the easy modification of the aptamer. (aptamer: black; modification: yellow; cell receptor: blue; cell: red) See also Color Insert.

Another method of conferring nuclease resistance *in vivo* is to produce unnatural Spiegelmers — mirror images of aptamers synthesized from L-oligonucleotides rather than natural D-nucleotides — because nucleases are unable to degrade Spiegelmers. Selection is performed against a mirrored target to select a natural D-nucleotide aptamer. A synthetic Spiegelmer derived from the aptamer sequence will then bind the unmirrored target.[9]

Aptamers can also be made with a higher affinity for their target via photo-SELEX. The incorporation of photoreactive nucleotides such as 5-bromo-2′-deoxyuridine that can form covalent bonds with sulfur-bearing amino acid residues, greatly increases the binding affinity.[10]

A number of strategies can be used to determine the progression of SELEX that establishes which SELEX cycle shows the greatest aptamer pool binding to the target molecule and should, therefore, be cloned and sequenced to obtain suitable aptamer clones. Most of these procedures are also used to determine the binding efficiency of cloned aptamers. Quantitative PCR, or qPCR, can determine aptamer concentration before and after SELEX via extrapolation of the qPCR standard curve.[11] Other methods utilize the detection of percentage of binding, such as nitrocellulose membrane filtration.[21] Parallel interrogation of fixed aptamer truncations can be used to determine binding consensus via microarray,[22] while flow cytometry can be used to determine aptamer binding to whole cells in suspension.[11] A standard method of determining the binding efficiency of an aptamer library as SELEX cycles become more stringent is via radiolabeling using ^{32}P.[14] The incorporation of radiolabeled nucleotide monophosphates allows for the direct determination of the percentage of binding for any round through scintillation counting before and after the binding reaction.

8.2 Applications of Aptamers in Diagnostics

The application of aptamers in analytical chemistry is a very promising and exciting field of research due to their capabilities to bind specifically with the target molecule.[23] The use of oligonucleotides as *in vitro* diagnostic tools has grown exponentially since the 1990s, becoming the basic tools for major molecular methods such as PCR, biochip arrays, and *in situ* hybridization.[24] The ability to engineer and chemically modify aptamers makes them ideal tools for applications that require precise and reliable molecular recognition.[25] Indeed, given their similarity to antibodies, aptamers can be used in assays and applications that were once solely the domain of antibodies. The first use of aptamers as molecular recognition elements in sensors was reported in 1996, when fluorescent-tagged aptamers were employed for the optical detection of human neutrophil elastase.[26] Assays such as western blot, flow cytometry, and enzyme-linked assays have all trialed the use of aptamers and shown to be equal, or even superior, to antibodies.[25,27] Targets of interest include enzymes, biomarkers overexpressed on cancer cell membranes, antibodies, growth factors, viruses, and biological toxins. They can provide the molecular recognition unit that is required as the first step in any sensor design or assay. Depending on how the aptamer sensor/array is constructed, aptamers can also provide the transduction and signal generation steps necessary to complete the sensor design. An aptamer is often required to be immobilized to the surface for integration into a device with the important goal being to maintain the binding affinity and selectivity that the aptamer displays in solution. This can be achieved by covalently tethering the aptamer to a surface-bound linker and in some cases, noncovalently through physisorption.[27,28]

The microarray, which has revolutionized the field of genomics, is now emerging as a very exciting and promising tool in the field of proteomics, given the ability of aptamers to recognize proteins and peptides. Multiplexed protein detection systems remain an extremely important goal in drug discovery and clinical diagnosis.[29] However, one of the problems with using antibodies in protein detection systems is their cross-reactivity with other proteins and the significant obstacles associated with antibody production, whereas aptamers can be designed such that they distinguish between proteins that differ by only a few amino acids.[27] In addition, biosensors utilizing aptamers can be chemically denatured, stripping off the affinity-bound analytes, and then refolded into their active conformations by washing in binding buffer, allowing the sensor to be reused, an ability limited to aptamers.[27] A variety of detection systems have been applied to aptamer arrays, including electrochemical, quartz crystal microbalance, microcantilevers, surface plasmon resonance (SPR) imaging, and acoustic and various optical methods.[26,30] Indeed, two companies are currently producing microarrays that utilize aptamers. Archemix used different fluorescently labeled RNA aptamers for the specific detection of corresponding targets in human serum and cellular extracts, while Somalogic selected aptamers containing photoreactive 5′-bromodeoxyuridine (BrdU) capable of covalently cross-linking bound protein targets to develop arrays with these aptamers.[25,29]

Biosensors are powerful functional tools for the rapid detection of hazards and threats associated with food, agriculture, environment, and biosecurity. Their application within the field of rapid diagnostics has gained considerable importance and popularity since the 1990s. A functional detection system is capable of reporting the presence of threat agents or substances in a physiologically relevant manner.[31] Aptasensors are self-contained devices constructed using aptamers that are capable of providing specific quantitative and semiquantitative analytical information using a biological recognition element.[26,32]

For example, biotinylated RNA aptamers immobilized onto strepavidin-coated microbeads have been developed against the biothreat ricin.[29] In addition, biosensors have been developed using semiconducting nanowires or nanotubes that can detect a single virus.[32] Aptamer-modified nanoparticles have also been developed for use in diagnostics. One successful application has been a two-part detection system using aptamer-labeled magnetic nanoparticles followed by aptamer-modified fluorescent nanoparticles, which provides a rapid method for the detection of leukemic cells.[33] SPR sensors have also been developed capable of detecting low levels of immunoglobin E (IgE) in body fluids, offering a simple and easy platform for use in the diagnosis of allergies.[34]

Aptamer beacons contain a fluorophore at one end and a quencher at the other end of the molecule. These beacons have one structure when free in solution, with the quencher blocking the fluorescent signal due to its proximity, while binding to the target forces a conformational change, allowing the fluorescent signal to be quantitated.[35] Conformation switching aptamers have been utilized in immunoPCR for the detection of thrombin or platelet-derived growth factor.[36]

While aptamers are capable of distinguishing between proteins differing by only a few amino acids, they have also been developed against the abnormal prion protein (PrP) associated with transmissible spongiform encephalopathies, which differs only in the secondary and tertiary structure compared to its normal counterpart.[37] These aptamers could have profound effects on both diagnosis and the ability to determine food safety when these are developed into diagnostic arrays.

These diagnostic assays are not the limit of the use of aptamers. The development of analytical tools requiring molecular recognition is a rapidly growing area, and simple single assays will soon be replaced with multianalyte detection systems for different biomarkers. Substrates can include gold, silica, and silicon surfaces, as well as carbon nanotubes, quantum dots, carbohydrates, and polymer substrates, which can be used in a number of different formats, such as monolayers, DNA tiles, chemisorption, covalent coupling, and biocoatings. The choice of substrate or format depends on the application area, though those currently available include electrochemical and fluorescent methods, capillary electrophoresis, affinity chromatography, cantilever-based methods, SPR, and quartz crystal microbalances.[28]

In the future, it is hoped that given the ability of SELEX to target unknown cell surface markers, it will also be possible to eventually personalize aptamers to a patient's cancer cells and thus use them in the detection of minimal residual disease.

8.3 The Use of Aptamers as Therapeutic Agents

While aptamers are showing much promise in the area of diagnostics, they are also showing a great deal of promise in the field of therapeutics. The ideal indication for a therapeutic aptamer, given the current state of aptamer technology, is an acute condition for which an important spatially confined, extracellular protein target has been identified and for which no good alternative therapy exists. In such a situation, the local delivery of even a small dose of aptamer may be effective, both in terms of clinical response and cost.[38] The small size and polyanionic nature of aptamers can lead to rapid clearance from the blood, quick uptake, and possible minimized residence in the liver and kidney.[39] One of the more attractive features of an aptamer is that it can be modified to have a half-life ranging from several minutes to more than a day, depending on the requirements for a given indication.[40]

The potential of aptamers as immunomodulators in the development of vaccines is an area receiving a lot of attention. For example, several aptamers have been shown to interact with viral coats that cause pandemic zoonotic viral respiratory infections.[40,41] Nucleic acids can elicit a broad-spectrum activity against a wide range of viruses or be designed against a specific viral strain. In the area of immunomodulators, aptamer-based drugs that stimulate the host's immune response can offer protection against viruses regardless of origin or genetic mutations. Studies have already been successfully completed using aptamers that inhibit viral enzymes, including proteolytic processing, reverse transcription, and chromosomal integration, as well as viral expression, packaging, and entry.[40] HIV is a popular target for aptamer research. Indeed, one aptamer that has entered clinical development inhibits HIV replication.[42] HIV uses its gp120 envelope glycoprotein to bind to the CD4 receptor to enter T cells. Due to its extensive glycosylation, gp120 enables HIV to escape the immune response. However, the small size of aptamers allows them to bind to the small conserved domains of gp120, whereas large molecules, such as antibodies, cannot. These aptamers were able to prevent the interaction between HIV and its receptor, thereby blocking the infection of cells *in vitro*.[43] HIV is not the only virus being targeted with aptamers, and two aptamers have been developed against hepatitis C, achieving a 70% inhibition of the maltose-binding protein-NS3 (MBP-NS3) protease activity.[1]

In addition to targeting viruses, aptamers can also be selected against bacteria, thus acting as antibiotics if selected to inhibit a crucial bacterial protein or to disrupt cell membrane formation. In addition, by linking the aptamer to an antibiotic agent, these molecules could be used as a "targeting system" directed against specific pathogens.[44]

Endemic diseases in developing countries are also in need of novel, effective, and rapid treatments. Parasitic infections have been shown to be interesting targets for aptamers, given that parasitic protozoa cause the majority of tropical diseases. Human African trypanosomiasis is known to cause sleeping sickness and is caused by the protozoan parasites of the genus *Trypanosoma*. RNA aptamers have been selected against the trypanosome cell surface and have demonstrated their feasibility as a therapeutic agent, at least *in vitro*.[35,45]

Cellular proteins can also be involved in disease, and aptamers have been raised against the insoluble amyloid conformer of PrP in transmissible spongiform encephalopathies, such as bovine spongiform encephalopathy and Creutzfeldt-Jakob disease, with cell-based assays showing these aptamers can prevent the accumulation of the insoluble form of PrP and can potentially be used as drugs.[41,44]

Aptamers have also been selected against cytotoxic T-cell antigen-4 (CTLA-4), with inhibition thought to enhance antitumor immunity. This inhibition of CTLA-4 by aptamers induces the antigen-dependent expansion of T cells by blocking inhibitory signals delivered by CTLA-4. The efficacy of CTLA-4 aptamer in tumor suppression has been demonstrated in murine cancer models in which several aptamers have been shown to have a similar, or superior functionality, to the anti-CTLA-4 antibody.[43,46]

The pathological formation of a clot in response to injury, stasis, or hypercoagulability follows abnormal coagulation. Aptamers with moderate affinity have been developed against thrombin to prolong the clotting time of human plasma. A DNA aptamer with a half-life of approximately one to two minutes was developed against thrombin for use in surgical indications requiring regional anticoagulation of an extracorporeal circuit. A number of factors and cofactors are involved in the clotting cascade, with the enzymatic cascade initiated by the protease FVIIa with the aid of its cofactor, tissue factor. An RNA aptamer with 2′-fluoropyrimidines has been generated against FVIIa, with a half-life of about 15 hours, and has been shown to inhibit the factor X activation by 95% by preventing the formation of an active FVIIa-tissue factor complex.[38]

Inflammatory bowel disease (IBD) is another area of medicine benefiting from the area of aptamer development. Mucosal biopsies in patients suffering from IBD are characterized by an increased expression of the inducible form of nitric oxide synthase (iNOS) and increased levels of the radical nitric oxide. Inhibition of iNOS expression with aptamers has been proven in animal studies in areas of encephalomyelitis, sepsis, cerebral, and renal ischemia, showing a potential therapeutic application in the treatment of IBD.[47]

Autoimmune diseases occur when patients develop antibodies against their own cells or tissues. Myasthenia gravis is a neuromuscular disorder characterized by muscular weakness and fatigue resulting from an antibody-mediated autoimmune response to the nicotinic acetycholine receptor (AChR). A modified RNA aptamer against these autoantibodies has been shown to inhibit the autoimmune response in animal models.[43,44]

The most successful therapeutic application of aptamers to date has been the adoption of an antivascular endothelial growth factor (anti-VEGF) aptamer in the treatment of age-related macular degeneration (AMD).[41] Angiogenesis is critical in numerous physiological and pathological states, though $VEGF_{165}$ is elevated and associated with promoting the growth of abnormal blood vessels in the eyes, which eventually leak blood and cause vision loss. Following conjugation to a polyethylene glycol moiety, this aptamer, Macugen, was shown to have a half-life of 9.3 hours and a clearance rate of 6.2 mL/h. Within a phase IA safety study, 80% of patients exhibited stable or improved vision three months after injection, and following a phase II study, no serious side effects were reported. The FDA approved this drug for use in 2004, making this the golden milestone in the field of aptamer technology and revitalizing a field that has shown much promise but limited applications in the 15 years since the first publications detailing this method.[1,48]

While Macugen is the only FDA-approved aptamer currently on the market, Aptanomics (Lyon, France) is working on therapeutic targets involved in signaling pathways that are deregulated in a broad range of cancers, including a Bcl antagonist and a unique kinase antagonist, whereas Archemix (Cambridge, Massachusetts, US) has nine therapeutic aptamers that are currently in phase I or phase II clinical trials spanning hematology, cardiovascular disease, oncology, and AMD. While the therapeutic aptamers reviewed here are nowhere near a complete list of all the aptamers currently being investigated as therapeutic molecules, it does provide an overview. Table 8.1 provides a list of other promising agents currently being investigated.

Table 8.1 A summary of therapeutically targeted aptamers[1,57,70]

Antiviral	TAR decoy/Tat aptamers
	HIV-1 Rev response element
	HIV reverse transcriptase
	HIV gp120
	Hepatisis C virus NS3
	Trypanosoma cruzi
	PrP^{Sc}
Anticoagulation	Thrombin
	Factor VIIa

	Factor IXa
	Activated protein C
Antiangiogenesis	Vascular endothelial growth factor (VEGF)
	Angiopoietin-2
	Angiogenin
Anti-inflammatory	Human neutrophil elastase
	Platelet-derived growth factor
	P-Selectin/ L-Selectin/ Sialyl Lewis X
	Human nonpancreatic secretory phospholipase A2
	Nuclear factor κ-B (NF- κ-B)
	Human complement C5
Antiproliferation	Transcription factor E2F
	Prostate specific membrane antigen
	VEGF
	Tenacin-C
Immune modulation	Insulin receptor
	Acetylcholine receptors
	Immunoglobulin E
	Human interferon-γ
	CTLA-4
	CD4
Cancer targeting	MUC-1
	EGFR-3
	Nucleolin
	Pigpen
	ERK2

8.4 Targeted Drug Delivery

The development of novel approaches for early cancer detection and effective therapy will significantly contribute to the improvement of patient survival.[49] The ability of nanoparticles to deliver drugs in the optimum dose range, with reduced side effects and increased therapeutic efficacy of the drugs, has led to increased interest from nearly every branch of medicine. Blood circulation residence, maximal tolerated dose, and selectivity are the most important factors for achieving a high therapeutic index and corresponding clinical success.[50,51] Nanoparticles possess unique chemical and physical properties due to their small sizes, varying from 1 to 100 nm. These constructs have been used in imaging, diagnosis, and therapy and are classed as powerful tools.[52] Nanoparticles are capable of carrying a large payload of drugs, while protecting them from degradation. In addition, with the payload of drugs located within the particles, their types and numbers do not affect the pharmacokinetic and biodistribution properties of the nanoparticles.[53] Nanoparticle-drug delivery systems are gaining application in the pharmaceutical industry due to improved solubility, pharmacokinetics, and biodistribution compared to small molecule drugs. In addition, targeting to specific cells can lower the amount of drug needed, leading to efficacy at lower doses with fewer deleterious side effects.[54]

There are currently numerous drug delivery and drug targeting systems in practice or under development.[51] However, these systems need to outwit the human immune system to be effective. One of the main problems with nanoparticles is protein absorption, which leads to opsonization when absorbed onto the surface of the particle. Following opsonization, nanoparticles aggregate and are rapidly cleared from the bloodstream by phagocytosis by the mononuclear phagocytic system (MPS), a process that can occur within a few minutes.[50,54] To overcome these problems, nanoparticles can be coated with hydrophilic polymers, effectively protecting these particles from macrophages, one of the main phagocytic cells of the MPS. In addition to protection, this increases hydration, making the nanoparticle more water soluble and, therefore, less sensitive to enzymatic degradation and enhancing biocompatibility.[49] In the last 10 years, polymer-based drug delivery systems have increased exponentially in oncology due to the arrival of biodegradable polymers.[49] Examples of these nanoparticles are natural and synthetic polymers, microcapsules, liposomes, and dendrimers.[51]

Tumor growth is associated with angiogenesis, a deficient hypervasculature and deficient lymphatic drainage system, leading to enhanced permeability and retention (EPR). The blood vessels in a tumor are irregular in shape, dilated, leaky, or defective, and the endothelial cells are poorly aligned or disorganized with large fenestrations. Also, the perivascular cells and the basement membrane, or the smooth-muscle layer, are frequently absent or abnormal in the vascular wall. Tumor vessels have a wide lumen, whereas tumor tissues have poor lymphatic drainage. This anatomical defectiveness, along with functional abnormalities, results in the extensive leakage of blood plasma components, such as macromolecules, nanoparticles, and lipidic particles, into the tumor tissue. Moreover, the slow venous return in tumor tissue and the poor lymphatic clearance mean that macromolecules are retained in the tumor, whereas extravasation into tumor interstitium continues. The EPR effect can be attributed to two phenomena: (1) long-circulating nanoparticulate drugs are able to escape the vasculature through abnormally leaky tumor blood vessels, and (2) they are subsequently retained in the tumor tissue due to a lack of effective tumor lymphatic drainage. Nanoparticulate drugs of a size greater than 10 nm avoid kidney clearance, resulting in prolonged and elevated levels in the blood stream. The upper limit for particle size is approximately 400 nm, although generally a size of 100~150 nm is preferred in order to allow the particles to pass out of the blood vessels and diffuse within the tumor tissue.[55] This EPR effect has been successfully utilized in passive targeting, which allows macromolecules or drug delivery nanoparticles to accumulate preferentially in these tissues. This approach can enhance drug bioavailability and efficacy.[49,50] However, while these monofunctional nanoparticles can transport drugs, they do not distinguish between healthy and nonhealthy tissues or cells and, therefore, limit their potential.[52,53] Indeed, recent work comparing nontargeted nanoparticles, such as lipid- or polymer-based, to targeted nanoparticles has shown that the primary role of the targeting moiety is to enhance cellular uptake into cancer cells rather than to increase the accumulation in the tumor.[53] The concept behind using a targeted delivery system is to combine a controlled release drug with a targeting ligand to control both the cellular and tissular distribution profiles and ensure the release of the drug in the appropriate environment, thereby limiting some of the side effects associated with conventional chemotherapy.[56]

Active targeting involves the conjugation of targeting ligands to the surface of nanoparticles, and these ligands can include antibodies, engineered antibody fragments, proteins, peptides, small molecules, and aptamers.[50] Monoclonal antibodies have been used as the targeting molecules with some success in the treatment of non-Hodgkin's lymphoma[51] and also in the treatment of breast cancer with Trastuzumab and anti-HER2 monoclonal antibody, which inhibits the proliferation of cancer cells.[57] While the progress with monoclonal antibodies as targeting moieties has been encouraging, they are limited by their large hydrodynamic diameters, leading to poorer diffusion throughout tumor tissues.[50] In addition, the heterogeneity of antigenic expression, antigenic modulation, and cross-reactivity with other tissues rather than the tumor are limitations that are difficult to overcome.[51] Proteins have been used as targeting molecules with some success, though it is sometimes desirable to use small targeting molecules. Small molecules are attractive as targeting ligands, given the ease of surface functionalization with multiple molecules on a single nanoparticle.[50] Indeed, the benefits of nucleic acid aptamers over proteins and antibodies are that they are much smaller in size and can be chemically synthesized rather than needing to be produced via cell culture or animal models and thus lack the batch-to-batch variations.[58]

Aptamers are the ideal small molecules for conjugation to nanoparticles. Larger molecules, such as antibodies or proteins together with the conjugated nanoparticles, can get "caught up" by the reticular endothelial system and/or mononuclear phagocyte system. In contrast, aptamer-nanoparticle conjugates are able to travel through the microvasculature as well as the tumor interstitium, a function that depends strongly and inversely on size.[59] Aptamers show superiority over other targeting ligands due to their smaller sizes, which allows for a superior tissue penetration. Aptamers can be used as either direct conjugates to an active chemotherapeutic drug or via encapsulation of the drug in an aptamer-coated vesicle such as a liposome.[57] A recent study has illustrated the power of aptamer-mediated drug delivery, in which an RNA aptamer targeting prostate-specific membrane antigen (PSMA) was conjugated to nanoparticles containing docetaxel or siRNAs targeting cancer cell survival genes. These nanoparticles were internalized by PSMA-expressing prostate cancer cells and resulted in cell death *in vitro* and retarded cancer cell growth *in vivo* using tumor xenograft models.[58]

8.5 The Role of Aptamers in Molecular Imaging

A molecular or metabolic imaging methodology provides more diagnostic information than a simple anatomical scan. Current technologies that are being utilized in the diagnosis and assessment of treatment in cancer include computed tomography (CT), ultrasonography (US), magnetic resonance imaging (MRI), and positron emission tomography (PET). CT provides an anatomical framework for molecular imaging and has had an immense impact on the practice of oncology, while MRI has improved the management of patients with disorders of the central nervous system, head and neck region, and joint disease. These two imaging technologies delineate morphological features of the tumor, tissue, and organs, providing information on the anatomical location, extent, and size of the tumor at various levels of contrast, with the best spatial resolution among all the imaging modalities. While these methods are still the mainstay of clinical imaging, there is a need to obtain more relevant molecular and biochemical information from imaging.[49,60,61]

Tumors exhibit alterations in gene expression, cellular metabolism, signal transduction, cell proliferation, perfusion, oxygenation, vascularization, apoptosis, and cell adherence, each of which may be a target for directed therapy.[60] Cellular metabolism is one area that has already been used in cancer diagnosis and management by using [^{18}F] fluoro-2-deoxy-D-glucose (FDG) PET and FDG PET/CT. Tumors with a high metabolism show an increased uptake of glucose, allowing the detection of those tumors, though tumors that are slow growing, such as prostate cancer, have a low metabolic rate and, thus, are not suitable for this imaging modality.[49,62]

A major challenge in the field of imaging is to design contrast agents that are both highly specific for a biologically relevant molecular target and also suitable for *in vivo* use.[63] Nuclear medicine imaging methods use tracers that target specific mechanisms in cancer cells and tissues and depending on their properties, can target and visualize various aspects of cancer cells. In addition, anticancer drugs can be radiolabeled and molecular imaging methods can generate information on biodistribution, metabolism, and treatment-induced changes in the targets of these drugs. However, the development of these specific tracers can be laborious. In addition, the level of uptake can affect the success of imaging. High background uptake in an organ may interfere with tumor visualization in that organ, while a large tumor with low uptake may be missed.[64] Antibodies have been used as targeting agents, though these are expensive and unstable and don't necessarily have a high affinity or selectivity for their cognate proteins.[65] In contrast, aptamers have been shown to be a promising alternative to antibodies in cancer targeting due to their lack of immunogenicity and smaller size and thus better tissue penetration capacity.[66] Combined with sensitive techniques such as PET or MRI, they can become an integral part of the diagnosis and management in a number of diseases, including cancer.[63] Aptamers are perfectly suited to escorting various types of molecules, such as radionuclides, chemotherapeutic agents, enzyme-linked chemotherapeutics, catalytic ribozymes, and toxins.[35] Hicke *et al.* (2001), who described these novel nucleic acids as "escort aptamers," produced an aptamer (TTA1) against tenascin-C, an extracellular matrix protein, and labeled the aptamer with either radiotracers or fluorescent molecules. Fluorescent microscopy of the rhodamine red-X-labeled aptamer showed rapid uptake (within 10 minutes) and diffusion throughout the tumor within three hours. Radiolabeling, using ^{99m}Tc chelated to mercapto-acetyl glycine and Diethylene triamine pentaacetic acid, showed rapid blood clearance, with a half-life of less than 10 minutes, and rapid tumor penetration at 10 minutes. A tumour:blood ratio of 50:1 was obtained after three hours.[67] This study demonstrates the superiority of aptamer-guided imaging over other techniques used in nuclear imaging, where ^{67}Ga citrate takes 48 to 72 hours to achieve imaging, and radiolabeled tumor-specific monoclonal antibodies take 24 to 72 hours. The prolonged time lag in conventional nuclear-imaging modalities is caused by a high blood background due to slow blood clearance of radiolabeled antibodies.[68]

The development of tumor-targeted contrast agents based on a nanoparticle formulation may offer enhanced sensitivity and specificity for *in vivo* tumor imaging using currently available clinical imaging modalities.[49] Multifunctional nanoparticles (MFNs) could allow not only the direct imaging of cancer cells, both within the main tumor and also metastases, but also targeted drug delivery at the same time.[52] These MFNs have already been trialed in prostate cancer using docetaxel conjugated with aptamers against PSMA for prostate cancer.[52] The conjugation of aptamers to optical-imaging agents such as fluorophores and quantum dots/nanocrystals or magnetic nanoparticles for MRI can enable the detection of small foci of metastases.[51,69] Current cancer-targeting aptamers include human epidermal growth factor-3, PSMA, nucleolin, sialyl Lewis X, CTLA-4, fibrinogen-like domain of tenascin-C, platelet derived growth factor receptor, and Pigpen.[69]

The usefulness of aptamers as imaging agents is not restricted to cancer detection. Aptamers have been developed to thrombin, involved in the clotting pathways, leading to the anatomical localization of thrombi such as in deep vein thrombosis and pulmonary embolism. Two other successful targets of aptamers include the amyloid peptide in Alzheimer's disease and human neutrophil elastase to image inflammation.[67] Several radiopharmaceuticals have been developed for neurological imaging, and by conjugating these to aptamers specific for the amyloid plaques associated with Alzheimer's disease, it would be possible to determine the progression of disease and also determine the effectiveness of treatment strategies.[35]

Acknowledgment

The authors are supported by grants from National Health & Medical Research Council and the Department of Innovation, Industry, Science and Research, Australia.

References

1. S. M. Nimjee, C. P. Rusconi, and B. A. Sullenger, *Ann. Rev. Med.*, 555–583 (2005).
2. A. D. Ellington and J. W. Szostak, *Nature*, 818–822 (1990).
3. C. Tuerk and L. Gold, *Science*, 505–510 (1990).
4. T. Hermann and D. J. Patel, *Science*, 820–825 (2000).
5. E. W. Ng, D. T. Shima, P. Calias, E. T. Cunningham, Jr., D. R. Guyer, and A. P. Adamis, *Nat. Rev. Drug Discov.*, 123–132 (2006).
6. R. C. Conrad, L. Giver, Y. Tian, and A. D. Ellington, *In vitro* selection of nucleic acid aptamers that bind proteins, in *Combinatorial Chemistry* (Academic Press Inc: San Diego. 1996).
7. R. Stoltenburg, C. Reinemann, and B. Strehlitz, *Biomol. Eng.*, 381–403 (2007).
8. K. A. Marshall and A. D. Ellington, *In vitro* selection of RNA aptamers, in *RNA-Ligand Interactions, Part B* (Academic Press Inc: San Diego. 2000).
9. D. Eulberg, K. Buchner, C. Maasch, and S. Klussmann, *Nucleic Acids Res.*, 10 (2005).
10. Y. Yang, D. L. Yang, H. J. Schluesener, and Z. R. Zhang, *Biomol. Eng.*, 583–592 (2007).
11. D. F. Bibby, A. C. Gill, L. Kirby, C. F. Farquhar, M. E. Bruce, and J. A. Garson, *J. Virol. Methods*, 107–115 (2008).

12. C. Pestourie, L. Cerchia, K. Gombert, Y. Aissouni, J. Boulay, V. De Franciscis, D. Libri, B. Tavitian, and F. Duconge, *Oligonucleotides*, 323–335 (2006).
13. J. J. Tang, J. W. Xie, N. S. Shao, and Y. Yan, *Electrophoresis*, 1303–1311 (2006).
14. R. K. Mosing, S. D. Mendonsa, and M. T. Bowser, *Anal. Chem.*, 6107–6112 (2005).
15. S. M. Shamah, J. M. Healy, and S. T. Cload, *Acc. Chem. Res.*, 130–138 (2008).
16. M. Famulok, and G. Mayer, *Chembiochem.*, 19–26 (2005).
17. M. Berezovski, M. Musheev, A. Drabovich, and S. N. Krylov, *J. Am. Chem. Soc.*, 1410–1411 (2006).
18. J. A. Bittker, B. V. Le, and D. R. Liu, *Nat. Biotechnol.*, 1024–1029 (2002).
19. P. E. Burmeister, C. H. Wang, J. R. Killough, S. D. Lewis, L. R. Horwitz, A. Ferguson, K. M. Thompson, P. S. Pendergrast, T. G. McCauley, M. Kurz, J. Diener, S. T. Cload, C. Wilson, and A. D. Keefe, *Oligonucleotides*, 337–351 (2006).
20. A. D. Keefe, and S. T. Cload, *Curr. Opin. Chem. Biol.*, 448–456 (2008).
21. D. A. Daniels, A. K. Sohal, S. Rees, and R. Grisshammer, *Anal. Biochem.*, 214–226 (2002).
22. N. O. Fischer, J. B. H. Tok, and T. M. Tarasow, *PLoS ONE*, e2720 (2008).
23. C. Ravelet, C. Grosset, and E. Peyrin, *J. Chromatogr. A*, 1–10 (2006).
24. C. K. Younes, R. Boisgard, and B. Tavitian, *Curr. Pharmaceut. Des.*, 1451–1466 (2002).
25. M. Famulok, J. S. Hartig, and G. Mayer, *Chem. Rev.*, 3715–3743 (2007).
26. J. O. Lee, H. M. So, E. K. Jeon, H. Chang, K. Won, and Y. H. Kim, *Anal. Bioanal. Chem.*, 1023–1032 (2008).
27. J. R. Collett, E. J. Cho, and A. D. Ellington, *Methods*, 4–15 (2005).
28. S. Balamurugan, A. Obubuafo, S. A. Soper, and D. A. Spivak, *Anal. Bioanal. Chem.*, 1009–1021 (2008).
29. E. J. Cho, J. R. Collett, A. E. Szafranska, and A. D. Ellington, *Anal. Chim. Acta*, 82–90 (2006).
30. W. Rowe, M. Platt, and P. J. R. Day, *Integr. Biol.*, 53–58 (2009).
31. P. Banerjee, and A. K. Bhunia, *Trends Biotechnol.*, 179–188 (2009).
32. T. Mairal, V. C. Ozalp, P. Lozano Sanchez, M. Mir, I. Katakis, and C. K. O'Sullivan, *Anal. Bioanal. Chem.*, 989–1007 (2008).
33. J. K. Herr, J. E. Smith, C. D. Medley, D. H. Shangguan, and W. H. Tan, *Anal. Chem.*, 2918–2924 (2006).

34. Y. Kim, Z. Cao, and W. Tan, *Proc. Natl. Acad. Sci. USA*, 5664–5669 (2008).
35. S. Missailidis, and A. Perkins, *Cancer Biother. Rad.*, 453–468 (2007).
36. L. Yang, and A. D. Ellington, *Anal. Biochem.*, 164–173 (2008).
37. K. Takemura, P. Wang, I. Vorberg, W. Surewicz, S. A. Priola, A. Kanthasamy, R. Pottathil, S. G. Chen, and S. Sreevatsan, *Exp. Biol. Med.*, 204–214 (2006).
38. R. R. White, B. A. Sullenger, and C. P. Rusconi, *J. Clin. Invest.*, 929–934 (2000).
39. B. J. Hicke, A. W. Stephens, T. Gould, Y. F. Chang, C. K. Lynott, J. Heil, S. Borkowski, C. S. Hilger, G. Cook, S. Warren, and P. G. Schmidt, *J. Nucl. Med.*, 668–678 (2006).
40. K. C. Becker and R. C. Becker, *Curr. Opin. Mol. Therap.*, 122–129 (2006).
41. J. F. Lee, G. M. Stovall, and A. D. Ellington, *Curr. Opin. Chem. Biol.*, 282–289 (2006).
42. D. Proske, M. Blank, R. Buhmann, and A. Resch, *Appl. Microbiol. Biotechnol.*, 367–374 (2005).
43. C. Pestourie, B. Tavitian, and F. Duconge, *Biochimie*, 921–930 (2005).
44. Y. Yang, D. Yang, H. J. Schluesener, and Z. Zhang, *Biomol. Eng.*, 583–592 (2007).
45. A. Adler, N. Forster, M. Homann, and H. U. Goringer, *Comb. Chem. High Throughput Screening*, 16–23 (2008).
46. M. Blank and M. Blind, *Curr. Opin. Chem. Biol.*, 336–342 (2005).
47. E. F. de Vries, J. Vroegh, G. Dijkstra, H. Moshage, P. H. Elsinga, P. L. Jansen, and W. Vaalburg, *Nucl. Med. Biol.*, 605–612 (2004).
48. D. H. Bunka, and P. G. Stockley, *Nat. Rev. Microbiol.*, 588–596 (2006).
49. X. Wang, L. Yang, Z. G. Chen, and D. M. Shin, *CA A Cancer J. Clinicians*, 97–110 (2008).
50. F. Alexis, J. W. Rhee, J. P. Richie, A. F. Radovic-Moreno, R. Langer, and O. C. Farokhzad, *Urol. Oncol.*, 74–85 (2008).
51. K. Kairemo, P. Erba, K. Bergstrom, and E. K. J. Pauwels, *Curr. Radiopharmaceut.*, 30–36 (2008).
52. N. Sanvicens, and M. P. Marco, *Trends Biotechnol.*, 425–433 (2008).
53. M. E. Davis, Z. Chen, and D. M. Shin, *Nat. Rev. Drug Discov.*, 771–782 (2008).
54. M. A. Dobrovolskaia, P. Aggarwal, J. B. Hall, and S. E. McNeil, *Mol. Pharm.*, 487–495 (2008).

55. K. Greish, *J. Drug Targeting*, 457–464 (2007).
56. M. Hamoudeh, M. A. Kamleh, R. Diab, and H. Fessi, *Adv. Drug Deliv. Rev.*, 1329–1346 (2008).
57. M. Das, C. Mohanty, and S. K. Sahoo, *Exp. Opin. Drug Deliv.*, 285–304 (2009).
58. L. Cerchia, F. Duconge, C. Pestourie, J. Boulay, Y. Aissouni, K. Gombert, B. Tavitian, V. de Franciscis, and D. Libri, *PLoS. Biol.*, 697–704 (2005).
59. E. Levy-Nissenbaum, A. F. Radovic-Moreno, A. Z. Wang, R. Langer, and O. C. Farokhzad, *Trends Biotechnol.*, 442–449 (2008).
60. J. Czernin, W. A. Weber, and H. R. Herschman, *Annu. Rev. Med.*, 99–118 (2006).
61. J. M. Hoffman, and S. S. Gambhir, *Radiology*, 39–47 (2007).
62. S. S. John, A. L. Zietman, W. U. Shipley, and M. G. Harisinghani, *Int. J. Rad. Onc., Biol., Phys.*, S43–S47 (2008).
63. R. Boisgard, B. Kuhnast, S. Vonhoff, C. Younes, F. Hinnen, J. M. Verbavatz, B. Rousseau, J. P. Furste, B. Wlotzka, F. Dolle, S. Klussmann, and B. Tavitian, *Eur. J. Nucl. Med. Mol. Imaging*, 470–477 (2005).
64. P. L. Jager, M. A. de Korte, M. N. Lub-de Hooge, A. van Waarde, K. P. Koopmans, P. J. Perik, and E. G. de Vries, *Cancer Imaging*, S27–S32 (2005).
65. J. R. Heath, and M. E. Davis, *Annul. Rev. Med.*, 251–265 (2008).
66. O. C. Farokhzad, S. Jon, A. Khademhosseini, T. N. Tran, D. A. Lavan, and R. Langer, *Cancer Res.*, 7668–7672 (2004).
67. A. C. Perkins, and S. Missailidis, *Q. J. Nucl. Med. Mol. Imaging*, 292–296 (2007).
68. I. Ogihara-Umeda, T. Sasaki, H. Toyama, K. Oda, M. Senda, and H. Nishigori, *Cancer Res.*, 463–467 (1994).
69. O. C. Farokhzad, J. Cheng, B. A. Teply, I. Sherifi, S. Jon, P. W. Kantoff, J. P. Richie, and R. Langer, *Proc. Natl. Acad. Sci. USA*, 6315–6320 (2006).
70. S. T. Cload, T. G. McCauley, A. D. Keefe, J. M. Healy, and C. Wilson, Properties of therapeutic aptamers, in *The Aptamer Handbook* (ed. S. Klussmann) (Wiley-VCH: Weinheim. 2006).

Chapter 9

Nanotechnology for Regenerative Medicine

Manasi Das, Chandana Mohanty, and Sanjeeb K. Sahoo

Laboratory of Nanomedicine, Institute of Life Sciences, Chandrasekharpur, Bhubaneswar 751023, Orissa, India

sanjeebsahoo2005@gmail.com

9.1 Introduction

Regenerative medicine represents a global, groundbreaking, and interdisciplinary biotechnological effort with tremendous potential to promote and extend the quality of human life. From an economic point of view, regenerative medicine is positioned to play a major role in health care and therapeutics. This field has made great strides in recent years and has ensured major contribution in upcoming therapy. The concept of regenerative medicine encompasses tissue engineering (TE) and stem cell therapy (SCT). TE is one of the major components, which, in turn, combines the fields of cell transplantation, materials science, and engineering to acquire medicinal tissues that could restore and maintain normal tissue/organ function, having endogenous regenerative capacity [1]. Similarly, stem cell research offers novel opportunities for developing new treatments for various devastating diseases for which there are few or no cures. Stem cells are basically undifferentiated cells in the human body that can

Nanotechnology in Health Care
Edited by Sanjeeb K. Sahoo

ISBN 978-981-4267-21-2 (Hardcover), 978-981-4267-35-9 (eBook)
www.panstanford.com

continue dividing forever and can change into other types of cells. As stem cells have the capacity to differentiate into various types of cells, including bone, muscle, cartilage, and other specialized types of cells, they have the potential to treat many diseases, including Parkinson's, Alzheimer's, diabetes, and cancer. Therefore, they act as an attractive tool in regenerative medicine due to their ability to be committed along several lineages either through chemical or physical stimulation. The combination of stem cells with TE principles enables the development of the stem cell–based therapeutic strategy to human diseases. This close interrelationship will play an important role in the development of regenerative medicine for health care and therapeutics.

Significant attention has been given to the so-far-developed implants, cell therapies, and engineered tissues, which indicates that the current understanding of the superstructure and the microstructure of biomaterial (used in scaffold) is no longer efficient to create successful regenerative therapies. It has been widely speculated that adding nanotopographies to the surfaces of conventional biomaterials may promote the functions of various cell types. For these reasons, biomaterials can be tailored by selectively varying both chemical and physical factors in order to maximize favorable cellular interactions (i.e., increasing functions of tissue-forming cells but decreasing immune cell and bacteria functions). In this light, nanotechnology plays a pivotal role in promoting specific function associated with regenerative health care. At the nanometer scale, where many biological processes operate, nanotechnology can provide the tools to probe and even direct these biological processes. Numerous studies have reported that nanotechnology accelerates various regenerative therapies, such as those for the bone, vascular, heart, cartilage, bladder, and brain tissue. Various nanostructured polymers and metals (alloys) have been investigated for their biocompatibility properties. This chapter discusses these nanostructured polymers and metals and latest nanotechnology findings in regenerative medicine as well as their relative levels of success.

9.2 Regenerative Medicine

Regenerative medicine is a new, multidisciplinary field that combines expertise in biology, chemistry, engineering, materials,

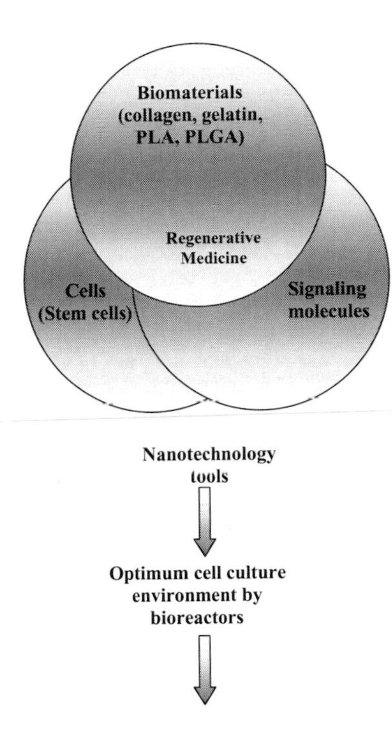

Figure 9.1 The combined effort of cells, biomaterials, the signaling molecule, and nanotechnology tools leads to the success of regenerative therapy.

and medicine to find solutions to some of the most challenging medical problems faced by humankind. It is the process of creating living, functional tissues to repair or replace tissue or organ function lost due to age, disease, damage, or congenital defects. Regenerative medicine empowers scientists to grow tissues and organs in the laboratory and safely implant them when the body cannot heal the damaged tissues and organs itself. Importantly, it has the potential to solve the problem of the shortage of organs available for donation compared to the number of patients that require life-saving organ transplantation. In this regard, it has the potential to impact the whole spectrum of health care, such as heart disease, emphysema, and diabetes. As previously discussed, the two main components of regenerative medicine are SCT and TE. The ultimate goal of regenerative medicine as a treatment concept is to replace or restore the anatomic structure and function of damaged, injured, or missing tissue or organs following any injury by combining biomaterials, cells (stem cell), and biologically active molecules. In this concept, the application of nanotechnology can have a significant impact by making TE or regenerative medicine more successful for repair or regeneration of tissue and organ function (Fig. 9.1).

9.3 Components of Regenerative Medicine

To achieve a successful regenerative therapy, the technology takes the support of many active factors like cell source, biomaterials, and bioreactor.

9.3.1 Cell Source

Cells for TE are obtained from a small piece of donor tissue, which is dissociated into individual cells. These cells are either implanted directly or expanded in culture, attached to a support matrix, and then implanted into the host after expansion. Cells used in TE can be derived from numerous sources, including primary tissues and cell lines [2, 3]. These cells may be autologous (self), allogenic (non-self, same species), or xenogenic (animal, other species). Autologous cells, besides being easy to isolate and expand *in vitro*, offer the advantage of manipulation with minimum risk of adverse host response and tissue manipulation. Allogenic cells offer the advantage of being bankable prior to need but are more likely to be complicated by the presence of disease-transmitting viruses. Moreover, both allogenic and xenogenic cells are more likely to generate an adverse response from the host [4, 5]. Ideally, the cells should be nonimmunogenic, highly proliferative, and easy to harvest and have the ability to differentiate into a variety of cell types with specialized functions [3].

Most of the strategies for TE depend on autologous cells from diseased organs of the host. However, in extreme circumstances, such as extensive end-stage organ failure, a tissue biopsy may not yield enough normal cells for expansion and transplantation. In view of this, further attention was focused on the potential use of stem cells for regenerative medicine. Stem cells have the capabilities of self-renewal and differentiation. Thus, stem cells hold great promise as an alternative source of cells for treating damaged tissue where the source of cells for repair is extremely limited or not readily accessible [6–8]. Adult bone marrow stem cells can be collected from circulation after mobilization with cytokines. These can then be used clinically to treat a range of hematological disorders. It has been reported that marrow-derived stem cells can give rise to multiple human cells, for example, immune cell, endothelial cell, neuron cell, hepatocytes, cardiac muscle cells, and lung tissues [9] (Fig. 9.2). This suggests that efficient recruitment of bone marrow stem cells to sites of injury or their injection into the target sites may provide a source of cells for tissue repair [10, 11]. Similarly, embryonic stem cells (ESC) are attractive because of their remarkable properties like the ability to proliferate in an undifferentiated but pluripotent state (self-renewal) and also the ability to differentiate into many specialized cell types. Human ESCs have been shown to differentiate *in vitro* into different tissues, but harvesting human ESC requires the destruction of the human embryos, which raises significant human and ethical concerns [12]. Therefore, the use of programmable stem cells is an emerging approach to TE or regenerative medicine–based therapies.

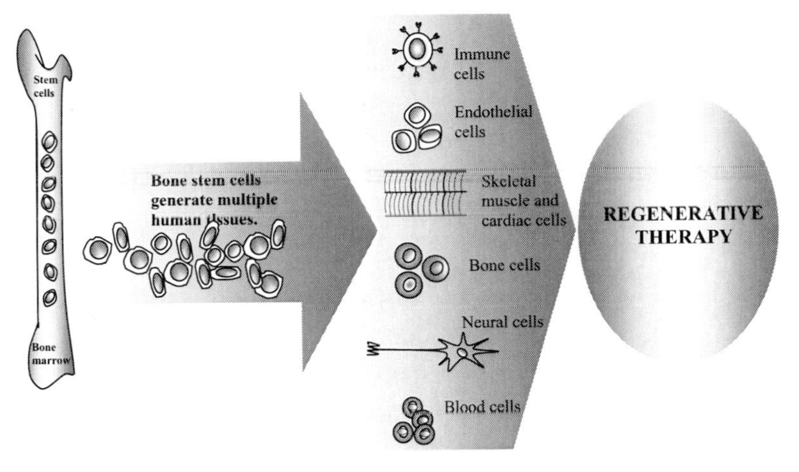

Figure 9.2 The bone marrow stem cell can generate several cell lineage, playing a significant role in regenerative therapy.

9.3.2 Biomaterials

Biomaterials are an important component of TE and involve the use of biodegradable, biocompatible, and cell- and tissue-specific scaffolds to modulate cellular phenotype and promote cellular integration and tissue formation *in vitro* and *in vivo*. Scaffolds aim to provide a three-dimensional (3-D) physical architecture and chemical environment wherein cells can grow to mimic the *in vivo* process. It is presumed that as the seeded cells proliferate and integrate into the recipient tissue bed, the scaffold will degrade, eventually dissolving completely and leaving behind a mature construct indistinguishable from the surrounding tissue. Scaffolds are typically fabricated by natural materials (bioactive but lacking mechanical strength) or synthetic materials (lacking bioactivity but having good mechanical strong and that can be fabricated with the desirable macro- (shape) and microarchitecture). Numerous types of biomaterials are continually being discovered, both man-made or from natural sources. Efforts are currently on to modify the surface of these materials to guide and enhance stem cell differentiation [13]. Initially, scaffolds were designed to be bioinert, but nowadays, biomaterials are made to interact with the cells, being able to release growth factors, genes, or other signals in a time-dependent manner [14, 15]. Scaffolds can be meshes, fibers, porous, solids, or hydrogels. The material should encourage the cells to attach, proliferate, and differentiate. The scaffold incorporates into the host and eventually provides support for seeded and native cells. So the seeding and expanding of the scaffold prior to implantation require *ex vivo* nutrient exchange for the developing construct. In this regard, novel bioreactor techniques play a significant role in making the process more successful [16, 17].

9.3.3 Bioreactors

To entice the cells to grow into the desired tissues/organs, the proliferating cells (in the scaffold) must be provided a similar *in vivo* growth environment. The *in vivo* growth conditions can be somewhat mimicked by the use of bioreactors. Bioreactors provide a system capable of controlling environmental factors such as pH, temperature, oxygen tension, and mechanical forces. The use of these dynamic *in vitro* culture systems results in the maintenance of sterility and reduction in labor as these bioreactors when utilized in a closed manufacturing system allow for the seeding of cells as well as the growth, freezing, and storage of the tissue-engineered products all within the same container [18–20]. Future challenges in TE will include upgrading the bioreactors to ensure that they put shear and mechanical forces on developing tissues and that are competent in handling multiple cell types.

9.4 Nanotechnology for Regenerative Medicine Applications

In the present scenario, regenerative medicine has a greater potential to enhance the quality of life but it has many obstacles to overcome. For example, the most common obstacle in current regenerative therapy approaches is the successful integration of different tissues to give a fully functional, mechanically competent structure. To achieve a successful technology, an extremely broad, interdisciplinary research field is needed, which can both unravel the mechanisms of tissue/cell and biomaterial interaction at the nano-scale. Current trends in nanotechnology have evolved very systematically, with direct applications to the current limitations of regenerative medicine. Using nanotechnology, biomaterial scaffolds can be manipulated at atomic, molecular, and macromolecular levels and constructed into specific geometrical and topological structures at the nano-scale (1–100 nm). It helps to create a unique nano-scale surface feature applicable to numerous medical fields. In this regards, TE has experienced great progress due to the recent innovative emergence of nanotechnology. TE approaches make use of biomaterials, cells, and factors either alone or in combination to restore, maintain, or improve tissue function. The TE strategy is illustrated in Figure 9.3 and generally involves the isolation of healthy cells from a patient, followed by their expansion *in vitro* with an aim to get cell-based organ/tissue replacement.

Nanotechnology touches SCT for improving regenerative medicine application. Stem cell nanotechnology refers to the application of nanotechnology in stem cell research. The approach of nanotechnology and stem cells will dramatically advance our ability to understand and control stem cell-fate decisions and develop novel stem cell technologies, which will eventually lead to stem cell-based therapeutics for the prevention, diagnosis, and treatment of human diseases. To this end, advancement in nanotechnology in stem cell research augurs well for stem cell microenvironment research, stem cell transfection, isolation and sorting, tracking and imaging, TE, and molecular detection. The combination of stem cells with TE principles enables the development of the stem cell-based therapeutic strategy for human diseases. Various micro-/nanofabrication technologies have been introduced to guide stem cells to develop into 3-D tissue constructs. For example, nanofibers are able to provide an

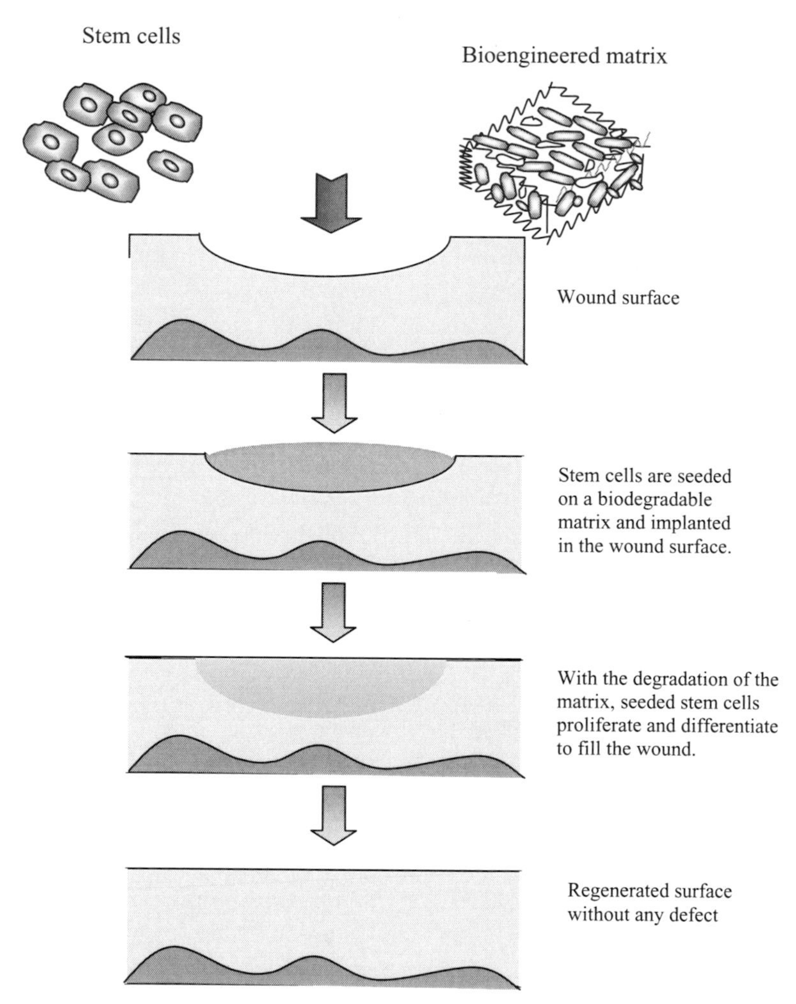

Figure 9.3 The general strategy of regenerative therapy.

in vivo-like extracellular scaffolding to promote the regeneration of specific tissues. Nanopatterned or nanostructured scaffolds are designed to trigger stem cells to become specific cell types comprising the tissues and organs in the body. In addition, nanofibers have also been used for nerve regeneration, vascular grafts, bone TE, among other things. It becomes evident that nanotechnology plays a vital function in regenerative medicine. The following section depicts the application of nanostructured polymers and metals used to make successful regenerative therapy.

9.4.1 Bone Regeneration

Skeletal disorders have become one of the major health concerns because of an ageing population and increased occurrence of sports-related injuries. Bone damage, due to pathologies or traumas, is a very common occurrence and represents a major problem in orthopedics. Many orthopedic disorders leave millions of people crippled due to inefficient therapeutic methods. The conventional methods of treatment of orthopedic disorders solve some, but not all, of the problems. In addition, several factors limit the use of transplanted grafts, including donor site morbidity, limited source, possible transmission of pathogens, and problems associated with tissue storage. Although autogenous grafts or allogenic bone has been used for many years, various problems such as failure of complete resorption of autologous bone, difficulties in shaping the bone grafts to fill the defects, and lack of sufficient parent material greatly limit their potential as bone substitutes. So the ability to generate new bones for skeletal use is a major clinical need.

Bone-forming cell (osteoblast) functions on various nanomaterials, such as nano-hydroxyapatite, electro-spun silk [21], anodized titanium [22], and nanostructured titanium surfaces work more proficiently compared to conventional orthopedic implant materials [23, 24]. Studies reveal that the difference is due to more bioactivity and availability of adsorbed proteins (such as vitronectin, fibronectin, and collagen) due to increased surface energy of nanostructured surfaces [25, 26]. Recent studies have also shown that bone cells respond differently on submicron and nanometer-scale titanium surfaces despite the minimal size difference between these two surface topographies [23]. In fact, it has been demonstrated that small changes in nanometer surface features can have larger consequences for bone regeneration [23]. Each of these studies provided clear evidence that bone cell behavior is strongly dependent upon the size of surface features where nanometer- and submicron-sized surface features can substantially improve long-term functions of bone cells. For these reasons, in the near future, it is strongly believed that these optimized nanotextured implant materials will enter commercialization in the orthopedic as well as dental markets; some nanomaterials have already received Food and Drug Administration (FDA) approval for human implantation [27].

9.4.2 Skin Regeneration

Skin is the body's largest organ and the body's first defense against disease-causing organisms. It prevents dehydration, holds extensive capillary networks and sweat glands, and maintains body temperature. Though skin cells can regenerate and repair themselves, the capacity for regeneration is very limited in the case of deep second-degree and third-degree burns. Chronic wounds also represent a different kind of challenge for wound healing. Furthermore, owing to a strong immune defense system, transplantation in skin is more intricate. TE is expected to have a great impact on wound repair and further its transplantation [28–30]. Replacement and regrowth of damaged skin have been considered two of the first successful TE applications. Several TE products have been approved by the FDA for use as a skin graft material, aimed toward patients suffering from severe burns or diabetic ulcers. A well-known version of these products is Apligraf® [31]. The primary goal of tissue-engineered skin is to achieve complete wound closure and restore normal skin function. The ideal tissue-engineered skin should be bilayered and shear resistant. The skin product must be nontoxic, and it should be minimally antigenic to reduce the risk of rejection. Recently, novel cost-effective electrospun nanofibrous membranes (NFMs) have been established for wound dressing and allogeneic cultured dermal substitute have been developed through the cultivation of human dermal fibroblast for healing skin defects. The large surface area with the microstructure of NFMs could quickly start signaling pathways and attract fibroblasts to the dermal layer, which can excrete important extracellular matrix components, such as collagen and several cytokines (e.g., growth factors and angiogenic factors), to repair damaged tissue. Wound dressing with electrospun nanofibrous membrane can also be useful as they meet requirements such as higher gas permeation and protection of wounds from infection and dehydration. Polycaprolactone nanofibres also support fibroblast-cell cultures. The ultimate goal of wound dressing is the production of an ideal structure — one that has higher porosity and is a good barrier. To reach this goal, several works have been done. For example, Chung *et al.* explored the use of poly(ε-caprolactone) (PCL) grafted with nanostructured chitosan (CS) as a TE scaffold for the growth of human dermal fibroblasts [32]. To create nanostructured CS, first PCL is cast as a flat surface and then acetone is applied to the surface at 40°C while spinning at 80 rpm. The resultant nanostructured PCL surface is used as a mold, over which a cross-linked form of CS is cast followed by an additional layer of PCL over the top smooth side of the CS film. This can yield an approximately 106 nm thick nanostructured CS film on top of a 100 μm thick PCL film. Resultant nano-CS/PCL surfaces exhibit significantly higher surface roughness values as compared to smooth CS/PCL surfaces: 106 nm compared to 3.6 nm, respectively. Furthermore, these nano-CS/PCL constructs exhibit significantly higher rates of fibroblast proliferation and viability as compared to smooth CS/PCL surfaces or nanorough PCL surfaces. The technique of solvent spin-etching for polymers may represent an inexpensive means to prepare nano-scale TE scaffolds as improved artificial skin grafts. Recently, a group developed an alternative approach to wound healing that they termed autologous layered dermal reconstitution (ALDR) [33]. This technique relies upon novel TE scaffolds that consist of electrospun fibers made of PCL and gelatin, between 300 and 600 nm in diameter, with a total thickness of only 28 μm. The scaffolds were seeded with human dermal fibroblasts, which remained viable in the scaffold for all time points tested (up to two weeks) and doubled in population approximately every three days. Although no *in vivo* results are currently available, ALDR using electrospun scaffolds should offer a distinct advantage over traditional techniques. For example, ALDR will allow for a rapid, layer-by-layer buildup of tissue in deep wounds, with dermal fibroblasts distributed throughout. This can occur because the electrospinning process takes place on top of a commercially available polyurethane wound dressing. As little as 48–72 hours after implantation, the wound dressing can be removed and another scaffold/wound dressing construct placed in the wound site. This is repeated until the wound area is fully repaired. Since each scaffold will be individually seeded with dermal fibroblasts prior to implantation, this layer-by-layer technique eliminates the long *in vivo* culture times needed for cellular infiltration and growth within larger, single-layer scaffolds. The end result is a continuous layer of tissue wherein the use of a porous, nanostructured scaffolds allows for rapid cellular proliferation and integration between layers.

Results of the preliminary study proved that the dermal fibroblast seeded on biocompatible synthetic or natural nanofiber matrices will support cell adhesion and proliferation and form extracellular matrix (ECM) within the confines of the matrices.

Electrospun nanofibrous membrane not only shows good and immediate adherence to wet wound surface but also attains uniform adherence to the wound surface without any fluid accumulation. The rate of epithelialization was increased, and the dermis got well organized into the electrospun nanofibrous membrane providing efficient support for dermal wound healing.

9.4.3 Cardiac Tissue Regeneration

Cardiac diseases remain a significant cause of morbidity and mortality in the Western world [34]. Successful treatment has been limited in many situations by the poor performance of synthetic materials used for tissue replacement. Application of nanotechnology toward TE has been explored for making significant contributions toward the development of functional heart tissue constructs in recent years. In this regard, a novel submicron-structured scaffold consisting of electrospun poly(L-lactide) (PLLA) and poly(lactic-co-glycolic) acid (PLGA) fibers was created for the *in vitro* culture of cardiac myocytes [35]. The scaffolds consisting of randomly oriented fibers were then subjected to a uniaxial stretching and heating process in order to achieve a higher degree of fiber alignment. Not only the cardiac myocytes adhere to and grow on the surface of the scaffolds but also they crawl inside and align with the local orientation of the fibers. After seven days of cell seeding onto PLLA scaffolds, cells had established a cohesive electrical unit and were able to respond to external pacing stimuli at rates up to 6 Hz. Recent research has focused on developing and growing *in vitro* TE heart valves. In conventional replacement practice, artificial valves require the use of chronic anticoagulant therapy, and animal-derived valves often calcify, harden, and must be replaced after several years. A successfully developed TE valve would not possess any such shortcomings. As an added advantage, it could grow to accommodate enlargement of the heart as pediatric patients mature [36].

In a study, Brody *et al.* characterized the decellularized basement membrane of porcine aortic valves and found specific nano-scale surface feature dimensions in all regions of the valve [37]. Specifically, analysis using both scanning electron microscopy and atomic force microscope revealed a matrix of fibers possessing diameters of approximately 30 nm. In fact, the sizes of the aortic basement membranes examined in this study were significantly smaller than those of the endothelial basement membrane found in both the cornea and the bladder of various mammals. As such, it would certainly follow that an optimum TE scaffold should possess similar scale surface features in order to optimize its interactions with endothelial cells, thus ensuring a confluent and healthy endothelium across the valve surface. Recently, Fred Schoen *et al.* described that artificial heart valves composed of resorbable synthetic polymer scaffolds containing cultured bone marrow–derived cells produce functional valves and further implanted cells are likely to be replaced during remodeling *in vivo*. Apparently, this denotes that the mechanical microenvironment of the leaflet induces ingrowth and differentiation of the tissue, which results in the regeneration of normal valve architecture [38].

9.4.4 Vascular Tissue Engineering

Successful treatment has been limited in many cases of peripheral vascular disease. Current surgical therapy for diseased vessels involves bypass grafting with autologous arteries or veins [39]. Vascular grafting is a common surgical practice, but it has significant limitations and complications. Arterial conduits have restricted dimensions and are limited in supply, while venous conduits may have various degenerative alterations that can lead to aneurysm formation during high-pressure arterial circulation. Moreover, allografts are problematic because of a high rate of rejection. Synthetic materials based on expanded polytetrafluoroethylene (ePTFE) and polyethylene terephthalate (Dacron) although used for the construction of heart valves, blood, vessels, and so on, may carry some risk of rejection and thromboembolic complications [40, 41]. Some other problems associated with synthetic vascular grafts include platelet adhesion and activation and a decreased compliance compared with the adjacent arterial tissues. Therefore, a severe limitation of all of the treatment modalities available is the inability to grow and remodel with the surrounding tissue. Because of these problems, significant efforts are being made in vascular TE. Advances in vascular TE have utilized both mesenchymal and hematopoietic stem cells as a cell source in an attempt to create a fully engineered small-diameter graft. Stem cells offer enormous potential as a cell source because of their proliferative and growth potential, and the application of stem cell technology has far-reaching implications for future applications. The advances in nanotechnology can bring additional functionality to vascular scaffolds, optimize internal vascular graft surface, and even help to direct the differentiation of stem cells into the vascular cell phenotype. The development of rapid nanotechnology-based methods of vascular tissue biofabrication represents one of most important recent technological breakthroughs in vascular TE because it dramatically accelerates vascular tissue assembly and, importantly, also eliminates the need for a bioreactor-based scaffold cellularization process.

The primary goal in the field of vascular TE is the development of a biologically and mechanically sound, thrombosis-resistant, and immunologically safe blood vessel substitute. Homograft availability is limited because allografts are hampered by immune rejection and potential disease transmission [42]. To address this shortage, research focused on the fabrication of small-diameter blood vessel substitutes that incorporate living smooth muscle cells (SMCs) embedded in an ECM composed of biological proteins, which could be lined with endothelial cells (ECs) to provide a living, responsive, and nonthrombogenic blood vessel. To congregate specific demands for sophisticated applications, modifications of nonwoven surfaces have received much attention in creating new chemistries to promote superficial functionalities such as hydrophilicity, biomedical-related affinities, permeability, or selectivity on or through the fabric surfaces [43]. Venugopal *et al.* reported the modified PCL/collagen nanofiber scaffolds having amino group. These amino groups facilitate the adherence and proliferation of SMCs on nanofibers, showing even cell distribution to form a blood vessel [44]. In a recent study, Lu *et al.* reported increased adhesion and proliferation levels of endothelial cells on titanium (Ti) stent surfaces, patterned with nanometer- as opposed to micron-scale surface features [45]. These surfaces consisted of periodic arrays of linear, rectangular cross-section grooves with width and spacings between 750 nm and 100 μm. Such grooves were produced using a novel plasma-etching technique known as titanium inductively coupled plasma deep etching (TIDE). Endothelial cell proliferation studies show that nanostructured Ti surfaces exhibit higher initial endothelial cell adhesion and proliferation than smooth Ti surfaces. Furthermore, endothelial cells reach confluence after five days in culture on surfaces with linear nano-scale surface patterns. For all time points, as the width and spacing between grooves decrease, the alignment of endothelial cells increases, with cells exhibiting a more linear rather than rounded morphology.

9.4.5 Bladder Tissue Engineering

There are numerous clinical trials underway that employ TE in order to address problems such as the eventual need for the transplantation of donor organs in case of bladder cancer. Unfortunately, many conventional synthetic biodegradable polymers and natural scaffolds investigated to date have shown limited success in bladder tissue regeneration applications due to their poor mechanical stability, adverse tissue, and immune responses [46, 47]. Thus, it is necessary to develop bladder organ replacement design strategies not with conventional biodegradable polymers but rather with advanced novel biodegradable polymers in which the synthetic material is quickly and efficiently replaced by healthy host tissue. Moreover, experiments provided evidence that, in general, scaffolds and resident cells experiencing a sustained pressure stimulus function similarly to those experiencing atmospheric pressures. Thus, these engineered scaffolds using nanotechnology hold great promise toward the development of *in vivo* replacements for the urinary bladder wall. It is reported that bladder cells respond differently to nanodimensional, micron, and flat surface features; this may be due to the fact that surfaces of these nanomaterials mimic their natural environment more efficiently. Recently, it was reported that PLGA and polyurethane (PU) with nano-scale surface features promote the growth of bladder smooth muscle cells more than conventional PLGA and PU [48]. Interestingly, tissue-engineered bladders often form a small number of calcium oxalate stones after successful implantation. A study of calcium stone recurrence showed a 14% return after 1 year, 35% after 5 years, and 52% after 10 years [49]. Recent data [50] indicates that submicron-pored, nanometer rough PU not only enhances the adhesion and proliferation of bladder urothelial cells but also leads to the formation of fewer calcium oxalate stones than conventional polymers. The pores in the surface of advanced polymers created using nanotechnology functioned to absorb calcium and oxalate separately, which prevented the interactions that lead to the formation of calcium oxalate stones. In addition, Pattison *et al.* showed that novel, 3-D, porous PLGA scaffolds promote increased adhesion, growth, and protein production by bladder smooth muscle cells as compared to what occurred on conventional, microdimensional scaffolds [51].

9.4.6 Neural Tissue Engineering

Autologous nerve graft remains the "gold standard" for peripheral nerve repair, but it creates donor site morbidity and size mismatch, additional surgery time, and incomplete functional nerve recovery. The limited availability of donor nerves and drawbacks of second operation for nerve harvesting lead to the idea of engineering novel grafts as a substitute for nerve regeneration [52]. Evans *et al.* utilized PLLA scaffolds in attempt to guide peripheral nerve regeneration [53]. PLLA tissue guidance conduits have proven 10 times stronger and stiffer than PLGA conduits of similar pore morphology over an eight-week *in vitro* degradation period. [54]. Yang *et al.* studied aligned and random PLLA polymer nanofibers (500–3,000 nm) supporting neural stem cell adhesion and differentiation for nerve regeneration [55]. Similarly, collagen is a major component of ECM proteins broadly used as material in various surgical prosthesis and thus in nerve repair [56]. Adhesiveness of this collagen for different cell types allows their long-time survival and proliferation [57]. Collagen plays a dual role, serving as a physical framework for regenerating nerves [58] providing ECM proteins and specific adhesion molecules facilitating attachment and movement of cells [59]. It also serves as a source of various tropic factors for regenerating axons, especially in early regeneration [60]. Nerve growth factor (NGF), brain derived neurotrophic factor (BDNF), fibroblast growth factor (FGF), glial growth factor, and ciliary neurtrophic factor (CNF) delivered within a conduit may significantly increase the morphological and functional recovery of transected and repaired nerves [61]. Xu *et al.* designed the polyphosphoesters (PPEs) scaffolds similar to PLGA polymers and controlled the degradation of polymer scaffold by introducing phosphate as a backbone [62]. These PPE tubes lead to the appearance of cracks as early as one to three days after implantation and increase porosity and permeability to facilitate the exchange of the nutrients and growth factors from surrounding environment and enhance the constitution of the matrix [63]. Successful nerve regeneration requires tissue-engineered scaffolds to provide mechanical support for growing neuritis and prevention from ingrowth of fiber scar tissue. ECM proteins are involved in specific interactions with neural tissues to produce biomimetic scaffolds for nerve regeneration [64]. Components of ECM have been mostly used among the natural polymers for nerve reconstruction such as laminin, fibronectin, and collagen [65]. Labrador *et al.* studied the influence of the concentration of collagen and laminin gels filling silicon nerve guides on the recovery of 4 mm and 6 mm gaps in mouse sciatic nerves [66]. Miller *et al.* showed that the microgrooved PLA substrates selectively adsorbed with laminin provided physical and chemical guidance to Schwann cells (SCs) and enhanced their addition and alignment on the substrates *in vitro*. Fibronectin and fibronectin-derived peptides containing arginine-glycine-aspartic acid (RGD)-binding motifs were immobilized on glass substrates to enhance neurite outgrowth [67].

In another study, Yang *et al* have studied the potential of PLLA-based electrospun nanofibrous scaffolds for the purpose of neural TE. Their study involved understanding the influence of the nanofibrous scaffolds on neural stem cells (NSCs). Their results indicated that randomly oriented nanofibers (150–350 nm) not only supported neural stem cell adhesion but also promoted NSC differentiation [68]. The authors attributed the aforementioned findings to higher surface area and roughness of the nanofibers. Yang *et al.* have recently reported another study wherein they tried to understand the role of aligned nanofibers in neural TE. They obtained aligned nanofibers by collecting nanofibers on the edge of a rotating disc. The 3-D scaffolds were fabricated to the desired thickness by adjusting the collecting time; however, after approximately 30 minutes, residual charges on the collecting fibers led to random collection of the fibers on top of the scaffold. The scaffolds with oriented nanofibers were then studied with NSCs to determine the influence of nanofiber orientation on NSCs. The results demonstrated that NSCs elongated and their neurites grew out along the direction of the fiber orientation of the aligned nanofibers. Further, it was observed that the NSCs show an increased rate of differentiation on aligned nanofibers compared with microfibers. Therefore, the aligned PLLA nanofibrous scaffolds show the potential to be developed for neural TE [55].

9.5 Conclusions

The promise of TE is great, but there exist major challenges that must be met for this new field to reach its potential. Although TE and SCT hold great potential for the treatment of many injury and degenerative diseases, repairing diseased or damaged tissue to restore normal function still represents one of the greatest challenges in modern-day science and medicine. A critical challenge in TE is to regenerate tissues that grow and/or remodel in concert with the changing needs of the human body. Another principle requirement for tissues engineered *in vitro* is the sufficient supply of oxygen and nutrients and the removal of carbon dioxide and waste, as they do not have their own blood supply. Additional challenges include the preservation of the products so that they have a long shelf life and the successful use of various approaches to prevent tissue rejection. Future challenges in TE include the upscaling of bioreactors that put shear and mechanical forces on the developing tissues and the production of final products involving multiple cell types. Despite the myriad of challenges, the field of TE endows a better health care system and will definitely pave the way toward better therapeutics in the near future. This technology will definitely go from being something closer to scientific fiction to become a scientific fact and have a major impact on future health care practice.

References

1. Atala, A: Recent applications of regenerative medicine to urologic structures and related tissues. *Curr. Opin. Urol.*, **16**, 305–309 (2006).
2. Fuchs, JR, BA Nasseri, and JP Vacanti: Tissue engineering: a 21st century solution to surgical reconstruction. *Ann. Thorac. Surg.*, **72**, 577–591 (2001).
3. Vacanti, JP, R Langer, J Upton, and JJ Marler: Transplantation of cells in matrices for tissue regeneration. *Adv. Drug Deliv. Rev.*, **33**, 165–182 (1998).
4. Faustman, DL, RL Pedersen, SK Kim, IR Lemischka, and RD McKay: Cells for repair: breakout session summary. *Ann. N. Y. Acad. Sci.*, **961**, 45–47 (2002).
5. Germain, L, F Goulet, V Moulin, F Berthod, and FA Auger: Engineering human tissues for *in vivo* applications. *Ann. N. Y. Acad. Sci.*, **961**, 268–270 (2002).

6. Atala, A: Recent developments in tissue engineering and regenerative medicine. *Curr. Opin. Pediatr.*, **18**, 167–171 (2006).
7. Giannoudis, PV, and I Pountos: Tissue regeneration. The past, the present and the future. *Injury* 36 Suppl 4, S2–S5 (2005).
8. Polak, JM, and AE Bishop: Stem cells and tissue engineering: past, present, and future. *Ann. N. Y. Acad. Sci.*, **1068**, 352–366 (2006).
9. Reubinoff, BE, P Itsykson, T Turetsky, MF Pera, E Reinhartz, A Itzik, and T Ben-Hur: Neural progenitors from human embryonic stem cells. *Nat. Biotechnol.*, **19**, 1134–1140 (2001).
10. Fleming, JE, Jr., CN Cornell, and GF Muschler: Bone cells and matrices in orthopedic tissue engineering. *Orthop. Clin. North Am.*, **31**, 357–374 (2000).
11. Lagasse, E, H Connors, M Al-Dhalimy, M Reitsma, M Dohse, L Osborne, X Wang, M Finegold, IL Weissman, and M Grompe: Purified hematopoietic stem cells can differentiate into hepatocytes *in vivo*. *Nat. Med.*, **6**, 1229–1234 (2000).
12. Assady, S, G Maor, M Amit, J Itskovitz-Eldor, KL Skorecki, and M Tzukerman: Insulin production by human embryonic stem cells. *Diabetes*, **50**, 1691–1697 (2001).
13. Solanki, A, JD Kim, and KB Lee: Nanotechnology for regenerative medicine: nanomaterials for stem cell imaging. *Nanomedicine*, **3**, 567–578 (2008).
14. Langer, R, and JP Vacanti: Tissue engineering. *Science*, **260**, 920–926 (1993).
15. Leor, J, Y Amsalem, and S Cohen: Cells, scaffolds, and molecules for myocardial tissue engineering. *Pharmacol. Ther.*, **105**, 151–163 (2005).
16. Down, JD, and ME White-Scharf: Reprogramming immune responses: enabling cellular therapies and regenerative medicine. *Stem. Cells*, **21**, 21–32 (2003).
17. Matsue, H, K Matsue, M Kusuhara, T Kumamoto, K Okumura, H Yagita, and A Takashima: Immunosuppressive properties of CD95L-transduced "killer" hybrids created by fusing donor- and recipient-derived dendritic cells. *Blood*, **98**, 3465–3472 (2001).
18. Bilodeau, K, and D Mantovani: Bioreactors for tissue engineering: focus on mechanical constraints. A comparative review. *Tissue Eng.*, **12**, 2367–2383 (2006).
19. Naughton, GK: From lab bench to market: critical issues in tissue engineering. *Ann. N. Y. Acad. Sci.*, **961**, 372–385 (2002).

20. Wang, D, W Liu, B Han, and R Xu: The bioreactor: a powerful tool for large-scale culture of animal cells. *Curr. Pharm. Biotechnol.*, **6**, 397–403 (2005).

21. Jin, HJ, J Chen, V Karageorgiou, GH Altman, and DL Kaplan: Human bone marrow stromal cell responses on electrospun silk fibroin mats. *Biomaterials*, **25**, 1039–1047 (2004).

22. Yao, C, EB Slamovich, and TJ Webster: Enhanced osteoblast functions on anodized titanium with nanotube-like structures. *J. Biomed. Mater. Res. A*, **85**, 157–166 (2008).

23. Khang, D, J Lu, C Yao, KM Haberstroh, and TJ Webster: The role of nanometer and sub-micron surface features on vascular and bone cell adhesion on titanium. *Biomaterials*, **29**, 970–983 (2008).

24. Webster, TJ, RW Siegel, and R Bizios: Osteoblast adhesion on nanophase ceramics. *Biomaterials*, **20**, 1221–1227 (1999).

25. Khang, D, SY Kim, P Liu-Snyder, GT Palmore, SM Durbin, and TJ Webster: Enhanced fibronectin adsorption on carbon nanotube/poly(carbonate) urethane: independent role of surface nano-roughness and associated surface energy. *Biomaterials*, **28**, 4756–4768 (2007).

26. Webster, TJ, LS Schadler, RW Siegel, and R Bizios: Mechanisms of enhanced osteoblast adhesion on nanophase alumina involve vitronectin. *Tissue Eng.*, **7**, 291–301 (2001).

27. Sato, M, and TJ Webster: Nanobiotechnology: implications for the future of nanotechnology in orthopedic applications. *Expert Rev. Med. Devices*, **1**, 105–114 (2004).

28. Falanga, V: Chronic wounds: pathophysiologic and experimental considerations. *J. Invest. Dermatol.*, **100**, 721–725 (1993).

29. Phillips, T, B Stanton, A Provan, and R Lew: A study of the impact of leg ulcers on quality of life: financial, social, and psychologic implications. *J. Am. Acad. Dermatol.*, **31**, 49–53 (1994).

30. Phillips, TJ: Chronic cutaneous ulcers: etiology and epidemiology. *J. Invest. Dermatol.*, **102**, 38S–41S (1994).

31. Eaglstein, WH, and V. Falanga: Tissue engineering and the development of apligraf(r), a human skin equivalent. *Clin. Ther.*, **19**, 894–905 (1997).

32. Chung, TW, YZ Wang, YY Huang, CI Pan, and SS Wang: Poly (epsilon-caprolactone) grafted with nano-structured chitosan enhances growth of human dermal fibroblasts. *Artif. Organs*, **30**, 35–41 (2006).

33. Chong, EJ, TT Phan, IJ Lim, YZ Zhang, BH Bay, S Ramakrishna, and CT Lim: Evaluation of electrospun PCL/gelatin nanofibrous scaffold for

wound healing and layered dermal reconstitution. *Acta. Biomater.*, **3**, 321–330 (2007).

34. Baguneid, MS, PE Fulford, and MG Walker: Cardiovascular surgery in the elderly. *J. R. Coll. Surg. Edinb.*, **44**, 216–221 (1999).
35. Zong, X, H Bien, CY Chung, L Yin, D Fang, BS Hsiao, B Chu, and E Entcheva: Electrospun fine-textured scaffolds for heart tissue constructs. *Biomaterials*, **26**, 5330–5338 (2005).
36. Neidert, MR, and RT Tranquillo: Tissue-engineered valves with commissural alignment. *Tissue Eng.*, **12**, 891–903 (2006).
37. Brody, S, T Anilkumar, S Liliensiek, JA Last, CJ Murphy, and A Pandit: Characterizing nanoscale topography of the aortic heart valve basement membrane for tissue engineering heart valve scaffold design. *Tissue Eng.*, **12**, 413–421 (2006).
38. Mendelson, K, and FJ Schoen: Heart valve tissue engineering: concepts, approaches, progress, and challenges. *Ann. Biomed. Eng.*, **34**, 1799–1819 (2006).
39. Niklason, LE, J Gao, WM Abbott, KK Hirschi, S Houser, R Marini, and R Langer: Functional arteries grown *in vitro*. *Science*, **284**, 489–493 (1999).
40. Campbell, JH, JL Efendy, and GR Campbell: Novel vascular graft grown within recipient's own peritoneal cavity. *Circ. Res.*, **85**, 1173–1178 (1999).
41. Edelman, ER: Vascular tissue engineering: designer arteries. *Circ. Res.*, **85**, 1115–1117 (1999).
42. Shinoka, T, D Shum-Tim, PX Ma, RE Tanel, N Isogai, R Langer, JP Vacanti, and JE Mayer Jr: Creation of viable pulmonary artery autografts through tissue engineering. *J. Thorac. Cardiovasc. Surg.*, **115**, (1998).
43. Tyan, YC, JD Liao, R Klauser, I Wu, and CC Weng: Assessment and characterization of degradation effect for the varied degrees of ultra-violet radiation onto the collagen-bonded polypropylene non-woven fabric surfaces. *Biomaterials*, **23**, 65–76 (2002).
44. Venugopal, J, YZ Zhang, and S Ramakrishna: Fabrication of modified and functionalized polycaprolactone nanofiber scaffolds for vascular tissue engineering. *Nanotechnology*, **16**, 2138–2142 (2005).
45. Lu, J, MP Rao, NC MacDonald, D Khang, and TJ Webster: Improved endothelial cell adhesion and proliferation on patterned titanium surfaces with rationally designed, micrometer to nanometer features. *Acta. Biomater.*, **4**, 192–201 (2008).

46. Agrawal, CM, A Pennick, X Wang, and RC Schenck: Porous-coated titanium implant impregnated with a biodegradable protein delivery system. *J. Biomed. Mater. Res.*, **36**, 516–521 (1997).
47. Kambic, H, R Kay, JF Chen, M Matsushita, H Harasaki, and S Zilber: Biodegradable pericardial implants for bladder augmentation: a 2.5-year study in dogs. *J. Urol.*, **148**, 539–543 (1992).
48. Thapa, A, DC Miller, TJ Webster, and KM Haberstroh: Nano-structured polymers enhance bladder smooth muscle cell function. *Biomaterials*, **24**, 2915–2926 (2003).
49. Uribarri, J, MS Oh, and HJ Carroll: The first kidney stone. *Ann. Intern. Med.*, **111**, 1006–1009 (1989).
50. Chun, YW, D Khang, KM Haberstroh, and TJ Webster: The role of polymer nanosurface roughness and submicron pores in improving bladder urothelial cell density and inhibiting calcium oxalate stone formation. *Nanotechnology*, **20**, 85104 (2009).
51. Pattison, MA, S Wurster, TJ Webster, and KM Haberstroh: Three-dimensional, nano-structured PLGA scaffolds for bladder tissue replacement applications. *Biomaterials*, **26**, 2491–2500 (2005).
52. Stoll, G, and HW Muller: Nerve injury, axonal degeneration and neural regeneration: basic insights. *Brain Pathol.*, **9**, 313–325 (1999).
53. Evans, GR, K Brandt, AD Niederbichler, P Chauvin, S Herrman, M Bogle, L Otta, B Wang, and CW Patrick Jr: Clinical long-term *in vivo* evaluation of poly(L-lactic acid) porous conduits for peripheral nerve regeneration. *J. Biomater. Sci. Polym. Ed.*, **11**, 869–878 (2000).
54. Widmer, MS, PK Gupta, L Lu, RK Meszlenyi, GR Evans, K Brandt, T Savel, A Gurlek, CW Patrick Jr, and AG Mikos: Manufacturing of porous biodegradable polymer conduits by an extrusion process for guided tissue regeneration. *Biomaterials*, **19**, 1945–1955 (1998).
55. Yang, F, R Murugan, S Wang, and S Ramakrishnan: Electrospinning of nano/micro scale poly(L-lactic acid) aligned fibers and their potential in neural tissue engineering. *Biomaterials*, **26**, 2603–2610 (2005).
56. Keilhoff, G, F Stang, G Wolf, and H Fansa: Bio-compatibility of type I/III collagen matrix for peripheral nerve reconstruction. *Biomaterials*, **24**, 2779–2787 (2003).
57. Chi, H, H Horie, N Hikawa, and T Takenaka: Isolation and age-related characterization of mouse Schwann cells from dorsal root ganglion explants in type I collagen gels. *J. Neurosci. Res.*, **35**, 183–187 (1993).
58. Hall, S: Nerve repair: A neurobiologist's review. *J. Hand. Surg. Br.*, **26**, 129–136 (2001).

59. Ide, C: Peripheral nerve regeneration. *Neurosci. Res.*, **25**, 101–121 (1996).

60. Lundborg, G, L Dahlin, N Danielsen, and Q Zhao: Trophism, tropism, and specificity in nerve regeneration. *J. Reconstr. Microsurg.*, **10**, 345–354 (1994).

61. Pu, LLQ, SA Syed, M Reid, H Patwa, JM Goldstein, DL Forman, and JG Thomson: Effects of nerve growth factor on nerve regeneration through a vein graft across a gap. *Plast. Reconstr. Surg.*, **104**, 1379–1385 (1999).

62. Xu, X, WC Yee, H Yu, PYK Hwang, H Yu, ACA Wan, S Gao, K-L Boon, H-Q Mao, KW Leong, and S Wang: Peripheral nerve regeneration with sustained release of poly(phosphoester) microencapsulated nerve growth factor with nerve guide conduits. *Biomaterials*, **24**, 2405–2412 (2003).

63. Wan, ACA, HQ Mao, S Wang, KW Leong, and H Yu: Fabrication of poly(phosphoester) nerve guides by immersion precipitation and the control of porosity. *Biomaterials*, **22**, 1147–1156 (2001).

64. Shin, H, S Jo, and M AG.: Biomimetic materials for tissue engineering. *Biomaterials*, **24**, 4353–4364 (2003).

65. Letourneau, PC, ML Condic, and DM Snow: Interactions of developing neurons with the extracellular matrix. *J. Neurosci.*, **14**, 915–928 (1994).

66. Labrador, RO, M Buti, and X Navarro: Influence of collagen and laminin gels concentration on nerve regeneration after resection and tube repair. *Exp. Neurol.*, **149**, 243–252 (1998).

67. Miller, C, H Shanks, A Witt, G Rutkowski, and S Mallapragada: Oriented Schwann cell growth on micropatterned biodegradable polymer substrates. *Biomaterials*, **22**, 1263–1269 (2001).

68. Yang, F, CY Xu, M Kotaki, S Wang, and S Ramakrishna: Characterization of neural stem cells on electrospun poly(L-lactic acid) nanofibrous scaffold. *J. Biomater. Sci. Polym. Ed.*, **15**, 1483–1497 (2004).

Index

Color Insert

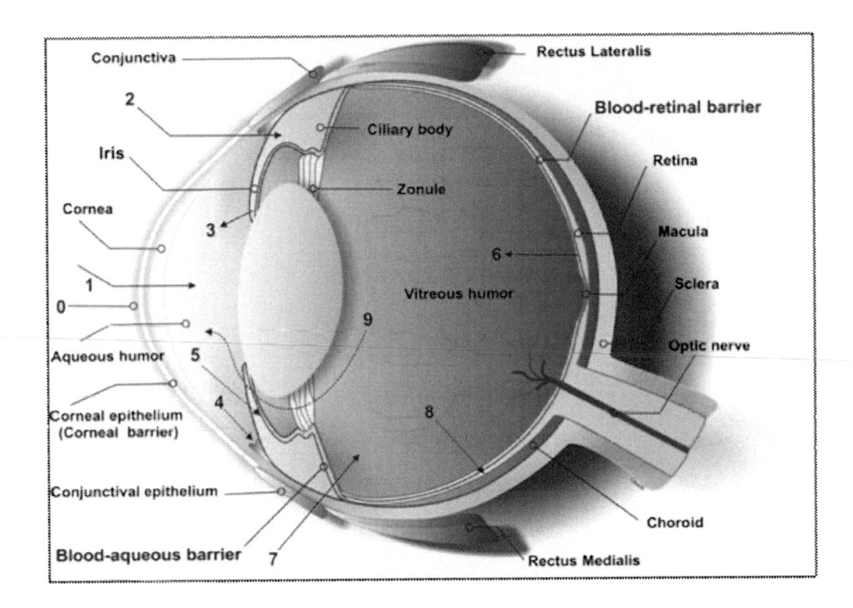

Figure 2.2

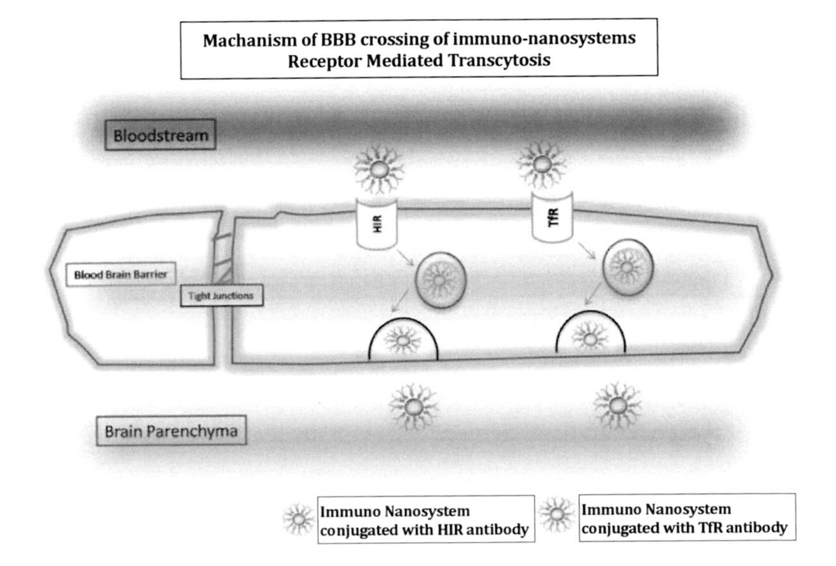

Figure 3.1

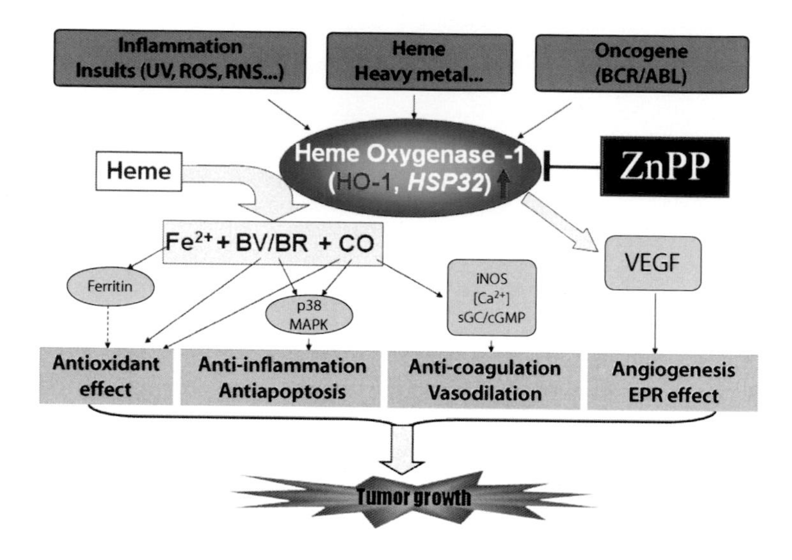

Figure 4.1

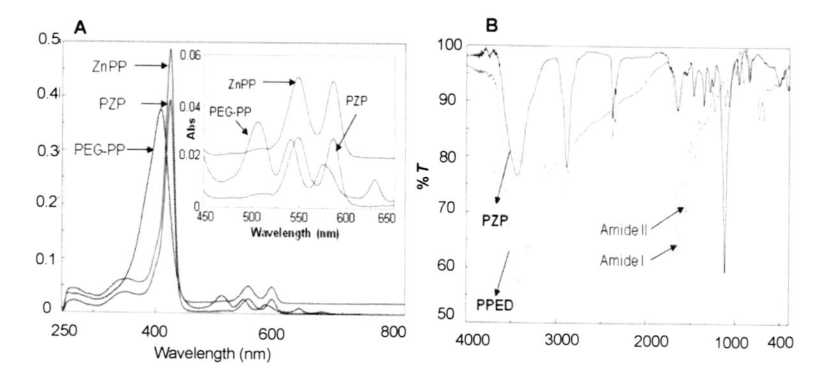

Figure 4.4

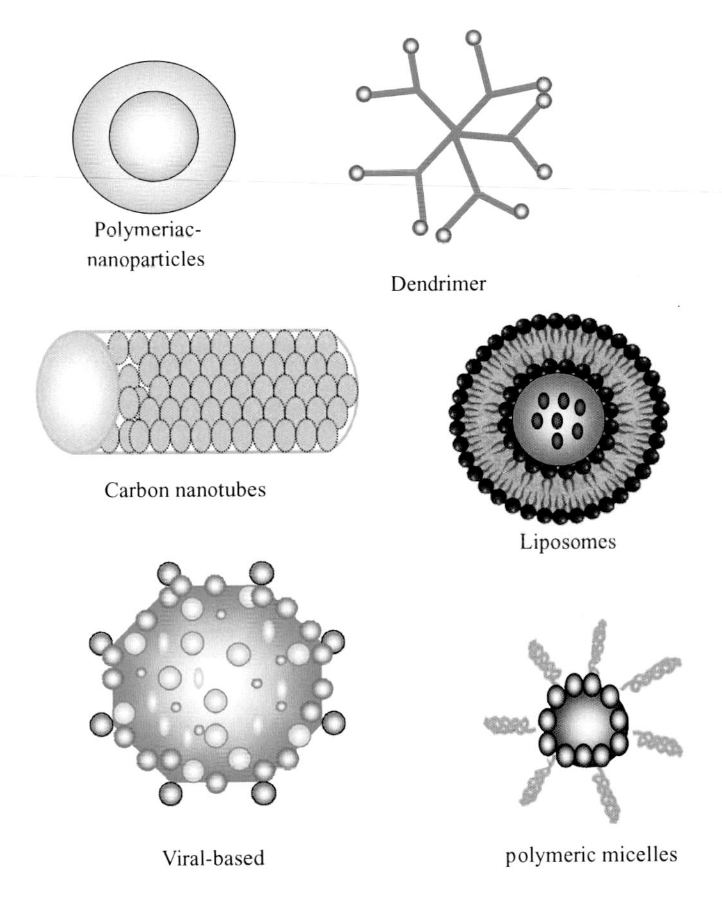
Polymeriac-
nanoparticles
Dendrimer
Carbon nanotubes
Liposomes
Viral-based
polymeric micelles

Figure 7.2

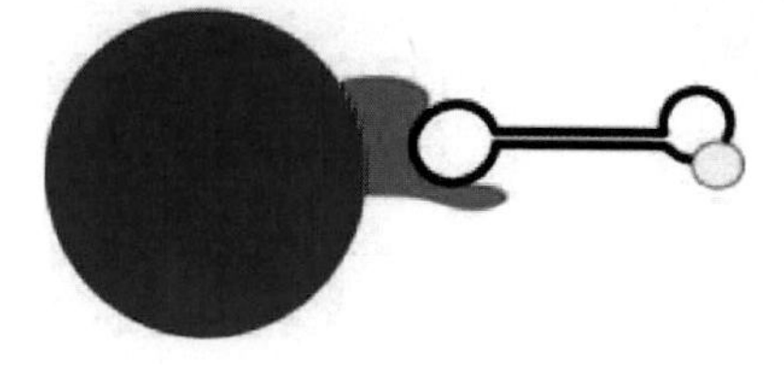

Figure 8.1